PERIOP

TRANSESOPHAGEAL ECHOCARDIOGRAPHY

Self-Assessment and Review

PERIOPERATIVE TRANSESOPHAGEAL ECHOCARDIOGRAPHY

Self-Assessment and Review

Roger L. Click, MD, PhD, FACC
Consultant, Division of Cardiovascular Diseases, Mayo Clinic, Rochester, Minnesota; Associate Professor of Medicine, College of Medicine, Mayo Clinic

Joy X. Cai, MD, FASE
Formerly, Fellow in Cardiovascular Diseases and Thoracic Anesthesia, Mayo School of Graduate Medical Education, College of Medicine, Rochester, Minnesota; Currently, Cardiac Anesthesiologist, The Heart Institute of Staten Island, Staten Island University Hospital, Staten Island, New York

Martin D. Abel, MBBCh, FRCA
Consultant, Department of Anesthesiology, Mayo Clinic, Rochester, Minnesota; Professor of Anesthesiology, College of Medicine, Mayo Clinic

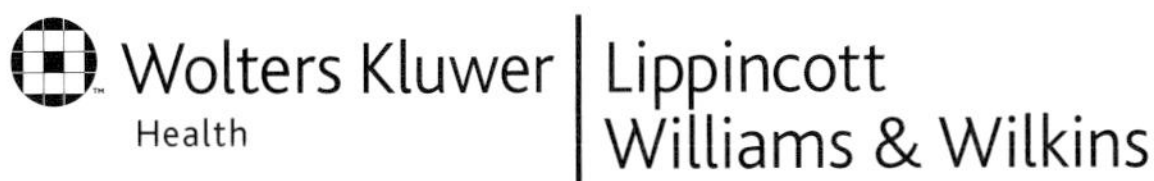

Lippincott Williams & Wilkins
a Wolters Kluwer business
Philadelphia • Baltimore • New York • London
Buenos Aires • Hong Kong • Sydney • Tokyo

Acquisitions Editor: Frances R. DeStefano
Managing Editor: Chris Potash
Project Manager: Jennifer Harper
Senior Manufacturing Manager: Benjamin Rivera
Marketing Manager: Kimberly Schonberger
Creative Director: Doug Smock
Production Services: Laserwords Private Limited, Chennai, India

---

Library of Congress Cataloging-in-Publication Data

Click, Roger L.
Perioperative transesophageal echocardiography self-assessment and review / Roger L. Click, Joy X. Cai, Martin D. Abel.
p. ; cm.
Includes bibliographical references and index.
ISBN-13: 978-0-7817-5576-4
ISBN-10: 0-7817-5575-X
1. Transesophageal echocardiography—Examinations, questions, etc. Roger, Click L. Cai, Joy X. II. Abel, Martin D. III. Perioperative transesophageal echocardiography self-assessment and review.
[DNLM: 1. Echocardiography, Transesophageal—Examination Questions. 2. Perioperative Care—Examination Questions. WG 18.2 C636p 2007]
RC683.5.T83C543 2007
616.1′2075430076—dc22

2007021830

---

10 9 8 7 6 5 4 3 2 1

Preface

Intraoperative or perioperative transesophageal echocardiography has become an integral part of most cardiac surgical procedures. Along with the increased use of echocardiography in the operating room, more formal training programs have developed. In addition, a certification process has been established (Aronson S, Thys DM. Training and certification in perioperative transesophageal echocardiography: a historical perspective. Anesth Analg. 2001;93:1422–1427).

Joy X. Cai, MD, did her cardiovascular/thoracic anesthesia training at Mayo Clinic in the late 1990s. At that time, Mayo Clinic did not have a formal echocardiography training program in the operating room, but she was persistent and learned most of what she wanted and needed to know on her own and from a number of cardiologists who were performing intraoperative echocardiography. She subsequently went into private practice and in 1999 took the Examination of Special Competence in Perioperative Transesophageal Echocardiography (PTEeXAM). This test, given by the National Board of Echocardiography, is the official certification examination for perioperative transesophageal echocardiography. It recognizes those physicians who have completed an approved training program in echocardiography and subsequently passed an examination that demonstrates special competence in echocardiography.

In preparing for this examination, Dr. Cai realized that no comprehensive review book or self-assessment guide was available to study for this test. With this background, she began to write and accumulate questions similar to those asked on the test. Martin D. Abel, MBBCh, FRCA, and I reviewed and edited the questions and added the supportive figures that have resulted in the current textbook. The purpose of this book is to provide a study and self-assessment guide for those preparing for the PTEeXAM. The audience for this book includes cardiologists and cardiology fellows, anesthesiologists and anesthesia fellows preparing for the test. It also provides an overview and review of transesophageal echocardiography for cardiologists and anesthesiologists already certified in perioperative transesophageal echocardiography. Finally, in cardiac surgical training programs today, the fellows have more exposure to transesophageal echocardiography, and this book offers a review of applications in the operating room.

I wish to thank other Mayo Clinic colleagues involved in the preparation of the manuscript and illustrations: Jane C. Wiggs (manuscript editor), Susan R. Miller (editorial assistant), Alissa K. Baumgartner (proofreader), Roberta J. Schwartz (production editor), Section of Scientific Publications; and Eunice A. Biel, Illustration and Design.

Roger L. Click, MD

Contents

Chapter 1

Ultrasound Physics

Questions

Multiple choice (choose the *one* best answer):

1. Ultrasound is defined as the sound with frequency
A. less than 20 Hz, which is below audible range.
B. less than 20 Hz, which is within audible range.
C. higher than 20,000 Hz, which is within audible range.
D. higher than 20,000 Hz, which is above audible range.
E. between 20 and 20,000 Hz, which is within audible range.

2. Rarefaction of a sound wave represents the region of
A. high density and low pressure.
B. low density and high pressure.
C. high density and high pressure.
D. low density and low pressure.
E. low density without pressure.

3. All of the following are true ***except***
A. Wavelength and frequency are inversely related.
B. Wavelength is the time from the onset of one cycle to the next.
C. Period is the time from the onset of one cycle to the next.
D. Frequency is the number of cycles in a given time.
E. Wavelength is the distance from the onset of one cycle to the next.

4. Which one of the following is true?
A. Pulse duration is the distance between the onset of one cycle to the next.
B. Spatial pulse length is the time between the onset of one cycle to the next.
C. Spatial pulse length is the distance from one cycle to the next.
D. Pulse repetition frequency is the number of pulses in a given time.
E. Pulse repetition frequency is the number of cycles in a given time.

5. Propagation speed in soft tissue is
A. 330 m/s.
B. 1,540 m/s.
C. 3,500 m/s.

D. determined by the ultrasound frequency.
E. not determined by the medium.

6. Amplitude
A. is equal to the difference between maximum and minimum value of an acoustic variable.
B. is doubled when the intensity or power is doubled.
C. is affected by changing the transmit control called output gain.
D. does not change as the sound travels through a medium.
E. increases as the sound travels though a medium.

7. Acoustic impedance
A. is a characteristic of the ultrasound that propagates through any medium.
B. is not a characteristic of the medium.
C. is very high when the medium is dense and the propagation speed is slow.
D. can be measured directly.
E. is important in the physics of reflection because reflection of an ultrasound wave depends on impedance mismatch.

8. Specular reflectors are best described as reflectors that
A. are small and smooth surfaced.
B. are large and smooth surfaced.
C. are small and rough surfaced.
D. are large and rough surfaced.
E. can have any type of surface.

9. Examples of specular reflectors include
A. cardiac structures.
B. red blood cells.
C. vessel walls.
D. A and C.
E. all of the above.

10. Attenuation is best described by which one of the following:
A. The only cause for attenuation is reflection.
B. Reflection and scatter are the main causes of attenuation in bone.
C. Reflection and absorption are the main causes of attenuation in air.
D. Absorption is the main cause of attenuation in soft tissue.
E. Absorption and scatter are the main causes of attenuation in air.

11. Attenuation is
A. increased when the ultrasound frequency is increased.
B. decreased when the distance that ultrasound travels is increased.
C. increased when the attenuation coefficient is decreased.
D. higher in soft tissues than in bones.
E. lower in lungs than in soft tissues.

12. Piezoelectric effect means the conversion of
A. electrical energy to heat.
B. mechanical energy to pressure.
C. mechanical energy to electrical energy.
D. heat to acoustic energy.
E. acoustic energy to pressure.

13. In clinical imaging ultrasound, reverse piezoelectric effect
A. occurs during the transmission phase.
B. occurs during the reception phase.
C. occurs during the transmission and reception phases.
D. does not occur during the transmission phase.
E. occurs in none of the above.

14. Piezoelectric materials
A. are found in nature, such as lead zirconate titanate and quartz.
B. are made synthetically, such as lead zirconate titanate and quartz.
C. are made synthetically but cannot be found in nature.
D. are depolarized and lose their piezoelectric property permanently when they are heated above Curie temperature.
E. are depolarized and lose their piezoelectric property when heated above Curie temperature. After cooling down, they regain their piezoelectric property because of repolarization.

15. Near field
A. is also called the Fraunhofer zone.
B. can be extended by increasing the transducer diameter.
C. can be extended by decreasing the transducer frequency.
D. can be extended by increasing the ultrasound wavelength.
E. is not determined by the transducer diameter, ultrasound wavelength, or frequency.

16. Focus or focal point
A. is the point of minimum beam intensity because it is the narrowest portion of the sound beam.
B. is the point of maximum beam intensity because it is the widest portion of the sound beam.
C. has the same beam intensity as the rest of the sound beam.
D. is located within the far field of an ultrasound beam. Therefore, one should focus when imaging the structures in far field but not those in near field.
E. provides the best lateral resolution because it is the narrowest portion of an ultrasound beam.

17. Far field is best characterized by which one of the following:
A. It is also called the Fresnel zone.
B. The beam diameter increases as sound travels through the far field.

C. The beam diameter decreases as sound travels through the far field.
D. The ultrasound amplitude decreases in the far field because the beam diameter is decreased.
E. The ultrasound amplitude increases in the far field because the beam diameter is increased.

18. The damping material
A. is bonded to the front side of the active element of the transducer.
B. is used to increase the ringing of the piezoelectric crystal.
C. improves picture quality.
D. increases the ultrasound pulse duration.
E. increases the spatial pulse length.

19. When the transducer diameter doubles, the near-field length
A. doubles.
B. quadruples.
C. decreases to one-half.
D. decreases to one-fourth.
E. does not change.

20. For continuous wave ultrasound, the transducer frequency is
A. identical to the electrical frequency that drives the piezoelectric crystals.
B. directly related to the speed of sound in the crystal.
C. directly related to the crystal thickness.
D. inversely related to the crystal thickness.
E. determined by the thickness of the crystal and the propagation speed of sound in the crystal.

21. For pulsed wave ultrasound, which one of the following about the transducer frequency is true?
A. The higher the propagation speed of sound in the crystal, the lower the frequency.
B. The thicker the piezoelectric crystal, the lower the frequency.
C. The lower the sound speed in the crystal, the higher the frequency.
D. The thinner the crystal, the lower the frequency.
E. The transducer frequency is identical to the electrical frequency that drives the piezoelectric crystal.

22. Bandwidth
A. is the difference between the resonant frequency and the highest frequency found in a pulse.
B. is the difference between the resonant frequency and the lowest frequency found in a pulse.
C. is decreased by damping material.
D. is narrower when the pulse is shorter.
E. is wider when the pulse is shorter, which yields high-quality images.

23. Methods of focusing include
A. mechanical focusing.
B. electronic focusing.
C. internal focusing.
D. external focusing.
E. all of the above.

24. As the degree of focusing is increased,
A. the lateral resolution is decreased.
B. the near-field length is increased.
C. the near-field length is not changed.
D. the divergence of sound beam beyond focus is decreased.
E. the focal depth is decreased.

25. The focal area
A. is located between the transducer and near field of a sound beam.
B. is located in the distal part of the far field of a sound beam.
C. provides decreased image quality because the beam is narrowed in this area.
D. provides increased image quality because the beam is wider in this area.
E. is the region surrounding the focus that has a narrow beam and gives better image quality.

26. Which one of the following best describes focal depth?
A. High-frequency waves have a shallow focus.
B. Low-frequency waves have a deep focus.
C. Large-diameter crystals produce a beam with a deep focus.
D. Small-diameter crystals produce a beam with a deep focus.
E. Focal depth is determined by ultrasound frequency but not determined by the crystal diameter.

27. Which one of the following about resolution is true?
A. Shorter pulses improve lateral resolution.
B. Narrow ultrasound beam improves longitudinal resolution.
C. Spatial resolution describes the overall ability of an ultrasound system to accurately create images of small structures in their correct anatomic positions.
D. Temporal resolution is the ability to distinguish two structures lying side-by-side.
E. Frame rate determines spatial resolution.

28. Lateral resolution
A. does not vary with image depth.
B. equals the ultrasound beam diameter.
C. is as good as longitudinal resolution when one wants to make diagnostic measurement.
D. is superior to axial resolution when one wants to make diagnostic measurement.
E. is not improved by focusing, which only improves longitudinal resolution.

29. Axial resolution
- A. is the ability to distinguish two structures close to each other front to back.
- B. is also called longitudinal resolution.
- C. is better when the spatial pulse length is shorter.
- D. equals half the spatial pulse length.
- E. is all of the above.

30. Range equation
- A. determines the distance from the transducer to a reflector.
- B. equals the product of propagation speed and pulse round-trip time.
- C. equals the pulse round-trip time in soft tissue.
- D. is the equation to calculate range resolution.
- E. is none of the above.

31. Which one of the following about attenuation is true?
- A. Attenuation is related to the property of a medium, not the frequency of ultrasound.
- B. Frequency and attenuation are inversely related.
- C. High frequency should be used to image deep structures because of attenuation.
- D. Low frequency should be used to image deep structures because of attenuation.
- E. Frequency and attenuation are not related.

32. Which one of the following about linear phased array is true?
- A. Multiple electronic signals are used to create a single acoustic pulse.
- B. Microsecond delays occur between electronic pulses delivered to the array elements.
- C. Ultrasound beam steering is electronic.
- D. Ultrasound beam focusing is electronic.
- E. All of the above.

33. Annular array transducers
- A. have concentric ring-shaped piezoelectric elements with a common center.
- B. have multiple foci which gives higher temporal resolution at all depth.
- C. use inner crystals for deep structures.
- D. use outer crystals for shallow structures.
- E. consist of inner and outer crystals which are not related to the depth of the structures.

34. Which one of the following is true about electronic steering and focusing?
- A. Beam focusing is determined by electronic slope.
- B. Beam steering is determined by electronic curvature.
- C. Upward electronic slope gives upward steering.
- D. Upward electronic slope gives downward steering.
- E. None of the above.

35. Temporal resolution is
A. better when the frame rate is decreased.
B. better when the number of scan lines per frame is decreased.
C. better when the beam diameter is decreased.
D. better when the scan line density is increased.
E. not related to frame rate, scan line density, or beam diameter.

36. Which one of the following provides information on the position of reflectors with respect to time?
A. A-mode.
B. B-mode.
C. M-mode.
D. All of the above.
E. None of the above.

37. Which one of the following about output power is true?
A. Output power is related to the output electrical impulse but not to the initial strength of an ultrasound wave.
B. Output power represents the intensity of the electrical impulse from transducer to the computer memory.
C. Transmit gain control should be minimized to decrease patient exposure to ultrasound intensity.
D. Output power should always be increased by increasing transmit gain control in order to obtain good image quality.
E. Output power is automatically set in an ultrasound system and cannot be controlled by the operator.

38. The correct sequence of the functions of an ultrasound receiver is
A. compensation, compression, amplification, rejection, and demodulation.
B. demodulation, amplification, compression, compensation, and rejection.
C. demodulation, amplification, rejection, compensation, and compression.
D. compression, compensation, amplification, demodulation, and rejection.
E. amplification, compensation, compression, demodulation, and rejection.

39. Amplification
A. enlarges all returned ultrasound signals for further processing.
B. is performed automatically by the ultrasound system and cannot be controlled by the operator.
C. enlarges output electrical signals but not returned signals.
D. enlarges both transmitted and returned signals.
E. results in regional expansion of an interested area with improved resolution.

40. Time gain compensation
A. makes echoes arising from identical structures appear at different brightness, depending on the depth of the structures.

B. means that ultrasound signals from deeper structures need extra time to return to receiver.
C. applies extra amplification for the echoes of deeper structures.
D. is related to phased array transmission with microsecond time delay of electrical impulse.
E. has a different function than that of depth gain compensation.

41. Which one of the following about time gain compensation is true?
A. Less time gain compensation is applied with high-frequency ultrasound waves.
B. More time gain compensation is applied with low-frequency ultrasound waves.
C. More time gain compensation is applied with shallower reflectors.
D. More time gain compensation is applied with high-frequency ultrasound waves.
E. Less time gain compensation is applied with deeper reflectors.

42. Dynamic range is the range of
A. the ultrasound frequencies emitted to image reflectors.
B. the highest to the lowest frame rate.
C. the dynamic depths of moving reflectors.
D. the signals that can be processed by an ultrasound system.
E. the dynamic numbers of scan lines per each frame at different times.

43. Compression
A. reduces all the returned signals and abolishes the difference between the large and small signals.
B. reduces all the returned signals and alters the relationship between the small and large signals.
C. reduces the total range of returned signals but does not alter the relationship between the signals.
D. reduces those returned signals that are too large to be processed, but it does not affect the small signals.
E. reduces the signals of electrical "noise" in order to minimize or remove them from the display screen.

44. Each of the following about reject is true ***except***
A. Reject is also called threshold or suppression.
B. Reject eliminates all the signals that are above and below the reject threshold.
C. Reject can be controlled by the operator.
D. Reject removes all the signals that are below a minimum strength.
E. Certain returned ultrasound signals are extremely weak and are therefore rejected.

45. Demodulation
A. does not change the shape of the electrical signals.
B. turns all the negative electrical signals into positive ones.
C. can be controlled by the operator.

D. does not include the smoothing process, which evens out the rough edges of the signals.
E. has five steps and occurs before the rectification process.

46. Zoom or regional expansion is
A. read magnification performed during postprocessing.
B. write magnification performed during postprocessing.
C. read magnification performed during preprocessing.
D. write magnification performed during preprocessing.
E. read magnification of an anatomic region of interest.

47. The advantages of write magnification include all the following ***except***
A. The ultrasound system rescans only the region of interest.
B. The scan line and pixel density in the region of interest are not changed.
C. There are more pixels in the region of interest.
D. Spatial resolution is improved in the region of interest.
E. The system collects new image data, and thus, more detailed information is used to create the magnified picture.

48. Signal processing is best described by which one of the following:
A. Preprocessing occurs before display but after data storage in the scan converter's memory.
B. Postprocessing occurs after receiver but before data storage in the scan converter's memory.
C. Preprocessing occurs before data storage in the scan converter's memory.
D. Postprocessing occurs after display.
E. Preprocessing occurs before receiver but after data storage in the scan converter's memory.

49. Spatial resolution is improved when
A. using read magnification.
B. the ultrasound frequency is decreased.
C. the pixel density is increased.
D. the number of display TV lines are decreased.
E. the field of view is increased.

50. Digital signal is best described by which one of the following:
A. Electrical signals sent by transducer to receiver are in digital form.
B. Digital signals are used for display on the CRT screen.
C. Digital signals are stored as very clear pictures.
D. Digital signals are stored as discrete numbers.
E. An ultrasound system uses digital signals only.

51. Image signals are converted from
A. analog to digital by an analog-to-digital converter before display.
B. digital to analog by a digital-to-analog converter before storage in the scan converter's memory.

C. analog to digital by a digital-to-analog converter before display.
D. digital to analog by an analog-to-digital converter before display.
E. analog to digital by an analog-to-digital converter before storage in the scan converter's memory.

52. A binary system is a number system that
A. uses both even and odd fields.
B. uses either even- or odd-numbered lines.
C. has either negative or positive value.
D. has both negative and positive symbols.
E. uses two symbols, either 0 or 1.

53. Which one of the following about pixel is true?
A. A pixel is the smallest amount of digital computer memory.
B. Pixel density is the number of pixels in a given time.
C. Decreased pixel density is associated with increased temporal resolution and improved image quality.
D. A pixel is the smallest element of a digital picture.
E. None of the above.

54. On an interlaced display, each field is created in 1/60th of a second. Therefore, the time to generate one frame
A. is 1/60th second.
B. is 1/30th second.
C. is 1/90th second.
D. is 1/120th second.
E. cannot be determined.

55. Advantages of a digital scan converter include
A. uniformity.
B. stability.
C. durability.
D. rapidity.
E. all of the above.

56. Which one of the following about display is true?
A. The display of one frame is called cine-loop.
B. A repeated display of several frames is called freeze frame.
C. An ultrasound system does not use a cathode ray tube for display.
D. One field makes up one frame on CRT display.
E. The electron beam moves from left to right and top to bottom with the odd-numbered lines and then the even-numbered lines.

57. All of the following about brightness and contrast are true ***except***
A. Underuse of the brightness control may not allow display of weak echoes.
B. Overuse of the brightness control increases overall image details.

C. Increasing contrast also increases the number of gray shades displayed.
D. Decreasing contrast also decreases the number of gray shades displayed.
E. The contrast control controls the brightness range of the image.

58. When the sector angle is narrowed,
A. the total scan lines are decreased.
B. the frame rate is decreased.
C. the field of view is increased.
D. the scan line density is decreased.
E. the resolution is improved.

59. Which one of the following about image depth is true?
A. Deep imaging results in shorter pulse duration.
B. Image depth cannot be controlled by the operator.
C. Shallow imaging results in longer listening time.
D. Decreasing image depth results in high pulse repetition frequency.
E. Image depth does not determine the pulse repetition frequency.

60. An increase in frame rate improves
A. axial resolution.
B. lateral resolution.
C. temporal resolution.
D. spatial resolution.
E. all of the above.

Answers & Discussion

1. Answer D

Ultrasound is a sound wave with a frequency higher than 20,000 Hz, which exceeds the upper limit of human hearing. A sound wave with frequency between 20 and 20,000 Hz is audible sound. A sound wave with frequency less than 20 Hz is infrasound, which cannot be heard by humans. **References** 9 *(p 10)*; 10 *(p 1)*; 26 *(p 2)*.

2. Answer D

A sound wave is a series of compressions and rarefactions. The combination of one compression and one rarefaction represents one cycle. Compression represents a region of high pressure and high density. In contrast, rarefaction represents a region of low pressure and low density. **References** 9 *(p 8)*; 10 *(p 2)*.

3. Answer B

Wavelength is the distance between the onset of one cycle to the next. Period is the time from the onset of one cycle to the next. Frequency is the number of cycles in a given time (cycles/second=Hertz). Frequency and wavelength are inversely related (wavelength=propagation speed/frequency). Higher-frequency waves have shorter wavelengths. In contrast, lower frequency waves have longer wavelengths. **References** 9 *(pp 8–11, 17–18)*; 10 *(p 3)*.

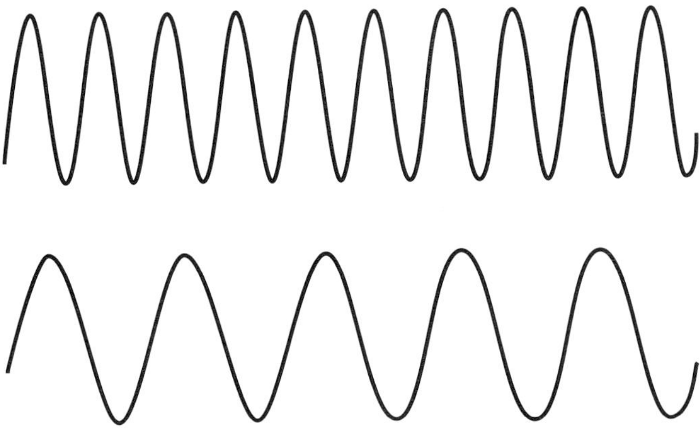

From Edelman SK (9). Used with permission.

4. Answer D

A pulse is a collection of cycles. Pulse repetition frequency is the number of pulses in a given time. Pulse duration is the time of a single pulse. Spatial pulse length is the length of a single pulse. **Reference** 9 *(pp 26–27, 32)*.

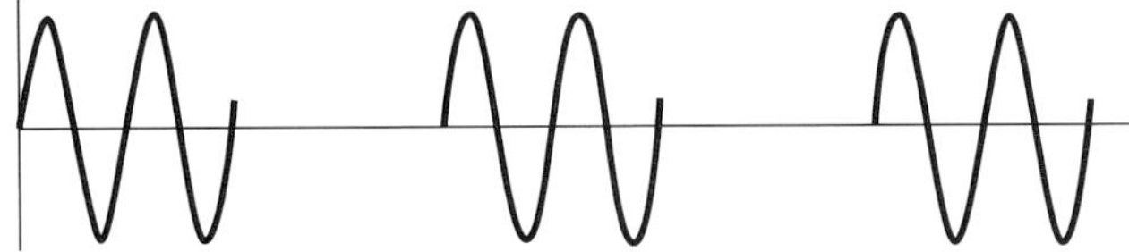

From Edelman SK (9). Used with permission.

5. Answer B

Propagation speed is the speed at which sound moves through a medium. It is also called sound speed, sound velocity, or acoustic velocity. Propagation speed is determined only by the characteristics of the medium and is not affected by the ultrasound frequency. Propagation speed in soft tissue is 1,540 m/s, whereas propagation speed is 330 m/s in air and 3,500 m/s in bone. **Reference** 9 *(pp 19–21)*.

6. Answer C

Three parameters are related to the size of a sound wave—amplitude, intensity, and power. Amplitude describes the magnitude of a sound wave. It equals the difference between the maximum and mean values of an acoustic variable (not the difference between the maximum and minimum values). As sound travels through a medium, its amplitude decreases because of attenuation. Amplitude can be affected by changing the transmit control called output gain. Intensity describes the concentration of energy in a sound beam. Power describes the rate at which work is performed or energy is transferred from the entire sound beam. Both intensity and power are proportional to the square of the sound wave's amplitude. If the amplitude is doubled, the intensity or power is increased by four times. **Reference** 9 *(pp 12, 15–16)*.

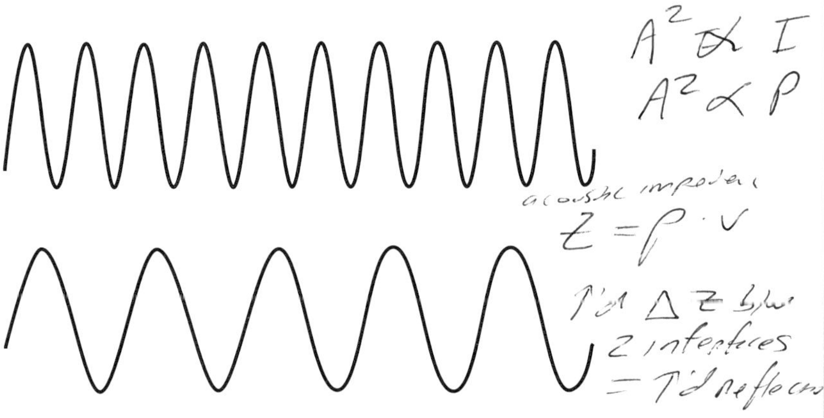

From Edelman SK (9). Used with permission.

7. Answer E

Impedance is the acoustic resistance of a medium to ultrasound that travels through the medium. Therefore, acoustic impedance is a characteristic of the medium only. High impedance occurs when a medium is very dense, has a fast propagation speed, or both. Acoustic impedance is derived from calculation and cannot be measured directly. The unit of acoustic impedance measurement is the rayl. Reflection occurs at the boundary of two media if their acoustic impedance is dissimilar; this is referred to as an impedance mismatch. **References** 9 *(p 57)*; 10 *(pp 1–2)*.

8. Answer B

Specular reflectors are mirrorlike reflectors that are large and smooth surfaced. A large reflector is at least two wavelengths in diameter. On a smooth surface, the reflector surface irregularities are larger than the wavelength of the ultrasound beam. In contrast, scatter reflectors are small and rough surfaced. **References** 9 *(p 60)*; 10 *(pp 2–3)*.

9. Answer D

Cardiac structures, vessel walls, and boundaries of the body's major organs are examples of specular reflectors. They are highly angle dependent. To optimize an ultrasound examination of specular reflectors, the angle of incidence should be perpendicular. Red blood cells are an example of a Rayleigh reflector or a Rayleigh scatterer, which reflects ultrasound energy concentrically and equally in all directions. **References** 9 *(pp 53, 60)*; 10 *(pp 2–3)*.

10. Answer D

Attenuation is the loss of sound energy when sound propagates through a medium. The three causes for attenuation are absorption, reflection, and scatter. Absorption is the conversion of sound energy to heat. Reflection represents the portion of sound energy returned from a boundary of two media with impedance mismatch. Scatter is diffusion or redirection of sound energy in multiple directions. Absorption is the main cause of attenuation in soft tissue. Absorption and reflection are the main causes of attenuation in bone. Scatter and reflection are the main causes of attenuation in air. **References** 9 *(pp 51–55)*; 10 *(p 3)*; 26 *(pp 4–5)*.

11. Answer A

Attenuation is lower in soft tissue than in bone or lung. Total attenuation is increased when the attenuation coefficient, ultrasound frequency, and path length are increased. Higher-frequency ultrasound penetrates poorly. Therefore, when imaging far-field objects, lower-frequency ultrasound is necessary. Attenuation is calculated as follows:

$$\text{Attenuation} = \text{attenuation coefficient} \times \text{path length}$$

$$\text{Attenuation coefficient} = 1/2 \times \text{frequency}$$

$$\text{Therefore, Attenuation} = 1/2 \times \text{frequency} \times \text{path length}$$

References 9 *(pp 51–55)*; 10 *(p 3)*; 26 *(pp 4–5)*.

12. Answer C

13. Answer A

Piezoelectric effect is also called pressure-electric or ferroelectric effect. It is a property of the piezoelectric materials to create an electrical voltage when they are mechanically deformed, as may occur with acoustic energy. The reverse is also true. As the electrical current passes through a piezoelectric crystal, the shape of the crystal varies with the electrical polarity. When the piezoelectric crystal expands and contracts, it produces a series of compressions and rarefactions, ie, sound waves. This is called the "reverse piezoelectric effect."

An ultrasound transducer contains piezoelectric material. It converts electrical energy into acoustic energy during transmission (reverse piezoelectric effect) and acoustic energy into electrical energy during reception (piezoelectric effect). **References** 9 *(p 72)*; 10 *(p 3)*; 26 *(p 5)*.

14. Answer D

Piezoelectric materials are found in nature or made synthetically. Natural piezoelectric materials include quartz, tourmaline, and Rochelle salts. Synthetic piezoelectric materials include lead zirconate titanate, barium titanate, and lead titanate.

Curie temperature is the temperature above which piezoelectric materials are depolarized and lose their piezoelectric property permanently. Therefore, ultrasound transducers should not be heat sterilized. The Curie temperature for lead zirconate titanate is about 300°–400°C or 600°–700°F. **References** 9 *(p 72)*; 10 *(p 3)*; 26 *(p 5)*.

15. Answer B

A sound beam is formed by near field, focus, and far field. The near field is also called the Fresnel zone. It is the area of the sound beam that extends from the front of the transducer to the beam focus. The near field is determined by the transducer diameter, ultrasound wavelength, or frequency. Near-field length is calculated as follows:

$$\text{Near-field length} = (\text{radius of transducer})^2/\text{wavelength} \textbf{ or}$$
$$= (\text{diameter})^2/(4 \times \text{wavelength})$$

Therefore, near-field length is extended by four times if the transducer diameter is doubled. Also, near-field length is inversely related to ultrasound wavelength. Because ultrasound wavelength and frequency are inversely related, near-field length is directly related to transducer frequency. A decrease in transducer frequency or an increase in ultrasound wavelength leads to a decrease in near-field length.

Because the beam diameter increases in the far field, the near field provides a better image than the far field. To obtain a better image for deep structures, the near field needs to be extended. Both increasing transducer diameter and frequency can extend the near field. However, because attenuation increases when ultrasound frequency increases, it virtually eliminates using high frequency. Therefore, the transducer diameter should be increased when near-field length needs to be extended for imaging deep structures. **Reference** 9 *(pp 81–83, 222–223)*.

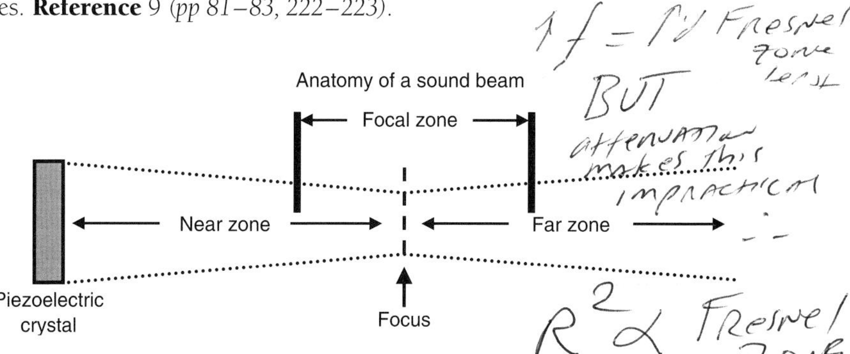

From Edelman SK (9). Used with permission.

16. Answer E

Focus is also called the focal point or transition point. It is located between the near field and the far field of an ultrasound beam. Focus is the narrowest portion of an ultrasound beam and the point of maximum beam intensity. Lateral resolution is better when the ultrasound beam diameter is smaller. (See also Question 28.) **References** 9 *(pp 81–83, 92, 222–223)*; 10 *(p 5)*.

17. Answer B

Far field is the area of the ultrasound beam beyond the focal point or focus. It is also called the Fraunhofer zone. As ultrasound travels through the far field, the beam diameter increases. The ultrasound amplitude and intensity decrease in far field because increasing ultrasound path length increases attenuation. **References** 9 *(pp 81–83)*; 10 *(p 5)*.

18. Answer C

Damping material is bonded to the back of the active element to decrease the "ringing" of the piezoelectric crystal. Because damping material shortens the pulse duration and the spatial pulse length, it provides better axial resolution, calculated as follows: Axial resolution = 1/2 × spatial pulse length. Thus, damping decreases the numerical value of the axial resolution and creates better images.

Without damping, the piezoelectric element has a sustained vibration and creates a long acoustic pulse. Increased pulse duration and spatial pulse length decrease axial resolution with lower image quality. **References** 9 *(pp 73, 90)*; 10 *(pp 3–4)*.

19. Answer B

Near-field length is directly proportional to the square of the diameter of the ultrasound transducer. Therefore, if the ultrasound transducer diameter is doubled, the near-field length is increased fourfold. If the ultrasound transducer diameter is halved, the near-field length is decreased to one-quarter. (See also Question 15.) **Reference** 10 *(p 5)*.

20. Answer A

21. Answer B

The ultrasound frequencies produced by piezoelectric crystals are different for continuous wave and pulsed wave ultrasound. For continuous wave ultrasound, the acoustic frequency is identical to the electrical frequency of the excitation voltage that drives the piezoelectric crystal.

For pulsed wave ultrasound, the number of electrical spikes delivered to piezoelectric crystal in a given time equals the pulse repetition frequency but not the ultrasound frequency. The ultrasound frequency of the pulsed wave transducer is determined by the thickness of the piezoelectric crystal and the propagation speed of ultrasound in the piezoelectric crystal. The pulsed wave frequency is inversely related to the thickness of the piezoelectric crystal and directly related to the speed of ultrasound in the crystal. Therefore, pulsed wave ultrasound frequency is higher if the piezoelectric crystal is thinner and the propagation speed in the crystal is higher. The pulsed wave ultrasound frequency is lower if the piezoelectric crystal is thicker and the propagation speed in the crystal is lower. **Reference** 9 *(pp 134–137)*.

22. Answer E

An imaging ultrasound transducer emits a sound pulse with a range of frequencies below and above the main or resonant frequency. The bandwidth is the difference between the highest and the lowest frequency found within an acoustic pulse. It is neither the difference between the highest and resonant frequencies nor the difference between the lowest and resonant frequencies.

Short pulses contain ultrasound with a wide range of frequencies and thus have broad bandwidth. Damping material shortens pulse duration, increases bandwidth, and provides better image quality. **References** 9 *(p 77)*; 10 *(pp 6–7)*.

23. Answer E

Focusing is a process whereby the lateral resolution of an ultrasound beam is improved by making the beam narrower. Focusing methods can be mechanical or electronic. Mechanical focusing is also called conventional focusing. There are two types of mechanical focusing: internal and external. Internal focusing is achieved with a curved piezoelectric element. External focusing is achieved by using a mirror or an acoustic lens placed on the front surface of the ultrasound transducer.

Electronic focusing uses the principle of phased array. It is accomplished by curving the electrical pulses to an array during transmission of the ultrasound energy. (See also Question 34.) **References** 9 *(p 88)*; 10 *(pp 5–6)*.

24. Answer E

Focusing affects the focal depth or the near-field length. As the degree of focusing increases, the focal depth or the near-field length is decreased. A strongly focused transducer has a shallower focal depth than that of an identical, but weakly focused transducer. Also, focusing increases the ultrasound beam divergence beyond the focal zone. Because the ultrasound beam is narrowed by focusing, its ability to identify two structures lying close together side-by-side is enhanced. Therefore, focusing improves lateral resolution by decreasing its numeric value, which results in superior image quality. **Reference** 9 *(pp 88–89, 92)*.

25. Answer E

The focal area is also called the focal zone. It is the region with narrow beam diameter surrounding the focus, which is located between the near field and the far field. The narrow beam diameter provides better lateral resolution and superior image quality. (See also the diagram accompanying Answer 15.) **Reference** 9 *(pp 81–83, 222–223)*.

26. Answer C

Focal depth is directly related to crystal diameter and the frequency of the sound. Large-diameter crystals and high-frequency waves produce a beam with a deep focus. In contrast, small-diameter crystals and low-frequency waves produce a beam with a shallow focus. (See also Question 15.) **References** 9 *(pp 81–83)*; 10 *(p 5)*.

27. Answer C

Resolution is the term used to describe image quality. It is the ability to distinguish or identify two objects that are close together. Lateral resolution is the ability to identify structures close to each other side-by-side. Narrower ultrasound beam gives better lateral resolution. Longitudinal, axial, range, or depth resolution is the ability to identify structures close to each other front to back. Shorter pulses provide better axial resolution. Spatial resolution describes the overall ability of an ultrasound system to accurately create images of small structures in their correct anatomic positions. Scan line density determines the spatial resolution. Temporal resolution is the ability to accurately locate the position of moving structures at particular instants in time. Rapid frame rate improves temporal resolution. (See also Questions 28, 29, and 35.) **References** 9 *(pp 89–90, 92, 100)*; 26 *(pp 7–9)*.

28. Answer B

Lateral resolution is the minimum distance that two side-by-side structures can be separated and still produce two distinct echoes on an ultrasound image. It is also called angular, transverse, or azimuthal resolution. Lateral resolution equals the ultrasound beam diameter, which varies with depth. Thus, the smaller the lateral resolution, the better the image. Because the ultrasound beam diameter is narrowest at focus, the lateral resolution is best at this point. As focusing narrows the waist of an ultrasound beam, it improves lateral resolution in the focal area. In general, longitudinal or axial resolution is superior to lateral resolution. Therefore, whenever possible, one should use axial resolution to make diagnostic measurements and diagnostic decisions. (See also Question 24.) **References** 9 *(pp 92, 223)*; 26 *(pp 7–9)*.

29. Answer E

Axial resolution describes the ability to distinguish two structures close to each other front to back. It is also called longitudinal, range, radial, or depth resolution. In diagnostic imaging, it ranges from 0.05 to 0.5 mm. Axial resolution equals half the spatial pulse length. A small numeric value of axial resolution is correlated with better axial resolution. Therefore, ultrasound with short spatial pulse length provides better axial resolution and superior image quality. (See also Question 27.) **References** 9 *(p 90)*; 26 *(pp 7–8)*.

30. Answer A

The range equation calculates the distance from a transducer to a reflector (structure of interest). It equals the product of propagation speed (velocity of sound in soft tissue) and pulse round-trip time (time from ultrasound pulse emission to its echo reception) divided by two.

Because the ultrasound propagation speed in soft tissue is 1.54 mm/μs, the range equation for soft tissue may be written as follows:

$$\begin{aligned}\text{Distance to a reflector (mm)} &= (1.54\ \text{mm}/\mu\text{s} \times 1/2) \times \text{pulse round} - \text{trip time } (\mu\text{s}) \\ &= 0.77 \times \text{pulse round} - \text{trip time}\end{aligned}$$

Reference 9 *(p 71)*.

31. Answer D

Attenuation is the decrease in intensity and amplitude as sound travels in a medium. It is determined by the frequency of a sound and the distance that the sound travels. Both frequency and distance are directly related to attenuation. The further the ultrasound travels, the greater the attenuation; also, the greater the frequency, the greater the attenuation. Therefore, one should use lower frequency to image deep structures in order to minimize ultrasound attenuation and obtain better image quality. **References** 9 *(p 51)*; 10 *(p 3)*.

32. Answer E

A linear array is a collection of piezoelectric elements arranged in a line within a single transducer housing. Each active element is connected to its own electronic circuitry and isolated from its neighboring crystals. In linear phased array, microsecond delays occur between electronic pulses delivered to the array elements. This time delay of electronic pulses makes electronic beam steering and focusing possible. Therefore, all answers are correct. **References** 9 *(pp 107–110)*; 10 *(pp 12–13)*.

33. Answer A

Annular array transducers have concentric ring-shaped piezoelectric elements with a common center. The transducer uses inner crystals for shallow regions and outer crystals for deep regions. Because small diameter rings have a shallow focus and large diameter rings have a deep focus, annular array transducers have multiple foci that give superior lateral resolution at all depths. However, because of the transducer's multiple foci, the time needed to make a single image or frame is longer; ie, the number of frames per given time is decreased. Therefore, annular phased array has low frame rates with reduced temporal resolution. **References** 9 *(pp 111–112)*; 10 *(pp 6, 42–43)*.

34. Answer C

In linear phased array transducers, both beam steering and focusing are electronic. Beam steering is determined by electronic slope, and beam focusing is determined by electronic curvature. When there is no electronic slope, there is no steering. An upward electronic slope gives upward steering, and a downward electronic slope gives downward steering. When there is no electronic curvature, there is no sound beam focusing. If there is electronic curvature, there is sound beam focusing. **Reference** 9 *(pp 107–110)*.

35. Answer B

Frame rate is the number of frames or images per each second. Each frame consists of individual scan lines. Line density is the number of scan lines per frame. In a given period, frame rate and line density are inversely related. The more scan lines per each frame, the lower the frame rate. In contrast, the fewer scan lines, the higher the frame rate. Temporal resolution is defined as the ability to accurately locate the position of moving structures at particular instants in time. To faithfully image moving structures, it is important to produce pictures (frames) as rapidly as possible. High frame rate provides better temporal resolution. Thus, lower scan lines per frame or lower line density is related to higher frame rate and better temporal resolution. **References** 9 *(p 100)*; 25 *(p 302)*.

36. Answer C

M-mode stands for motion mode. It is also called time-motion mode, which displays the motion of a reflector over time. M-mode has a high temporal resolution and is the only mode that provides information on the position of reflectors with respect to time. Combining M-mode with color flow Doppler is useful when examining cardiac structures and blood flow in terms of timing.

A-mode stands for amplitude mode. It displays returning echoes as spikes. The height of the spikes relates to the amplitude of the returning echoes. The location of the spikes relates to the depth of the reflecting structures.

B-mode stands for brightness mode. In B-mode display, the returning echoes show on the screen as bright dots. The brightness of the dot is related to the strength of the returning echo. The location of the dot is related to the depth of the reflecting structure. **References** 9 *(pp 96–97)*; 10 *(pp 8–12)*; 26 *(pp 9–10)*.

37. Answer C

The output power of a transducer is also called transmitter output, output gain, acoustic output, or energy output. Output power supplies the electrical impulse to the piezoelectric crystal and determines the initial strength of an ultrasound wave. The greater the electrical excitation voltage, the stronger the acoustic output. In contrast, the lower the electrical excitation voltage, the weaker the acoustic output.

The output power can be controlled by the operator using the transmit gain control. Since the transducer output controls the amount of ultrasonic energy that is directed into the patient, one should limit transmit gain to reduce the ultrasound dose to the patient. To optimize image quality, it is best to increase the receiver gain first because this process does not increase patient exposure to ultrasound. One should only increase output power after failing to optimize image quality by increasing receiver gain. **References** 9 *(p 166)*; 26 *(p 11)*.

38. Answer E

The returned ultrasound signals are transformed to electrical signals via piezoelectric elements of the transducer. These electrical signals produced by the transducer are very small. To be displayed on a screen, the small electrical voltages are sent to a receiver for further processing. The five functions of an ultrasound receiver are operated in the following sequence: 1) amplification, 2) compensation, 3) compression, 4) demodulation, and 5) rejection. A helpful tip to remember this sequence is that they are in alphabetical order. **Reference** 9 *(pp 164, 167–171)*.

39. Answer A

Amplification increases all returned ultrasound signals and has no effect on the transmitted ultrasound intensity that is determined by output power. The returned signals from the ultrasound transducer to the receiver are in the microvolt to millivolt range. They must be enlarged for further processing. Typically, signals are amplified by 100,000 to 10 billion times. Amplification can be controlled by the operator using receiver gain or overall gain control. When too little amplification is applied, some of the signals are too small for further processing. When too much amplification is applied, saturation occurs, and all echoes in the image become too bright to distinguish different tissues or structures. Problems attributable to inadequate amplification usually affect the entire image rather than just a portion of the picture. Regional expansion of an interested area with improved spatial resolution is called zoom or write magnification, not amplification. **Reference** 9 *(p 167)*.

40. Answer C

The receiver's compensation function is also called time gain compensation, depth gain compensation, or swept gain compensation. Because attenuation is directly related to the ultrasound path length, identical reflectors produce echoes with different strengths when they are located at different depths. Therefore, to display identical reflectors with similar echo brightness, the signal attenuation attributable to different path length needs to be compensated. Time gain compensation adjusts the degree of amplification, depending on the depth of the reflectors. It applies extra amplification for deeper echoes to make all echoes arising from identical structures appear at the same brightness, regardless of the depth of the reflector. **Reference** 9 *(pp 168–169)*.

41. Answer D

Time gain compensation can be controlled by the operator to optimize image quality. Because high frequency is associated with greater attenuation, more time gain compensation needs to be applied with high-frequency ultrasound waves. In contrast, less time gain compensation is needed with low-frequency ultrasound waves because they undergo less attenuation.

The time gain compensation curve displays the degree of compensation according to the depth of the reflectors. Near gain represents the depth at which no additional amplification is needed to compensate for attenuation because the image is shallow and the attenuation is not significant. Delay marks the depth at which the time gain compensation begins to compensate for attenuation. Slope is the range of depth where the amount of extra amplification is directly proportional to the increasing depth of the image. Thus, deeper structures require more time gain compensation, and shallower ones require less time gain compensation. The knee represents the depth at which the ultrasound system reaches its maximum amplification. Far gain is the region where the ultrasound system has already amplified all incoming signals maximally and cannot apply more time gain compensation, even though the image depth increases further. **References** 9 *(pp 168–169)*; 10 *(pp 17–18)*.

42. Answer D

Dynamic range is the range of the largest to smallest returned signals that can be processed by the different components of an ultrasound system. Because the range of the returned signals is too large to be managed, it must be compressed to be further processed and displayed by the ultrasound system. **References** 9 *(p 169)*; 10 *(pp 16–17)*.

43. Answer C

Compression is the process of reducing the total range of returned signals proportionally, without altering the relationships among the signals. The purpose of compression is to adjust returned signals to the dynamic range for the ultrasound system to further process these signals. During compression, the relative strengths of the signals are maintained. The largest signal remains the largest and the smallest one is still the smallest. **References** 9 *(pp 169–170)*; 10 *(p 19)*.

44. Answer B

Reject eliminates all returned signals that are below a minimum strength. Frequently, the low-level signals are associated with noise and, thus, decrease the image quality. To decrease this noise and improve image quality, reject processes and removes those signals below the reject threshold level. Reject is also called threshold or suppression. It can be controlled by the operator. **References** 9 *(p 170)*; 10 *(p 19)*.

45. Answer B

Demodulation changes the shape of the electrical signals to make them more acceptable for display. This function is automatically set by the ultrasound system and cannot be controlled by the operator.

Demodulation has two steps: rectification and smoothing. Rectification turns all the negative electrical signals into positive ones. Smoothing is also called enveloping. Smoothing eliminates the jagged, rough, or spiked portions of the electrical signals and creates a signal with smooth voltage transitions. **Reference** 9 *(p 171)*.

46. Answer D

47. Answer B

Zoom or regional expansion is also called write magnification. It is a special preprocessing form of image enlargement. Write magnification does not use the original data but collects new image information. Since the new image data are exclusively from the expanded region of interest, the magnified picture contains more scan lines and pixels. Therefore, the magnified region of interest is created using more detailed information with increased scan line density and pixel density, which lead to improved spatial resolution of the image.

In contrast to write magnification, read magnification is an example of postprocessing. Although the region of interest is expanded by read magnification, only the original data are used to create the new image. Thus, the scan line and pixel density in the enlarged region of interest are not increased by read magnification. This explains why the level of detail is similar in the expanded region of interest and the spatial resolution is not improved by read magnification. Write magnification is preferred over read magnification for expanding a region of interest in a clinical image. **Reference** 9 *(pp 186–188)*.

48. Answer C

Returned image signals must be processed by the ultrasound system in order to be displayed on a CRT screen. Preprocessing describes any manipulation of image data before they are stored in the scan converter's memory. Examples of preprocessing include amplification, time gain compensation, and write magnification. Postprocessing describes any manipulation of image data after the data are stored in the scan converter's memory but before display. Examples of postprocessing include read magnification and contrast enhancement. **Reference** 9 *(pp 180, 185–188)*.

49. Answer C

The spatial resolution of an ultrasound system is determined by the ultrasound frequency, pixel density, number of television lines, scan line density, and field of view. Increased ultrasound frequency, pixel density, number of TV lines, and scan line density are associated with improved spatial resolution. Decreased field of view increases the pixel density and number of scan lines per sector image. Thus, the spatial resolution is improved when the field of view is decreased. In contrast, the spatial resolution is decreased when ultrasound frequency is low, pixel density is decreased, number of display TV lines is decreased, field of view is increased, and scan line density is decreased. Read magnification does not rescan the image. The scan line and pixel density are not changed with read magnification. Therefore, spatial resolution is not improved by read magnification. **References** 25 *(pp 301–302)*; 42 *(pp 231–232)*.

50. Answer D

51. Answer E

Digital variables are discrete values and analog variables are a continuum of values. An ultrasound system uses both analog and digital signals. The electrical signals sent by transducer to receiver are in analog form. They are converted into digital form by an analog-to-digital converter to store the image information into the digital scan converter's memory. These digital signals are not actual pictures but use two discrete numbers, zero and one. However, digital signals cannot be displayed on a conventional display screen. After processing, the image data in digital form are converted to analog form by a digital-to-analog converter in order to be presented on a display screen. **Reference** 9 *(pp 180–185)*.

52. Answer E

A binary system is a number system that uses two symbols. In a digital system, a binary digit is called a bit, which is the smallest amount of digital computer memory. Each bit has a value of either zero or one. A group of bits represents a binary number that is assigned to a pixel to store the gray shade of that pixel. An image gray scale is determined by the number of bits per pixel. The more bits per pixel, the greater the selection of gray shades that can be represented. A binary system does not use negative and positive values or symbols. It is not related to odd- and even-numbered lines or fields, which are used for CRT display. **References** 9 *(pp 182–183)*; 42 *(pp 57–58)*.

53. Answer D

A pixel is the smallest element of a digital picture. The smallest amount of digital computer memory is called a bit. A group of bits is assigned to each pixel to store the gray shade of that pixel. The more bits assigned per pixel, the more extensive the choice of gray shades. Thus, an image has more shades of gray if the pixel has more bits. An image has fewer shades of gray if the pixel has fewer bits.

Pixel density is the number of pixels per a given area, but not per a given time. Decreasing pixel density decreases spatial resolution and thus decreases image quality. In contrast, increasing pixel density improves spatial resolution and provides superior image quality. Temporal resolution is determined by frame rate. It is not determined by pixel density. **Reference** 9 *(p 182)*.

54. Answer B

On interlaced display, each frame is formed by the combination of one odd field and one even field. If each field is created in 1/60 second, each frame requires 1/30 second (1/60 second+1/60 second). Frame rate is the number of frames per a given time. Since each frame lasts 1/30 second, there are 30 frames in a second. Therefore, the frame rate is 30 frames per second or 30 Hz. **Reference** 9 *(pp 178–179)*.

55. Answer E

Digital scan converters are used to digitize images. The advantages of digital scan converters are uniformity, stability, durability, and rapidity. Uniformity represents the consistent gray-scale qualities throughout the image. Stability indicates the absence of fade or drift. Durability means consistent pictures with time. Rapidity is the near-instantaneous data processing. **References** 9 *(p 181)*; 42 *(pp 59–60)*.

56. Answer E

An ultrasound system uses a CRT display, a sophisticated device capable of persistence and gray scale. The inner surface of the CRT screen is coated with phosphors that glow when struck by electrons. The image presented on a standard CRT screen comprises 525 horizontal lines. An electron gun fires an electron beam that strikes the phosphors across the screen from left to right and top to bottom with the odd-numbered lines (1, 3, 5, ... 525). This is the odd field. Then, the electron beam sweeps across the phosphor screen with the even-numbered lines (2, 4, 6, ... 524). This is the even field. Thus, the display is interlaced and two fields make up one frame. Freeze frame is the display of one frame. Cine-loop is a repeated display of several frames. **References** 9 *(pp 178–179)*; 23 *(p 91)*.

57. Answer B

Brightness is related to the brilliance of the image. The stronger the echo received by the transducer, the brighter the spot on the CRT screen. However, the overall brightness displayed on the screen can also be controlled by the operator. The brightness control regulates the intensity of the signals seen on the CRT display. Overuse of the brightness control in an attempt to bring in the picture actually decreases the overall image details because of the snowy appearance of the image with too many echoes. Underuse of the brightness control may not allow the display of weak echoes.

Contrast is related to the range of brilliance that is displayed. A high-contrast image has a broad range of brilliance. It greatly differs from the brightest to the dimmest regions on the image. A low-contrast image has a narrow range of brilliance. Contrast can be controlled by the operator. The contrast control regulates the range of brightness. An increase in contrast increases the number of gray shades displayed. A decrease in contrast decreases the number of gray shades displayed. **Reference** 9 *(p 179)*.

58. Answer E

Sector angle indicates the width of the sector on the display screen and determines the size of the image field. When the sector angle is narrowed, the field of view becomes smaller and the scan line density is increased, even though the total scan lines per frame are not changed. To a large extent, the image quality is determined by the scan line density. When the scan lines are widely spread, reconstruction of the image is difficult because of a deficiency of information. In contrast, increased scan line density results in a visually pleasing image. Therefore, the image with narrowed sector angle provides improved resolution with superior quality. An image with wide sector angle has the advantage of visualizing everything at the expense of image quality. **References** 9 *(pp 122–124)*; 10 *(pp 12–15)*; 25 *(pp 295–296)*; 42 *(pp 35–36)*.

59. Answer D

Image depth can be controlled by the operator using the depth control. Deep imaging results in more time for each imaging scan line and longer listening time. Thus, the pulse duration is prolonged and the pulse repetition frequency is decreased. Decreasing the image depth shortens the pulse duration and increases the pulse repetition frequency. **References** 9 *(pp 122–124)*; 25 *(p 297)*.

60. Answer C

An increase in frame rate improves temporal resolution. Frame rate is important when one is attempting to resolve the motion of rapidly moving structures. Increasing frame rate allows more detailed motion analysis, although this greater detail occurs at the price of decreased scan line density. Starting with a fixed number of lines of information, an increase in frame rate decreases the scan lines available for individual frames. As the scan lines per frame are reduced, the spatial resolution is decreased. Therefore, very high frame rates result in a trade-off between frame rate and image quality. However, when the frame rate is too low (fewer than 20 frames per second), the image appears to flicker because of decreased temporal resolution.

Both axial and lateral resolution are not determined by frame rate. Axial resolution is determined by spatial pulse length, lateral resolution, and ultrasound beam width. **References** 9 *(pp 100, 122–124)*; 25 *(p 302)*; 42 *(pp 230–232)*.

Chapter 2

Basic Principles of Doppler Ultrasound

Questions

Multiple choice (choose the *one* best answer):

1. The Doppler effect
   A. states that sound frequency increases as a sound source moves toward the observer and decreases as the sound source moves away from the observer.
   B. states that if a receiver is moving in relation to a stationary sound source, a shift in sound frequency is observed.
   C. states that if the sound source is moving in relation to a stationary receiver, a shift in sound frequency is observed.
   D. is observed when the red blood cells approach the ultrasound transducer or move away from it.
   E. is all of the above.

2. Positive Doppler shift indicates that
   A. the transmitted frequency is equal to the received frequency.
   B. the transmitted frequency is greater than the received frequency.
   C. the red blood cells are approaching the transducer.
   D. the red blood cells are moving away from the transducer.
   E. the red blood cells are not moving.

3. During a diagnostic Doppler examination, which one of the following is true?
   A. The sound wave emitted by the transducer is ultrasonic.
   B. The sound wave received by the transducer is ultrasonic.
   C. The Doppler shift is ultrasonic.
   D. A and B.
   E. All of the above.

4. Which one of the following best describes what the Doppler shift is used to measure?
   A. The speed of the red blood cells.
   B. The number of the red blood cells.
   C. The velocity of the red blood cells.
   D. The concentration of the red blood cells.
   E. The speed of the blood flow.

5. The Doppler equation

A. states that an increase in transmitted frequency results in a decrease in the Doppler shift.

B. describes the relationship among the flow velocity, ultrasound attenuation, and image depth.

C. states that Doppler frequency is inversely related to the velocity of the red blood cells.

D. is the mathematical relationship of the transmitted frequency, the frequency shift, and the velocity of the red blood cells.

E. indicates that the Doppler shift is overestimated when the angle of interrogation moves toward 90°.

6. The Doppler equation can be rearranged. Which one of the following is true about the rearranged Doppler equation?

A. Most frequently, the Doppler equation is rearranged to solve the propagation speed.

B. The rearranged Doppler equation is more useful because the propagation speed can be calculated instead of the Doppler shift frequencies.

C. The Doppler equation can be rearranged to solve the direction of flow instead of the Doppler shift frequencies.

D. The rearranged Doppler equation is less useful because the primary interest is usually the calculated Doppler frequency shift, not the flow velocity.

E. The Doppler equation is rearranged to calculate the velocity of the red blood cells instead of the frequency shift.

7. In diagnostic ultrasound, the range of Doppler shift frequencies is

A. 2.5 MHz to 7 MHz.

B. −2.5 MHz to −7 MHz.

C. 2 MHz to 10 MHz.

D. −2 MHz to −10 MHz.

E. −10 kHz to +10 kHz.

8. According to the Doppler equation, all of the following factors influence Doppler shift ***except***

A. the depth of reflectors.

B. the angle of interrogation.

C. the flow velocity.

D. the transmitted frequency.

E. the velocity of the red blood cells.

9. Doppler effect detects the velocity of red blood cells. Which one of the following situations limits the ability to successfully perform a diagnostic Doppler examination?

A. A patient with anemia due to decreased red blood cells.

B. A patient with a normal red blood cell level.

C. A patient with polycythemia.
D. A and C.
E. None of the above.

10. The Nyquist limit
A. is the Doppler frequency below which aliasing occurs.
B. equals half the pulse repetition frequency.
C. is present during continuous wave Doppler examination.
D. is not related to pulse repetition frequency.
E. is the threshold above which the flow velocity disappears on the Doppler spectral display.

11. To avoid aliasing, one should
A. avoid using continuous wave Doppler.
B. increase transmitted frequency.
C. decrease sector depth.
D. decrease velocity scale or avoid baseline shift on the Doppler spectral display.
E. decrease pulse repetition frequency.

12. The pulsed wave Doppler transducer
A. uses the same output power as that of clinical imaging.
B. uses split piezoelectric crystals in the transducer.
C. has two piezoelectric crystals in the transducer, one continuously transmits and the other continuously receives the ultrasound pulse.
D. uses one piezoelectric crystal in the transducer, alternating between transmitting and receiving ultrasound pulse.
E. does not use ultrasound because Doppler frequency is within an audible range.

13. A continuous wave Doppler transducer
A. uses more output power than a pulsed wave Doppler transducer.
B. uses split piezoelectric crystals in the transducer.
C. has multiple piezoelectric crystals in the transducer, alternating between transmitting and receiving ultrasound pulse.
D. uses one piezoelectric crystal in the transducer, alternating between transmitting and receiving ultrasound pulse.
E. does not use ultrasound because Doppler frequency is within an audible range.

14. The current method for spectral analysis of pulsed wave and continuous wave Doppler signals is
A. autocorrelation.
B. time interval histograms.
C. fast Fourier transform.
D. chirp z-transforms.
E. zero-crossing detection.

15. Autocorrelation is
- A. the current method for spectral analysis of color flow Doppler.
- B. faster than fast Fourier transform.
- C. less accurate than fast Fourier transform.
- D. all of the above.
- E. none of the above.

16. The Doppler spectral display is composed of
- A. the x-axis which represents time or duration of flow.
- B. the y-axis which represents the Doppler frequency shift or velocity.
- C. the z-axis which represents the gray scale.
- D. A and B.
- E. all of the above.

17. Doppler spectral display provides all the following graphic information ***except***
- A. the character of blood flow.
- B. the volume of blood flow.
- C. the magnitude of blood flow.
- D. the velocity of blood flow.
- E. the duration of blood flow.

18. Spectral broadening can be caused by
- A. turbulent flow.
- B. small sample volume size.
- C. narrow beam width.
- D. laminar flow.
- E. small sample volume size located in the near field.

19. The major advantage of pulsed wave Doppler is
- A. the ability to correctly measure high velocity of blood flow.
- B. range discrimination.
- C. the ability to avoid aliasing.
- D. range resolution.
- E. B or D.

20. The major disadvantage of continuous wave Doppler is best described as
- A. range discrimination.
- B. the inability to avoid aliasing.
- C. range ambiguity.
- D. range resolution.
- E. the inability to accurately measure high velocity of the blood flow.

21. When the sample volume is shallower (closer to the transducer),
- A. the pulse repetition frequency is decreased.
- B. the Nyquist limit is increased.
- C. aliasing is more likely to occur.

D. the pulse repetition frequency is not changed.
E. the Nyquist frequency is decreased.

22. The components of the Doppler spectrum include
A. the mean velocity.
B. the peak velocity.
C. the modal velocity.
D. A and B.
E. all of the above.

23. Color flow imaging
A. is the combination of two-dimensional imaging and color flow Doppler, which uses the continuous wave Doppler principle to assign the colors to the Doppler shift frequencies.
B. can depict maximum velocity as well as mean velocity.
C. uses the pulsed wave Doppler principle.
D. is not useful in characterizing blood flow.
E. is the two-dimensional image with the assignment of a special color.

24. The sampling method of color flow Doppler is
A. single gated.
B. double gated.
C. multiple gated.
D. not gated.
E. none of the above.

25. The sampling method of pulsed wave Doppler is
A. single gated.
B. double gated.
C. multiple gated.
D. not gated.
E. none of the above.

26. Packet size is
A. the number of ultrasound pulses in a packet at a particular gate.
B. the diameter of each packet.
C. the average volume of packets in one frame.
D. the number of packets per image.
E. the average size of packets per image.

27. An increase in packet size
A. improves temporal resolution.
B. improves estimation of peak velocity.
C. improves estimation of mean velocity.
D. increases frame rate.
E. B and C.

28. The variance mode map has
A. the color bar with red color at the top and blue color at the bottom.
B. the colors designating turbulent flow above the black stripe and those designating laminar flow below the black stripe.
C. the colors designating laminar flow above the black stripe and those designating turbulent flow below the black stripe.
D. the colors designating turbulent flow on the left and laminar flow on the right side of the color map.
E. the colors designating laminar flow on the left and turbulent flow on the right side of the color map.

29. Which one of the following about color maps is true?
A. Red color always indicates that the blood flow is moving toward the transducer.
B. Blue color always indicates that the blood flow is moving away from the transducer.
C. Blackness always depicts a no-flow region.
D. Green color is added to indicate areas of variance.
E. All of the above.

30. To preserve temporal resolution during color flow imaging, one should
A. decrease the frame rate.
B. increase the image depth.
C. use a narrow color sector.
D. increase the scan line density.
E. use a large packet size.

31. The most accurate velocity measurement is obtained when the red blood cells travel
A. in a direction with an acute angle between the blood flow and the ultrasound beam.
B. in a direction with an obtuse angle between the blood flow and the ultrasound beam.
C. in a direction perpendicular to the ultrasound beam.
D. in a direction parallel to the ultrasound beam.
E. in any direction relative to the ultrasound beam.

32. Which one of the following is a limitation of color flow imaging?
A. Color flow imaging systems generally have reduced temporal resolution.
B. Color flow images are subject to the aliasing artifact.
C. The optimal views for imaging are often different from the optimal views for Doppler.
D. Superior operator skills are required for optimal use and interpretation of color flow Doppler when compared with other ultrasound imaging techniques.
E. All of the above.

33. Comparing myocardial tissue motion with blood flow,
A. the tissue motion has lower Doppler velocity with higher Doppler signal intensity.
B. the blood flow has higher Doppler velocity with higher Doppler signal intensity.
C. the blood flow has lower Doppler velocity with higher Doppler signal intensity.
D. the tissue motion has lower Doppler velocity with lower Doppler signal intensity.
E. the blood flow has lower Doppler velocity with lower Doppler signal intensity.

34. During Doppler tissue imaging,
A. the Doppler system rejects high frequencies to measure wall motion velocities.
B. the high velocity of myocardial wall motion is detected by a conventional color flow Doppler system.
C. the Doppler system filters low frequencies with high-pass filter in order to measure wall motion velocities.
D. only the low-amplitude signals are analyzed.
E. the myocardium cannot be color coded according to the direction and velocity of its motion.

35. Tissue Doppler velocities
A. cannot be displayed in two-dimensional format.
B. cannot be displayed in M-mode format.
C. can be displayed in M-mode format, but not in two-dimensional format.
D. can be autocorrelated to a color scheme and displayed in two-dimensional format, but not in M-mode format.
E. can be autocorrelated to a color scheme and displayed both in M-mode and two-dimensional formats.

Answers & Discussion

1. Answer E

The Doppler effect or Doppler shift was named after the Austrian physicist Christian J. Doppler who first described this principle in 1842. The Doppler effect states that the frequency of a sound wave changes relative to the motion of the sound source or observer. If a sound source is moving in relation to a stationary receiver, a shift in frequency is observed. If a receiver is moving in relation to a stationary sound source, a shift in frequency also is observed. The sound frequency increases as a sound source moves toward the observer and decreases as the sound source moves away from the observer.

In daily life, a moving source of sound, such as a train, sounds higher in pitch to an observer whom it is approaching and sounds lower in pitch to an observer from whom it is receding. This phenomenon is attributable to the sound frequency shift or Doppler shift.

In clinical diagnosis, if ultrasonic energy encounters a moving particle, the energy reflected by those moving particles returns to the transducer at an altered frequency because of the Doppler effect. This phenomenon is observed when red blood cells approach the ultrasound transducer or move away from it. **References** 8 *(p 183)*; 9 *(pp 127–129)*; 10 *(pp 26–27)*; 18 *(pp 2–3)*; 26 *(pp 15–16)*.

2. Answer C

The Doppler shift is the difference between the frequency received by the transducer after striking red blood cells and the frequency initially produced by the ultrasound transducer. Therefore, a positive Doppler shift indicates that the received frequency is greater than the transmitted frequency. This occurs when the red blood cells are approaching the transducer. In contrast, a negative Doppler shift indicates that the received frequency is less than the transmitted frequency. This occurs when the red blood cells are moving away from the transducer. **References** 8 *(p 183)*; 9 *(pp 127–129)*; 10 *(pp 26–27)*; 18 *(pp 2–3)*; 23 *(p 16)*; 26 *(pp 15–16)*.

3. Answer D

During a diagnostic Doppler examination, the sound wave transmitted by the transducer is ultrasonic. The sound wave received by the transducer after it strikes the red blood cells also is ultrasonic. The difference between the received and transmitted frequencies is within the audible range. Therefore, the Doppler shift is audible, not ultrasonic. **References** 9 *(pp 127–129)*; 10 *(pp 26–27)*; 23 *(p 16)*; 26 *(pp 15–16)*.

4. Answer C

The Doppler shift or Doppler effect is used to measure the velocity of the red blood cells, not the speed. Velocity describes both the speed and the direction of a moving object. Speed describes only how fast an object is moving with no information about its direction. The Doppler shift is related to the speed and direction of the red blood cells. The faster the speed of the red blood cells, the greater the Doppler shift. Also, the red blood cells moving toward the transducer result in a positive Doppler shift and those moving away from the transducer result in a negative Doppler shift. **References** 9 *(pp 127–129)*; 10 *(pp 26–27)*; 23 *(p 16)*; 26 *(pp 15–16)*.

5. Answer D

The Doppler equation is the mathematical relationship of the transmitted ultrasound frequency, the frequency shift, and the velocity of the moving target, ie, red blood cells. Thus, $Fd = 2Fo \times V \times \text{cosine } \theta / C$. In this equation, Fd is the Doppler shift expressed in Hertz, Fo is the transducer frequency in Hertz, V is the velocity of the moving particles (red blood cells) in meters per second, C is the propagation speed of sound in soft tissue (1,540 m/s), and θ is the angle between the Doppler sound beam and the wall of the blood vessel, which is approximately the same as the direction of the blood flow. The 2 in the equation is necessary because the ultrasound must complete a round trip between the transducer and the moving blood cells, and thus, the amount of Doppler shift caused by a moving particle is doubled.

According to the Doppler equation, the Doppler frequency is increased when the transmitted frequency or the velocity of the red blood cells is increased. Because cosine θ equals one, the Doppler frequency is maximal when the angle θ is equal to $0°$; that is, the sound beam is parallel to the direction of the blood flow. The Doppler shift for the moving red blood cells at any velocity is zero if the angle θ is $90°$. When the angle of interrogation moves from $0°$ toward $90°$, the Doppler shift is progressively underestimated. **References** 8 *(p 185)*; 9 *(p 131)*; 10 *(p 27)*; 18 (pp 2–3); 23 *(p 16)*; 26 *(pp 15–16)*.

6. Answer E

The form of the Doppler equation is rearranged to calculate the velocity of the red blood cells instead of the frequency shift. Thus, V = Fd × C/2 × Fo × cosine θ. Usually, the velocity of the moving target rather than the Doppler shift frequency is the variable of primary interest. In general, the propagation speed is assumed constant (1,540 m/s), and the transmitted frequency is determined during the Doppler study. They are not the primary reasons to rearrange the Doppler equation. This rearranged Doppler equation is more useful because the unknown V (the velocity of the moving target) can be solved easily. Blood flow velocities determined by Doppler echocardiography are used subsequently to derive various hemodynamic data. **References** 9 *(p 131)*; 10 *(p 27)*; 18 *(pp 2–3)*; 23 *(p 16)*; 26 *(pp 15–16)*.

7. Answer E

In diagnostic ultrasound, the typical range of Doppler shift frequencies is −10 kHz to +10 kHz, using an ultrasound transducer with frequency range of 2 MHz to 10 MHz. This means that the reflected frequency that returns to the transducer after bouncing off a red blood cell falls in a range from 10 kHz below to 10 kHz above the frequency emitted by the ultrasound transducer. This range of Doppler shift frequencies is within the audible range. **Reference** 9 *(pp 127–129)*.

8. Answer A

As expressed in the Doppler equation, the factors influencing Doppler shift are the transmitted ultrasound frequency, the angle of interrogation, the flow velocity, and the red blood cell velocity. In general, the propagation speed of sound is the speed in soft tissue (1,540 m/s), which is assumed constant. According to the Doppler equation, an increase in the transmitted frequency or the velocity of the red blood cells results in an increase in the Doppler shift. The angle of interrogation is the angle between the ultrasound beam and the direction of a moving target. Because cosine θ is one, a 0° angle of interrogation results in the maximal Doppler shift. A 20° angle of interrogation results in a 6% underestimation of the true Doppler shift. A 60° angle results in a Doppler shift that is only half the true Doppler shift. A 90° angle results in no Doppler shift because cosine 90° is zero. Therefore, as angle θ increases, the corresponding cosine becomes progressively less than one. This results in underestimation of the Doppler shift. The depth of reflectors is not part of the Doppler equation. **References** 8 *(pp 186–187)*; 9 *(pp 129–130, 242)*; 10 *(p 27)*; 18 *(p 3)*.

9. Answer E

In clinical diagnosis, the Doppler effect detects the velocity of red blood cells. However, changes in red blood cell concentration do not limit the ability to successfully perform a diagnostic Doppler examination. Even in patients with anemia with decreased red blood cells, the number of red blood cells sufficient to support life is enough for successful performance of a diagnostic Doppler examination. Normal red blood cell levels, anemia, or polycythemia does not limit the ability to successfully perform a Doppler study. **Reference** 9 *(p 141)*.

10. Answer B

The Nyquist limit or Nyquist frequency is the Doppler frequency at which aliasing occurs during pulsed wave Doppler. The Nyquist limit (measured in Hertz) equals half the pulse repetition frequency. The Nyquist limit and aliasing are present during pulsed wave Doppler examination, but not during continuous wave Doppler. When aliasing occurs, the flow that exceeds the Nyquist limit does not disappear but appears as if it were flowing in the opposite direction; that is, the Doppler spectrum is cut off at the Nyquist limit and the remaining frequency shift is recorded on the opposite side of the baseline. This phenomenon is commonly called "signal wraparound." **References** 8 *(p 188)*; 10 *(pp 29–30, 32)*; 24 *(p 293)*; 26 *(p 19)*.

11. Answer C

Aliasing is recognized on conventional pulsed wave Doppler and color flow Doppler that uses the pulsed wave Doppler principle. To avoid aliasing, the examiner should do four things:

1. Decrease sector depth and increase pulse repetition frequency. When decreasing the sector depth, the go-return time required for the pulse to travel away from and back to the transducer is shortened. Thus, the pulse duration is decreased and the pulse repetition frequency is increased. Because the Nyquist limit equals half the pulse repetition frequency and is the frequency at which aliasing occurs, increasing pulse repetition frequency leads to an increase in Nyquist limit and a decrease in the chance of aliasing.
2. Shift the baseline position or increase the velocity scales on the Doppler spectral display. The zero baseline may be moved up or down by the operator to allow the ultrasound system to electronically unwrap the aliased signal. Mild aliasing can be resolved by shifting the baseline to the edge of the display, effectively allowing resolution of velocities up to twice the Nyquist limit. Similarly, the velocity scale can be increased to improve the velocity range that can be displayed without aliasing. However, these manipulations of velocity display can unwrap only mild aliasing signals. When the flow velocity is so high that the Doppler signals wrap around many times, aliasing cannot be avoided, even by shifting the baseline position or by increasing the velocity scale.
3. Decrease the transmitted frequency. As the transmitted frequency decreases, the Doppler shift frequency decreases. This may lower the Doppler shift below the Nyquist limit and, thus, eliminate aliasing.
4. Use continuous wave Doppler. Aliasing is the major disadvantage of pulsed wave Doppler. In contrast, continuous wave Doppler does not have this problem. In the continuous wave mode, the transducer has two piezoelectric crystals: one to send and the other to receive the ultrasound waves continuously. Therefore, the maximal frequency shift that can be recorded by continuous wave Doppler is not limited by the pulsed repetition frequency or the Nyquist limit. If range resolution is not important, using continuous wave Doppler resolves the problem of aliasing. **References** 10 *(pp 29–30, 32)*; 25 *(p 293)*; 26 *(p 19)*; 42 *(pp 274–275)*.

12. Answer D

13. Answer B

The pulsed wave Doppler uses a single piezoelectric crystal in the transducer, alternating between transmitting and receiving ultrasound pulse. The pulsed wave transducer sends an ultrasound pulse to the interested target located by sample volume and then becomes deaf to returning echoes. At the exact moment when the echo would return from the target as calculated by the ultrasound system, the transducer listens for a reflection. Therefore, only the returned signal from the interested target located by the sample volume is recorded. The output power used for pulsed wave Doppler is greater than that used for clinical imaging or for continuous wave Doppler. In contrast to pulsed wave Doppler, the continuous wave Doppler uses split piezoelectric crystals; that is, two pieces of piezoelectric crystal are used in the transducer: one continuously transmits and the other continuously receives the ultrasound pulses. Although Doppler shift is within an audible range, it is the difference between the transmitted and the received ultrasound frequencies. Therefore, both pulsed wave and continuous wave Doppler must have an ultrasound transducer to emit and receive the ultrasound frequencies. **References** 8 *(pp 188–191)*; 10 *(pp 28–29)*; 18 *(pp 3–5)*; 23 *(pp 16, 18–19)*; 26 *(p 17)*.

14. Answer C

The current method for spectral analysis of pulsed wave and continuous wave Doppler signals is the fast Fourier transform, a computerized, mathematical technique used to identify various frequencies that combine to form the complex Doppler waveform. Old methods of spectral analysis include zero-crossing detection, time interval histograms, and chirp z-transforms. Autocorrelation is the current method for color flow Doppler. **References** 9 *(pp 138, 141)*; 26 *(p 16)*; 42 *(pp 209–211)*.

15. Answer D

Autocorrelation is the current method for spectral analysis of color flow Doppler. During color flow Doppler, signal acquisition is based on repetitive transmission of an ultrasound burst along the scan line. The mean frequency along the scan line is estimated. This process is repeated for each scan line of the image. Then, the signals of the mean frequencies are digitized and automatically correlated (autocorrelation) with a preset color scheme. Color flow Doppler acquires an enormous amount of information related to blood velocities. The fast Fourier transform technique of spectral analysis used for both pulsed and continuous wave Doppler is not fast enough to process the huge quantity of data from color flow Doppler. Autocorrelation has the advantage of being faster than the fast Fourier transform technique. However, its disadvantage is that it is less accurate than the fast Fourier transform technique. **References** 9 *(p 156)*; 10 *(p 101)*; 18 *(p 8)*; 23 *(pp 20–21)*.

16. Answer E

The Doppler spectral display is composed of three axes, x, y, and z. The x-axis represents the duration or time of the flow. The y-axis represents the Doppler frequency shift or velocity. The z-axis is the gray scale of the spectral analysis, which represents the amplitude of the Doppler shift. Shades of gray are assigned to returning Doppler shift frequencies according to their amplitude. In other words, the gray scale is used to judge the intensity or, to some extent, the number of red blood cells in the moving column of blood being interrogated. **References** 8 *(p 187)*; 9 *(p 138)*; 10 *(p 32)*; 18 *(pp 5–6)*; 26 *(pp 16–17)*.

17. Answer B

Doppler spectral analysis displays the graphic information about the duration, velocity, magnitude, and character of the blood flow. The duration of the blood flow is presented on the x-axis of the spectral display. The velocity is the speed and direction of the blood flow. The y-axis indicates the speed of the blood flow. By convention, positive Doppler shifts are displayed above the zero baseline, and negative Doppler shifts are displayed below the zero baseline. The magnitude of the blood flow is demonstrated on the spectral display by the modal velocity. The character of the blood flow is demonstrated by pulsed wave spectral display as either laminar or turbulent by the degree of spectral broadening and spectral window fill-in. However, the spectral analysis does not directly display any graphic information about the volume of the blood flow. **References** 8 *(p 187)*; 9 *(p 138)*; 10 *(p 32)*; 18 *(pp 5–6)*; 26 *(pp 16–17)*.

18. Answer A

Spectral broadening is the widening of the Doppler shift display. It can be caused by turbulent flow, large sample volume size, and wide beam width. Because turbulent flow moves in multiple directions with multiple velocities, it creates a wide range of Doppler shift frequencies and, hence, spectral broadening. A large sample volume introduces spectral broadening because the sample gate detects Doppler shift frequencies over a greater anatomic area. Beam diameter is determined by the distance from the transducer. When the sample gate is placed in the far field, the beam width is wide, and thus, the Doppler shift information is detected over a broad anatomic area. This may result in spectral broadening. **Reference** 31 *(p 283)*.

19. Answer E

The major advantage of pulsed wave Doppler is the ability to determine the Doppler shift at a precise location by using a sample volume or range gate. This ability is called range discrimination or range resolution. In pulsed wave Doppler, a single piezoelectric crystal emits an ultrasound pulse to the interested area located by the sample volume and awaits the return of reflected ultrasound wave from that area. Only the Doppler shift information corresponding to the location of the sample volume is received and processed. Therefore, one can place the pulsed wave Doppler sample volume at an interested area and receive Doppler shift information from that location only. (See also Questions 12 and 20.) **References** 8 *(p 188)*; 9 *(p 134)*; 26 *(p 18)*.

20. Answer C

The major disadvantage of continuous wave Doppler is range ambiguity. With continuous wave Doppler, the Doppler shift information is detected all along the sound beam, and the spectrum displays Doppler shift created by any blood flow intersecting the path of the sound beam. Therefore, the precise location of the Doppler shift cannot be detected. This lack of range resolution is called range ambiguity. Range discrimination or range resolution is the major advantage of pulsed wave Doppler. The major advantage of continuous wave Doppler is the ability to accurately measure high velocities of blood flow. Since the continuous wave transducer has two piezoelectric crystals with one to send and the other to receive the ultrasound waves continuously, continuous wave Doppler does not cause aliasing in the presence of high velocities. Answers B and E are wrong because the inability to accurately measure high velocity due to aliasing is the major disadvantage of pulsed wave Doppler.

In summary, for continuous wave Doppler, the major advantage is the capability of high-velocity measurement; the major disadvantage is the range ambiguity or lack of range resolution. For pulsed wave Doppler, the major advantage is the range discrimination or range resolution; the major disadvantage is the inability of high-velocity measurements due to aliasing. (See also Question 19.) **References** 8 *(p 188)*; 9 *(p 132)*; 10 *(pp 28–29)*; 18 *(pp 3–5)*; 26 *(pp 22–23)*.

21. Answer B

Pulsed wave Doppler measures flow velocities at a specific location within a sample volume. The pulse repetition frequency and Nyquist limit vary inversely with the depth of the sample volume. The shallower the location of the sample volume, the higher the pulse repetition frequency and Nyquist limit. In contrast, the deeper the sample volume, the lower the pulse repetition frequency and Nyquist limit. Aliasing occurs when the Doppler shift frequency of the blood flow with high velocity exceeds the Nyquist limit. An increase in pulse repetition frequency and Nyquist limit reduces the chance of aliasing. In other words, higher velocities may be recorded without aliasing by pulsed wave Doppler if the sample volume is closer to the transducer. (See also Question 19.) **References** 8 *(p 188)*; 26 *(pp 18–19, 134)*.

22. Answer E

The components of the Doppler spectrum are mean, peak, and modal frequencies or velocities. Mean frequency or velocity represents the average Doppler shift frequency or velocity. Peak frequency or velocity is the maximum Doppler shift frequency or velocity. Modal frequency or velocity is the frequency or velocity with the highest amplitude. Modal frequency or velocity is less affected by the noise level than either the mean or the peak frequency or velocity. **Reference** 42 *(pp 212–215)*.

23. Answer C

Color flow imaging is the combination of two-dimensional imaging and color flow Doppler, which uses the pulsed wave Doppler principle to assign the colors to the Doppler shift frequencies. It provides real-time, color-coded blood flow velocity information superimposed on a two-dimensional image. Because color flow Doppler is based on pulsed wave Doppler principles, aliasing occurs when the Nyquist limit is exceeded. Color flow imaging has gained wide acceptance for the evaluation of intracardiac flow disturbances. It is useful in characterizing blood flow as laminar or turbulent. However, color flow Doppler displays mean velocity flow information only and cannot depict the maximum velocity. **References** 9 *(pp 146–155)*; 23 *(pp 20–22)*; 25 *(pp 291–305)*; 42 *(pp 218–233)*.

24. Answer C

25. Answer A

Color flow Doppler uses multiple sampling sites or gates along each scan line to detect Doppler shift information. At each sampling site or gate, the frequency shift is measured, converted to a digital format, automatically correlated with a preset color scheme, and displayed as color flow superimposed on two-dimensional imaging.

Pulsed wave Doppler detects a Doppler shift using one gate along the scan line. Analyzing sound received only at specific times (gating) localizes and analyzes reflections from a specific depth. Therefore, the sampling method of color flow Doppler is multigated and that of pulsed wave Doppler is single gated. The accompanying drawing illustrates how color flow imaging is performed and displayed. Dots indicate multiple sampling sites (gates). The frequency shift measured at each gate is automatically correlated (autocorrelation) and converted to a preset color scheme (red for flow toward and blue for flow away from the transducer). **References** 9 *(pp 132–135)*; 23 *(pp 16, 18–19)*.

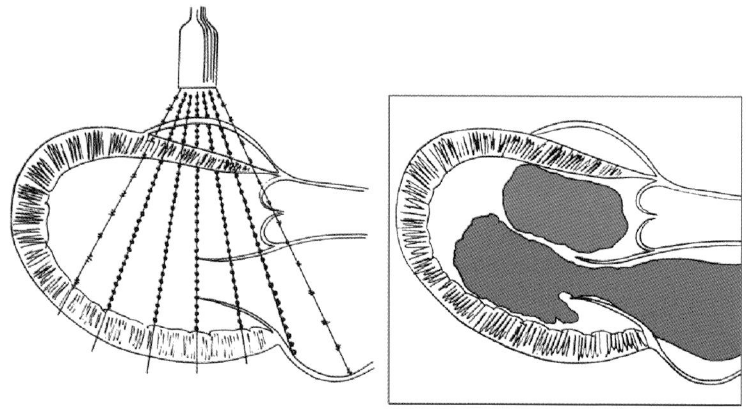

Figure from Oh et al. (23). Used with permission of Mayo Foundation for Medical Education and Research.

26. Answer A

Accurate measurement of the red blood cell velocity is impossible using only a single ultrasound Doppler pulse, and information from a number of pulses is required to estimate the velocity of blood flow at a particular gate. This group of ultrasound pulses is called a packet or a pulse train. The number of ultrasound pulses in the packet at a particular gate is called the packet size. Obviously, the larger a packet size, the more data that are integrated and the more accurate the mean frequency. **References** 9 *(p 153)*; 18 *(p 12)*; 42 *(p 224)*.

27. Answer C

The accuracy of Doppler velocity measurements depends on the packet size. When the packet size is increased, estimation of the Doppler shift is more accurate. However, as packet size increases, more time is required to collect Doppler information from each scan line. Thus, the disadvantage of increasing packet size is that the frame rate decreases. Because color flow Doppler provides information on mean velocity only, an increase in packet size improves the estimation of mean velocity but at the cost of decreasing the frame rate and reducing temporal resolution. **References** 9 *(p 153)*; 18 *(p 12)*; 42 *(p 224)*.

28. Answer E

In color flow imaging, there are two types of color maps, the velocity mode and the variance mode. The velocity mode map has the colors displayed above and below the black stripe on the color bar according to the velocity of the blood flow. The black stripe indicates that no Doppler shift was measured. In general, the color designating blood flow directed toward the transducer appears above the black stripe, and the color designating blood flow directed away from the transducer appears below the black stripe. Each color has multiple shades, and the lighter shades within each primary color are assigned to higher velocities within the Nyquist limit. When flow velocity is higher than the Nyquist limit, color aliasing occurs and is depicted as a color reversal.

The variance mode map allows color flow Doppler systems to display both laminar and turbulent flows. As the velocity mode map, the variance mode map displays the colors above and below the black stripe according to the direction of the blood flow in relation to the transducer. In addition, the variance mode map varies from side to side, depending on the character of the blood flow. The colors designating laminar flow appear on the left side of the color map and those designating turbulent flow appear on the right side. **References** 9 *(pp 147–155)*; 23 *(pp 20–22)*; 25 *(pp 291–305)*; 42 *(pp 218–233)*.

29. Answer D

Red or blue color does not always indicate that the blood flow is moving toward or away from the transducer, for two reasons:

1. The color map used to display flow velocity is somewhat arbitrary. Although many echocardiography laboratories use red to denote flow toward the transducer and blue for flow away from the transducer, there is actually no standardization of color format. Thus, for proper interpretation, one must always study the color map on the image.
2. Because color flow Doppler is based on the pulsed wave Doppler principle, its major disadvantage is aliasing at very high velocity. Aliasing is displayed on color flow Doppler as color reversal. Therefore, very high-velocity blood flow toward the transducer may be encoded in blue because of aliasing and that away from the transducer may appear in red.

An absence of color or blackness is used to depict areas where no Doppler shift is detected, which indicates either no flow or blood flow directed at a 90° angle to the path of the ultrasound beam. Because the cosine of 90° is zero, the Doppler shift is zero according to the Doppler equation. Therefore, any blood flow moving perpendicular to the ultrasound beam does not have detectable Doppler shift and is encoded in black.

Both turbulent flow and signal aliasing result in an apparent wide range of velocities. Thus, flow disturbance and very high-velocity flow are characterized by the presence of variance. The degree of variance from the mean velocity can be coded as a variance color. Typically, a shade of green is added to indicate areas of variance. Therefore, turbulent blood flow and flow acceleration are easily recognized by the combinations of multiple colors according to the degree of variance. **References** 9 *(pp 147–155)*; 23 *(pp 20–22)*; 25 *(pp 291–305)*; 42 *(pp 218–233)*.

30. Answer C

Temporal resolution is important when examining rapidly moving structures. To preserve temporal resolution, the frame rate is preserved by using a narrow color sector, low scan line density, small packet size, and shallow image depth. Scan line density is the number of scan lines per frame. It affects both the spatial and temporal resolution of the color flow display. Closely spaced scan lines provide optimal spatial resolution but decrease frame rate by the finite amount of time needed to interrogate each scan line. Similarly, a wide color sector with a large number of scan lines decreases frame rate. In contrast, lower scan line density results in a higher frame rate with improved temporal resolution at the cost of spatial resolution. To some extent, the trade-off between frame rate and scan line density can be optimized by narrowing the sector width to include only the region of interest. If the color sector width is decreased, the line density increases while the frame rate is preserved. During color flow Doppler, the accurate measurement of mean velocity depends on the packet size. As the packet size increases, the estimation of mean velocity is improved, but more time is required to obtain the Doppler information. This leads to a reduced frame rate and decreased temporal resolution. In contrast, smaller packet size decreases the time required for data collection and increases the frame rate, although flow measurements are less accurate. Therefore, the color flow system must balance the desire for accurate Doppler with the need for a diagnostic frame rate. Maximum depth is the greatest depth at which color flow Doppler is displayed. An increase in the maximum image depth reduces the frame rate and thus decreases temporal resolution. In contrast, a decrease in image depth increases the frame rate and therefore improves temporal resolution. **References** 9 *(pp 100, 153)*; 10 *(pp 40, 102–104)*; 18 *(pp 11–12)*; 42 *(pp 224, 230–232)*.

31. Answer D

Mathematically, the Doppler effect can be represented by the following Doppler equation: $Fd = 2Fo \times V \times \text{cosine}\ \theta / C$. The angle of interrogation θ is the angle between the ultrasound beam and the wall of the blood vessel in which the red blood cells travel. Because cosine θ is one, the most accurate velocity measurement is obtained when the red blood cells travel in a direction parallel to the ultrasound beam. The Doppler shift for moving red blood cells at any velocity is zero when the angle of interrogation is 90° because cosine 90° is zero. **References** 8 *(pp 185–187)*; 9 *(pp 129–131, 242)*; 10 *(p 27)*.

32. Answer E

Color flow imaging has several limitations:

1. Reduced temporal resolution. The time required for the ultrasound system to make a single color flow image is relatively long. Therefore, color flow imaging generally reduces temporal resolution.
2. Aliasing artifact. Because color flow Doppler is based on the pulsed wave Doppler principle, color flow images are subject to aliasing artifact.
3. Differing views. The optimal views for imaging are often different from the optimal views for Doppler. During two-dimensional imaging, in order to obtain more accurate measurement and better image quality, the ultrasound beam is best oriented perpendicular to the anatomic structure of interest, because the axial resolution is superior to the lateral resolution. However, the Doppler frequency shift is measured

most accurately when the ultrasound beam is parallel to the direction of the moving target. Therefore, the examiner should balance these considerations to produce the most clinically relevant images.

4. Need for superior operator skills. Although the color flow images are alluring, superior operator skills are a prerequisite for the optimal use and interpretation of color flow Doppler compared with other ultrasound imaging techniques. **References** 9 *(p 159)*; 10 *(pp 40–42)*; 42 *(pp 228–232)*.

33. Answer A

Doppler tissue imaging or tissue Doppler measures and displays cardiac wall motion velocities. Comparing myocardium with blood flow, the myocardium is a strong reflector of ultrasound with low velocity (5–20 cm/s); red blood cells are weak reflectors of ultrasound with higher velocity. Therefore, the myocardial tissue motion has lower Doppler velocity with higher Doppler signal intensity. In contrast, blood flow has higher Doppler velocity with lower Doppler signal intensity. **References** 13 *(pp 7–20)*; 23 *(p 22)*.

34. Answer A

Doppler tissue imaging or tissue Doppler is a technique to image the velocities of the myocardium using the color flow method. During conventional Doppler recording of blood flow velocities, tissue velocities with low frequency are filtered by a high-pass filter. The conventional color flow Doppler system was modified to detect low wall motion velocity. Therefore, during Doppler tissue imaging, the signals of blood flow with high frequencies and low amplitude are rejected, and the signals of tissue motion with low velocities and high amplitude are analyzed. The myocardium is color coded according to the direction and velocity of its motion. Then, the color flow imaging of wall motion velocity is superimposed on the two-dimensional images. **References** 13 *(pp 7–20)*; 23 *(p 22)*.

35. Answer E

Tissue Doppler velocities can be autocorrelated to a color scheme and displayed both in M-mode and two-dimensional formats. In general, the myocardial wall moving toward the transducer is color coded in red, and that moving away from the transducer is color coded in blue. Akinetic segments are represented by the absence of color because the wall motion velocity is zero. Wall motion velocity over time can be demonstrated by color M-mode. Movement and velocities of cardiac structures are related to underlying systolic and diastolic function of the heart. The potential applications of Doppler tissue imaging include the quantitative analysis of wall motion in patients with impaired systolic or diastolic ventricular function and the assessment of regional ventricular function in patients with ischemic cardiac disease. The mitral anulus velocity measured by tissue Doppler is an indicator of myocardial relaxation, relatively unaffected by preload or afterload. Another potentially useful approach is to enhance the detection of the endocardium. Further investigation is needed to establish the clinical applications of this unique technology. **References** 13 *(pp 23–42)*; 23 *(pp 22, 43)*.

Chapter 3

Artifacts and Pitfalls of Imaging

Questions

Multiple choice (choose the *one* best answer):

1. Which one of the following statements about artifacts and pitfalls of imaging is true?
   A. Ultrasound systems operate on certain assumptions of imaging.
   B. Artifacts can be caused by equipment malfunction or the physics of ultrasound.
   C. Pitfalls of imaging are errors in interpretation of normal and abnormal anatomy.
   D. Both operator and interpreter errors may cause artifacts and pitfalls of imaging.
   E. All of the above.

2. Which one of the following is one of the important assumptions made during the creation of images by ultrasound systems?
   A. Sound travels at a variable speed in the body, depending on the propagation speed in each medium.
   B. The amplitude of returning echoes is influenced by several factors such as attenuation.
   C. Pulses travel directly to a reflector and then may go to a second reflector before they return to the transducer.
   D. Reflections arise only from structures along the main axis of the sound beam.
   E. Sound travels in directions that can change as degrees of refraction change.

3. Reverberations
   A. are multiple, unequally spaced echoes or reflections that may occur when two strong reflectors lie in the line of the ultrasound beam.
   B. are multiple, equally spaced echoes on the display.
   C. are always created from multiple real anatomic structures.
   D. can be created either front to back or side to side.
   E. place too many echoes on the image, thus making it impossible to distinguish which one is real.

4. If suspecting reverberation, one should
   A. readjust the angle of the transducer.
   B. increase the gain setting.
   C. decrease the gain setting.
   D. change the contrast setting.
   E. tell the surgeon that there is no way to eliminate the artifact.

5. Which one of the following about color gain setting is true?
   A. During color flow imaging, the jet area is determined by the amount of the flow but not affected by different color gain setting.
   B. Setting the gain level just below the level of random background noise optimizes the flow signal.
   C. Different gain settings may be used when looking for serial changes over time in an individual patient.
   D. Gain settings do not affect the size of the color flow display.
   E. Too low a gain setting displays a larger flow area than is actually present.

6. Ghosting may be produced by
   A. rapidly moving structures.
   B. slowly moving structures.
   C. stationary structures.
   D. all of the above.
   E. none of the above.

7. Mirror image
   A. is a duplicate of an anatomic structure because of an embryologic abnormality.
   B. always appears deeper than the true anatomic structure.
   C. always appears shallower than the true anatomic structure.
   D. always appears on the side of the true anatomic structure.
   E. may appear at any position.

8. Near-field clutter arises from
   A. inappropriate contrast enhancement.
   B. gain control dysfunction.
   C. high-amplitude oscillations of the piezoelectric elements.
   D. inappropriately increased gain setting.
   E. a higher reject threshold in the near field than in the far field.

9. The accompanying image is obtained during cardiac surgery. The artifact that affects the whole image is

A. damaged display screen.
B. insufficient scan line density.
C. dysfunctional ultrasound equipment.
D. side lobes.
E. electronic interference.

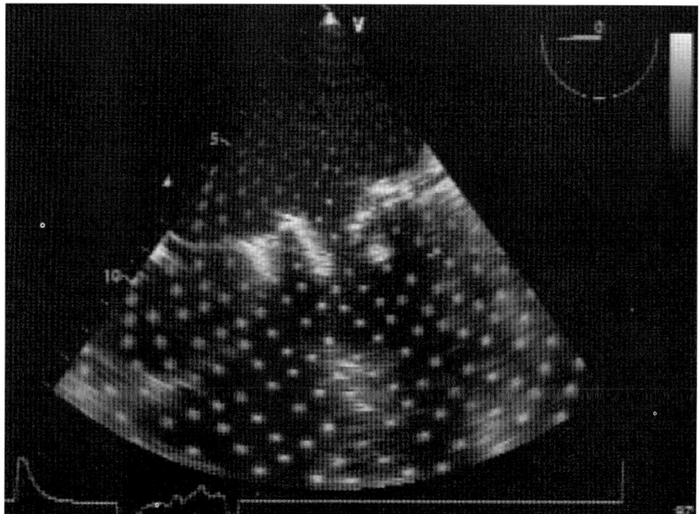

10. The accompanying picture shows

A. double aorta.
B. aortic dissection.
C. reverberation.
D. ghosting.
E. side lobes.

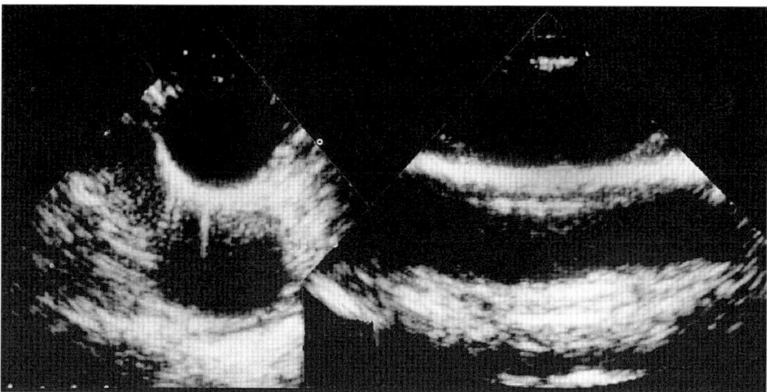

Figure from Seward et al. (35). Used with permission.

11. Shadowing is
- A. the echo drop-out before a strong reflector.
- B. the echo drop-out before a weak reflector.
- C. the echo drop-out behind a weak reflector.
- D. the echo drop-out behind a strong reflector.
- E. none of the above.

12. Which one of the following best describes the cause of shadowing?
- A. The structure within the shadow has high acoustic impedance.
- B. The structure within the shadow has high attenuation.
- C. The strong reflector in front of the shadow has high attenuation.
- D. A low-intensity ultrasound beam was emitted by the transducer.
- E. The resolution within the shadow is poor.

13. Shadow artifact always
- A. appears black.
- B. appears white.
- C. has the same shade of gray as the background of the ultrasound scan.
- D. has variable colors.
- E. has colors undetermined.

14. Snell's law defines the physics of
- A. refraction.
- B. reflection.
- C. reverberation.
- D. mirror image.
- E. ghosting.

15. Refraction
- A. generally causes an artifactual duplicate positioned side by side from the true anatomy, at almost the same depth.
- B. occurs when there is a right angle between the sound wave and the boundary of two media with different propagation speeds.
- C. is a change in direction, or a bending away from a straight-line path, of a sound wave traveling within a medium.
- D. is a change in direction, or a bending away from a straight-line path, of a sound wave traveling through two media with the same propagation speeds.
- E. places a second copy of the anatomic structure on the image, always deeper than the true reflector.

16. Side lobes
- A. produce stronger echoes of a true anatomic structure at its correct position because side lobes have greater acoustic energy.
- B. produce artifactual echoes displayed as a curved line at the same level as the true anatomic structure.
- C. produce artifactual echoes at the side of the true anatomy but at incorrect depth.
- D. produce artifactual echoes at a deeper position than the true anatomy.
- E. produce artifactual echoes at a shallower position than the true anatomy.

17. Which one of the following statements about side lobes is true?
A. Side lobes are usually evident and conflict with the echoes of true reflectors.
B. Many side lobes are not actually seen.
C. Side lobes usually produce artifactual echoes that overshadow true echoes.
D. Side lobes usually have the same acoustic energy as that in the primary ultrasound beam.
E. Side lobes have stronger acoustic energy than that in the primary ultrasound beam.

18. Trabeculations
A. are more prominent in the left atrium than in the right atrium.
B. can be seen only in the left atrial appendage.
C. usually have different texture or echo density than thrombus or tumor.
D. can never be distinguished from thrombus.
E. are diminished or vanished if the right ventricle is hypertrophied.

19. The arrowheads in the accompanying image (AS, atrial septum; AV, aortic valve; LA, left atrium; RA, right atrium) indicate
A. benign tumor masses.
B. trabeculations.
C. metastatic tumor masses.
D. vegetations.
E. thrombi.

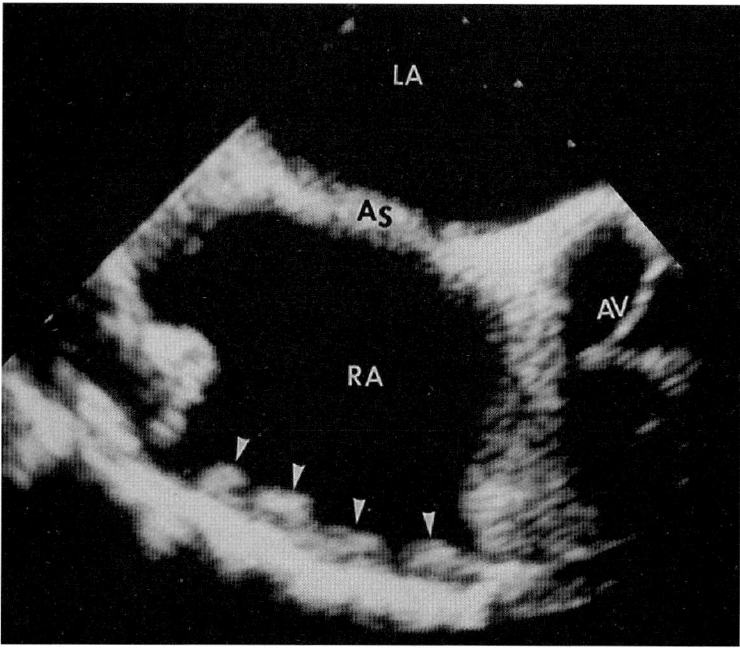

Figure from Seward et al. (35). Used with permission.

20. Usually, the Chiari network
   A. originates from the coronary sinus.
   B. originates from the left upper pulmonary vein.
   C. originates from the superior vena cava.
   D. originates from the right atrial wall.
   E. is associated with the orifice of the inferior vena cava, although its primary origin may vary.

21. The Chiari network
   A. has not been reported to be a site of entrapment of a right heart catheter.
   B. is a frequent site of vegetation formation.
   C. is a prominent coronary sinus valve with fenestrated fibrous extensions.
   D. is seen as filamentous structures with rapid chaotic motion in the right atrium.
   E. has not been reported to be a site of thrombus formation.

22. The accompanying transesophageal echocardiographic image is obtained during a preoperative cardiac evaluation. The surgeon told that this structure (arrow)
   A. is a linear thrombus with high risk of embolization.
   B. frequently causes obstruction.
   C. does not need to be removed surgically, but the patient should be treated with heparin.
   D. does not need to be removed surgically, but the patient should be treated with antibiotics for 6 weeks.
   E. is nonpathologic.

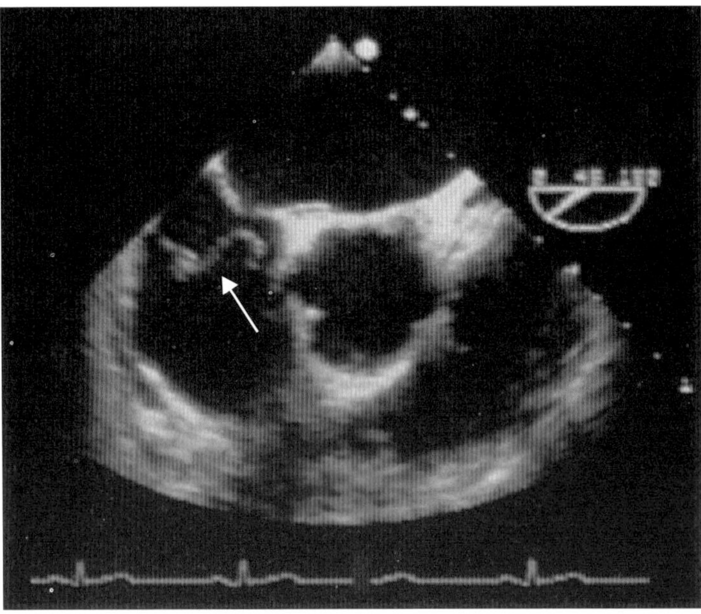

Figure from Redberg RF. Echocardiographic evaluation of the patient with a systemic embolic event. In: Otto CM, ed. The Practice of Clinical Echocardiography. Philadelphia: WB Saunders, 1997;639. Used with permission.

23. Frequently, the patient with the structure shown in the preceding transesophageal echocardiographic image

A. also has an associated atrial septal aneurysm.
B. also has thrombi in the right ventricle.
C. also has vegetations in the right ventricle.
D. has a decreased incidence of patent foramen ovale.
E. has a decreased incidence of associated cardiac abnormality.

24. The accompanying transesophageal echocardiographic image is obtained intraoperatively (LA, left atrium; RA, right atrium). Your diagnosis is

A. a malignant tumor of the atrial septum.
B. a large thrombus on the atrial septum.
C. lipomatous hypertrophy of the atrial septum.
D. an atrial myxoma.
E. a tumor mass with unknown pathology.

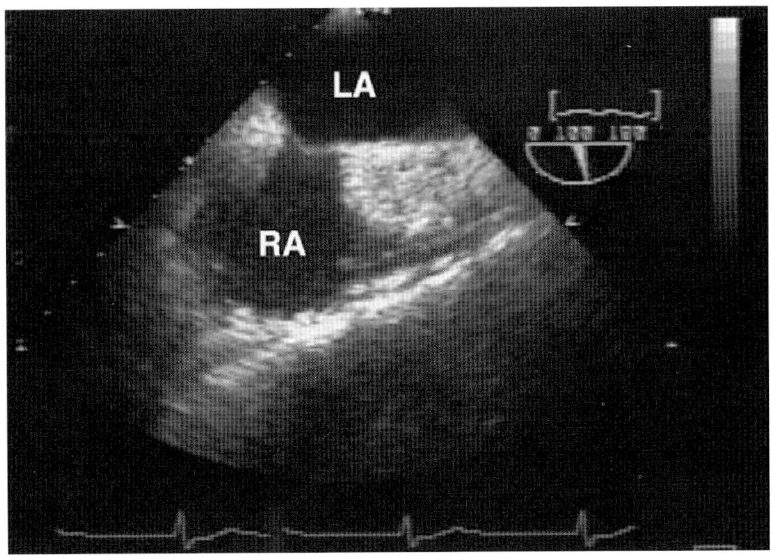

25. In the accompanying transesophageal echocardiographic image (AV, aortic valve; LA, left atrium), the arrow indicates

A. a tumor mass in the left atrium.
B. normal partition between the left atrium and the left upper pulmonary vein.
C. a large vegetation.
D. a thrombus in the left atrium.
E. a structure that cannot be determined.

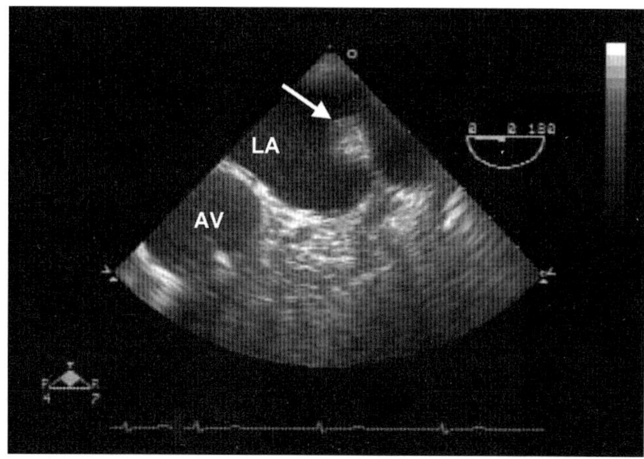

26. The accompanying transesophageal echocardiographic image (LA, left atrium; LAA, left atrial appendage) suggests that this patient

A. most likely has a dissected left upper pulmonary vein.
B. has persistent left superior vena cava.
C. has a cyst in the left atrium.
D. has an abscess in the left atrium.
E. does not have persistent left superior vena cava.

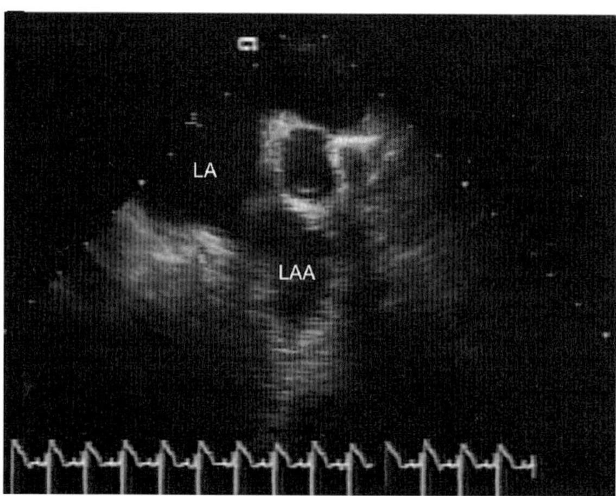

27. The patient's transesophageal echocardiogram appears as shown before cardioversion for atrial fibrillation of less than 48 hours. The clinician should

A. treat the patient with a tissue-type plasminogen activator before proceeding to cardioversion.

B. treat the patient with heparin three days before cardioversion.

C. treat the patient with warfarin three days before cardioversion.

D. recommend surgical removal of the left atrial appendage thrombi before cardioversion.

E. proceed to cardioversion.

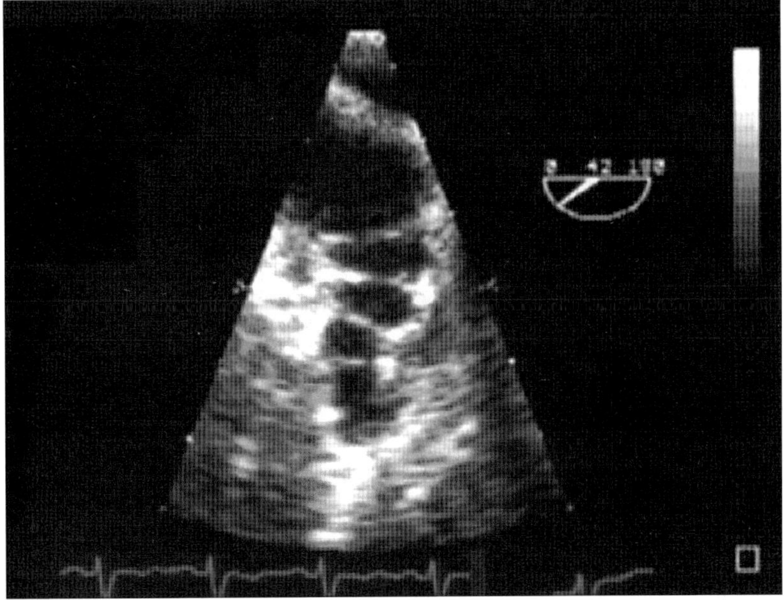

28. The accompanying transesophageal echocardiographic image of the aortic valve shows

A. a large vegetation on the noncoronary cusp.
B. a tumor mass on the left coronary cusp.
C. a papillary fibroelastoma on the noncoronary cusp.
D. a large thrombus on the right coronary cusp.
E. a normal aortic valve.

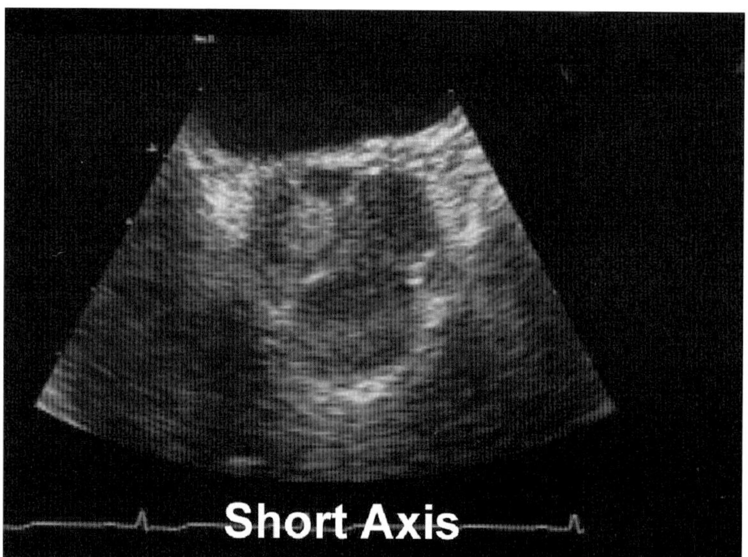

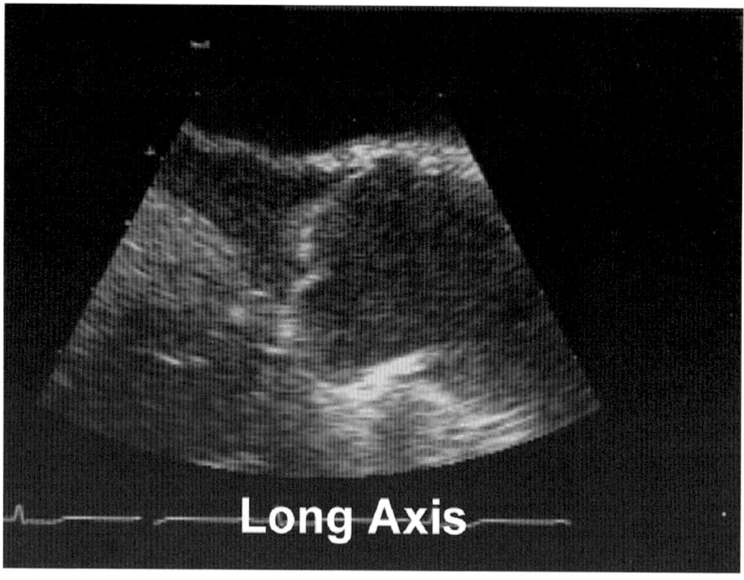

29. A moderator band is found in
A. the right ventricle.
B. the left ventricle.
C. the right atrium.
D. the left atrium.
E. the left atrial appendage.

30. The accompanying image is obtained during cardiac surgery. The large white arrow points to
A. an artifact.
B. a thrombus of the eustachian valve.
C. a pulmonary artery catheter.
D. a moderator band.
E. a small papillary fibroelastoma.

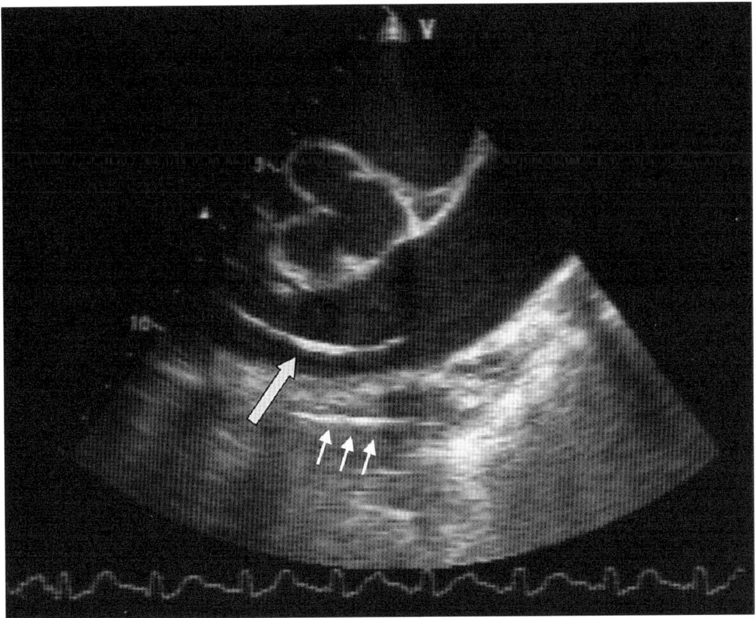

31. The three small arrows in the preceding image indicate
A. reverberation.
B. shadowing.
C. an enhancement artifact.
D. an image defect caused by machine dysfunction.
E. a side lobe.

32. False tendons represent
A. the reverberation of a true linear structure outside the image.
B. the reverberation of a real specular reflector in the image.

C. ghosting.
D. a mirror image.
E. filamentous structures in the left ventricle.

33. The arrow in the accompanying transesophageal echocardiographic image indicates
A. a linear thrombus in the left atrium.
B. linear vegetation in the left atrium.
C. the membrane of the fossa ovalis.
D. a false tendon in the left atrium.
E. a linear reverberation artifact.

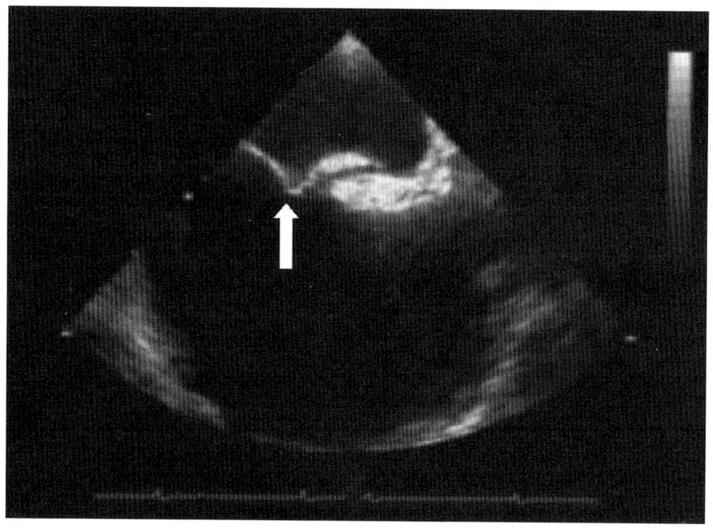

34. The transverse sinus is best described as
A. the venous drainage system of the heart that enters the right atrium.
B. a part of the lymphatic drainage system of the heart.
C. a fluid-filled space between the left atrium and the esophagus.
D. a pericardial reflection between the left atrium and the great vessels.
E. a posterior pericardial reflection between the pulmonary veins.

35. Most likely, the structure indicated by the arrows in the accompanying transesophageal echocardiographic image (Asc Ao, ascending aorta; LA, left atrium; PA, pulmonary artery) is

A. a tumor mass.

B. epicardial fat.

C. a thrombus.

D. the left atrial appendage.

E. B or D.

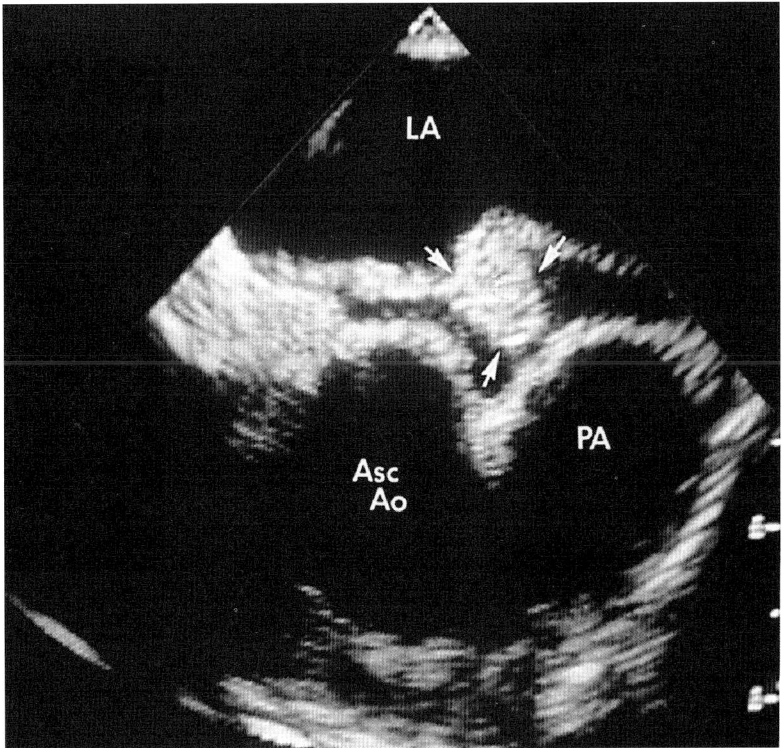

Figure from Seward et al. (35). Used with permission.

36. The accompanying images show transverse and longitudinal views of the aorta. Which one of the following statements is true?

A. This is a type A aortic dissection.
B. This is a type B aortic dissection.
C. The patient should be brought to the operating room for emergency surgery.
D. This is linear reverberation.
E. A and C.

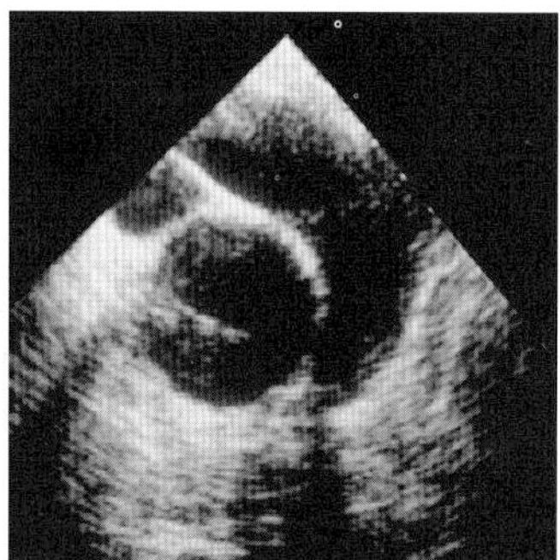
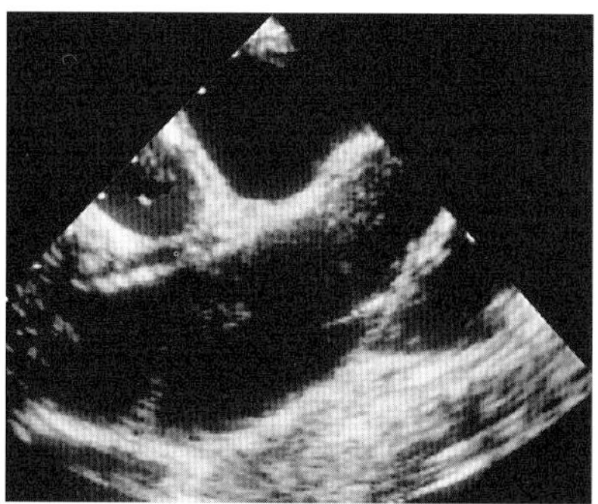

Figure from Seward et al. (35). Used with permission.

37. In the accompanying transesophageal echocardiographic image, the arrow indicates

A. the left atrium with multiple thrombi.
B. the left atrium with multiple papillary fibroelastoma.
C. the descending aorta with multiple plaques.
D. the stomach.
E. a pathologic cavity.

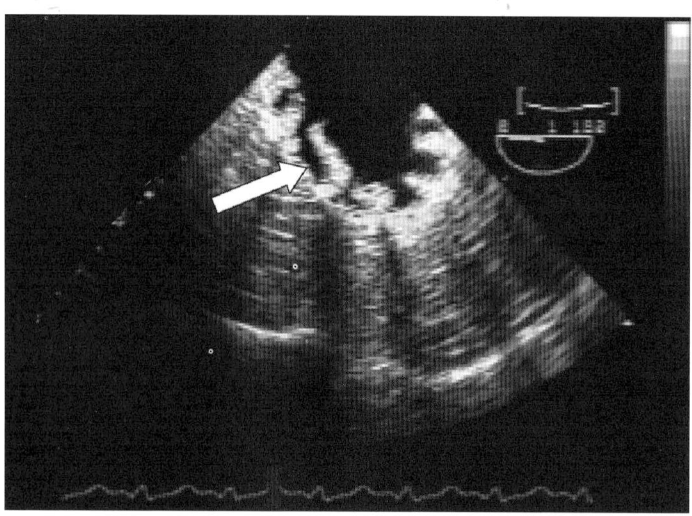

38. The eustachian valve

A. originates from the margin of the inferior vena cava.
B. is also called the valve of the inferior vena cava.
C. directs blood returning from the inferior vena cava across the fossa ovalis in the fetus.
D. may simulate vegetation, thrombus, or tumor when it is large and mobile.
E. is all of the above.

39. The arrows in the accompanying transesophageal echocardiographic image (AS, atrial septum; LA, left atrium; LV, left ventricle; MV, mitral valve; RA, right atrium; RV, right ventricle; TV, tricuspid valve; VS, ventricular septum) indicate

A. a benign tumor mass in the right atrium.
B. a tumor mass of unknown pathology at the tricuspid valve anulus.
C. a malignant tumor mass in the tricuspid atrioventricular groove.
D. a pseudomass of the tricuspid valve anulus.
E. a ring abscess.

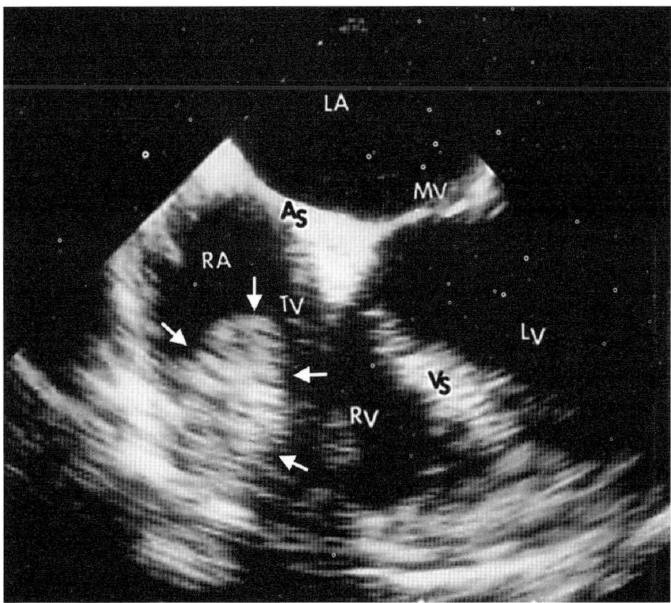

Figure from Seward et al. (35). Used with permission.

Answers & Discussion

1. Answer E

An artifact is defined as an error in imaging. An ultrasound image contains artifacts when the reflections do not represent the true anatomy of the patient. Artifacts may be caused by violations of certain basic assumptions of acoustic imaging, equipment malfunction or poor design, the physics of ultrasound, operator error, or interpreter error. Although ultrasound systems make images of true reflectors, they operate on the basis of certain basic assumptions of imaging. Pitfalls of imaging are potential erroneous diagnoses resulting from misinterpretation of normal and abnormal anatomy. (See also Question 2.) **Reference** 9 *(p 199)*.

2. Answer D

Ultrasound systems are designed to operate on the basis of several basic assumptions of acoustic imaging. Artifacts occur when any of these assumptions are violated. There are six basic assumptions during ultrasound imaging:

1. Sound travels in a straight line. In reality, sound may be refracted. When this assumption is violated, refraction artifact occurs.
2. Reflections arise only from structures along the main axis of the sound beam. However, echoes may result from side lobes or grating lobes.
3. The strength of a reflection is related to the scattering strength of the anatomic structure that produces it. In reality, the amplitude of the returning echoes are affected by several factors such as attenuation.
4. Pulses travel directly to a reflector and then back to the transducer. In mirror image or reverberation, this assumption is violated.
5. Sound travels at a speed of 1,540 m/s in the body. However, 1,540 m/s represents an average speed. The true propagation speed may be slower or faster than this average speed, depending on the individual structure being imaged. When propagation speed errors occur, reflectors are placed in improper positions or at incorrect depth.
6. The imaging plane is extremely thin, but the ultrasound beam has some thickness in the perpendicular beam plane. Reflections from the structures above or below a reflector may be placed with this reflector on the display screen. **References** 9 *(pp 199–212)*; 10 *(pp 22–26)*; 11 *(pp 129–148)*.

3. Answer B

Reverberations are multiple, equally spaced echoes or reflections that appear on the image at ever-increasing depth. Reverberation occurs when two strong reflectors lie in the line of the ultrasound beam. The ultrasound pulse may actually bounce back and forth between the two reflectors, sending multiple echoes back to the transducer. The first and second echoes arise from true anatomic structures in their correct position. The subsequent echoes arise as the sound pulse bounces between the reflectors, and they do not represent true anatomic structures. (See also Question 4.) **References** 9 *(pp 91, 203)*; 10 *(pp 24–25)*; 26 *(pp 12–13)*.

4. Answer A

If a reverberation artifact is suspected, one should readjust the angle of the transducer. Reverberations arise when two strong reflectors lie along the main axis of the ultrasound beam. If a different imaging angle is used, the reverberation may disappear because the reflectors are not in line with the sound beam. Therefore, changing the imaging plane or readjusting the angle of the transducer eliminates reverberation. Changing the gain setting or the contrast setting does not eliminate reverberations. **References** 9 *(p 203)*; 10 *(pp 24–25)*; 26 *(pp 12–13)*.

5. Answer B

Color Doppler gain settings have a dramatic effect on the color flow image. Color gain settings can greatly affect the size of the color flow display. Extensive gain settings result in a uniform speckled pattern across the two-dimensional image plane because of background noise. Conversely, too low a gain setting results in a smaller displayed flow area than is actually present, an effect colloquially known as "dial-a-jet." To optimize the flow signal, the gain level should be set just below the level of random background noise. One approach to setting color gain is to increase gain until excess background noise is seen and then reduce the gain to the level just below excess background noise. Significant variation in jet area occurs with different color gain settings. Obviously, consistency in color gain setting and other instrument settings is needed when looking for serial changes over time in an individual patient. **Reference** 26 *(p 24)*.

6. Answer A

During color flow imaging, ghosting may occur as brief flashes of color that overlay anatomic structures and do not correspond to underlying flow patterns. Typically, ghosting is a uniform red or blue color. This artifact is inconsistent from beat to beat. Ghosting is produced by rapidly moving structures such as valves. Slowly moving or stationary structures do not produce ghosting. **References** 10 *(p 41)*; 11 *(p 145)*; 26 *(p 23)*.

7. Answer B

Mirror image is the artifactual duplicate of a real anatomic structure on the display screen because the sound beam bounces off a strong reflector (the true anatomic structure). During ultrasound imaging, the ultrasound beam strikes a strong, mirrorlike (specular) reflector, such as pericardium or diaphragm. This structure acts as a mirror and redirects the ultrasound beam toward a second reflector. Then, the ultrasound beam retraces its steps to the transducer. Ultrasound systems assume that sound waves travel directly to the reflector and back to the transducer. The transducer "thinks" the sound is coming from the original direction in which it sent sound out toward the mirror, but it takes longer to return that sound from the mirror itself, so it "sees" the object behind the mirror. Therefore, the mirror image duplicate always appears deeper than the true anatomic structure. Mirror image artifact occurs only under the conditions described above. If the relative orientation of the sound beam, the mirror, and the imaged structure is altered, the mirror image artifact may disappear. Hence, to eliminate mirror image artifacts, one should try a different imaging orientation. **References** 9 *(p 204)*; 26 *(p 23)*.

8. Answer C

Near-field clutter is acoustic noise near the transducer. This artifact arises from high-amplitude oscillations of the piezoelectric elements. Near-field clutter prevents the operator from clearly identifying echogenic structures in the near field. Near-field clutter is not caused by higher reject threshold in the near field than that in the far field. Inappropriate gain control or contrast enhancement affects the whole image, not just the near field. **Reference** 10 *(p 26)*.

9. Answer E

In this intraoperative transesophageal echocardiographic image, the linear "dot" artifact affecting the whole image is electronic interference caused by electrocautery. **Reference** 26 *(pp 23–24)*.

10. Answer C

This transesophageal echocardiographic image shows reverberation artifact of the aorta. The aorta close to the transducer is the true anatomic structure, and the second "aorta" is a reverberation artifact. This reverberation artifact of the aorta may be mistakenly identified as a double aorta or dissected aorta. (See also Questions 3 and 4.) **Reference** 11 *(p 148)*.

11. Answer D

12. Answer C

Shadowing is the loss of echoes or echo drop-out behind a strong reflector. It is caused by high ultrasound attenuation due to the intervening structure with high density, such as calcium and prosthetic valves. When an ultrasound pulse travels through a structure with very high attenuation, the ultrasound beam is weakened. The echo signals arising from deeper structures are correspondingly weak and, hence, may be rejected and not displayed on the image. This results in shadowing. Shadow artifact can be a problem when trying to visualize a structure or flow behind a strong reflector. An example of acoustic shadowing is produced by prosthetic mechanical valve that causes high ultrasound attenuation and echo drop-out behind it. Poor resolution within the shadow is not the cause, but the result of shadowing. (See also Question 13.) **References** 9 *(p 207)*; 10 *(pp 25–26)*; 26 *(p 12)*.

13. Answer C

Shadow artifact always has the same color as the background of the image. Although an ultrasound image is commonly white on black, it can be black on white. On a white-on-black image, shadow artifact appears black; on a black-on-white image, shadow artifact appears white. (See also Questions 11 and 12.) **References** 9 *(p 207)*; 10 *(pp 25–26)*; 26 *(p 12)*.

14. Answer A

Snell's law defines the physics of refraction: Sine transmission angle/sine incident angle = propagation speed of medium 2/propagation speed of medium 1. According to Snell's law, when the propagation speed of medium 2 is greater than that of medium 1, the transmission angle is greater than the incident angle. When propagation speed of medium 2 is less than that of medium 1, the transmission angle is less than the incident angle. **Reference** 9 *(pp 67–68)*.

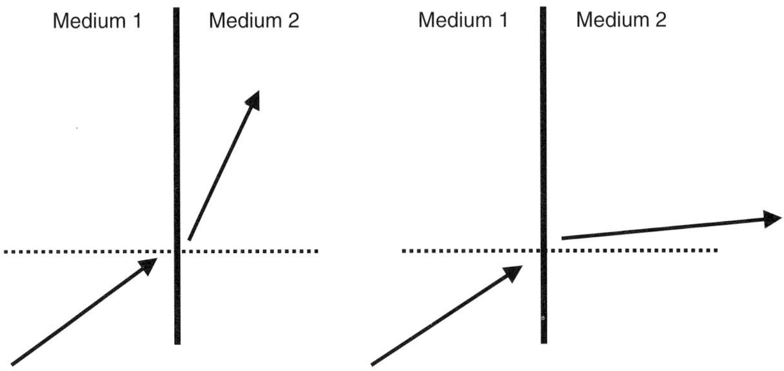

Figure from Edelman (9). Used with permission.

15. Answer A

Refraction is a change in direction, or a bending away from a straight-line path, of a sound wave traveling from one medium to another. Refraction occurs only when the propagation speeds in the two media are different and there is an oblique incidence between the sound wave and the boundary of two media.

In daily life, refraction causes a straight drinking straw in a glass of water to appear bent. In ultrasound imaging, refraction generally causes an artifactual duplicate A positioned side by side from the true anatomy B, at almost the same depth. The basic assumption of acoustic imaging violated by refraction artifact is that the sound wave travels in a straight line. **References** 9 *(pp 67–68, 202)*; 10 *(pp 1–2)*; 26 *(pp 3–4, 12, 14)*.

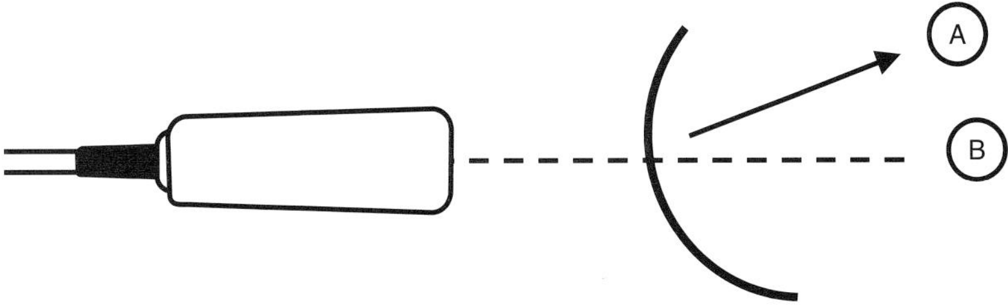

Figure from Edelman (9). Used with permission.

16. Answer B

Side lobes are generated from the edges of the transducer elements and do not occur in the direction of the main ultrasonic beam. Side lobes produce artifactual echoes of the true reflector at its correct depth but laterally from the true anatomy. The violated assumption is that reflections are produced by structures located only along the main axis of the sound beam. The accompanying figure illustrates how side lobes can produce artifactual information on a two-dimensional echocardiogram. When the main ultrasonic beam strikes an object, the echoes of the object are displayed on the oscilloscope (A). When the main ultrasonic beam is directed away from the object and the side lobe hits the object, the echoes of the object are recorded at the direction of the main ultrasonic beam because the ultrasound system assumes they are originated from the main beam (B). If the beam is oscillating rapidly, the multiple artifactual echoes produced by the side lobes are displayed as a curved line at the same level as the true object (C). **References** 9 *(p 205)*; 10 *(pp 22–24)*.

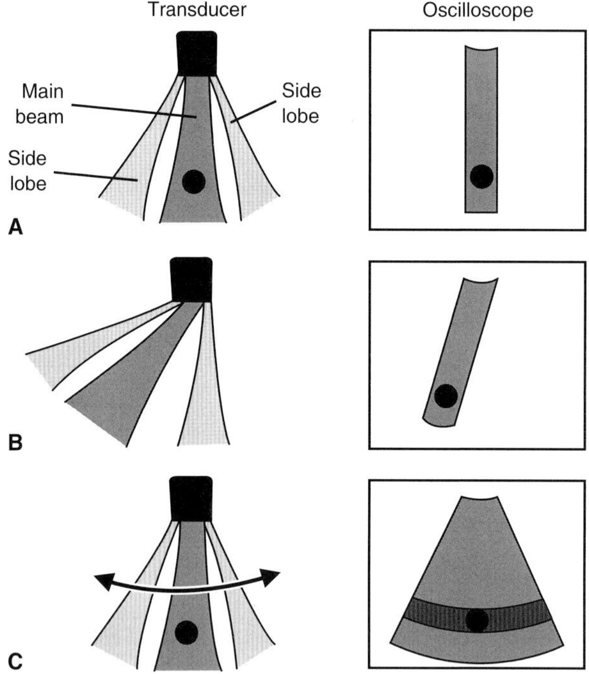

Figure from Feigenbaum (10, p 23). Used with permission.

17. Answer B

Side lobes are considerably weaker than the main beam and hence, have less acoustic energy than the primary beam. Thus, the returning echoes are clearly weaker than the dominant, real echoes. In fact, many side lobe echoes are not actually seen because they are overshadowed by true echoes in the same vicinity. Side lobes usually become evident when they do not conflict with real echoes. Another prerequisite for a dominant side lobe artifact is that the artifactual echoes must originate from a fairly strong reflecting surface. **References** 9 *(p 205)*; 10 *(pp 22–24)*.

18. Answer C

Trabeculations are normal muscle ridges (pectinate muscles) that are more prominent in the right heart and the walls of both atrial appendages. These muscle ridges are small, refractile, and multiple. Usually, thrombus can be differentiated from trabeculations or pectinate muscles because it has different texture or echo density and is uniform in consistency. Also, thrombus typically occurs in severe atrioventricular valve disease, low-output state, or atrial fibrillation. Tumors are also distinctly different in echo density from normal muscle ridges. Right ventricular hypertrophy accentuates trabeculations in the right ventricle and may produce confusing echocardiograms. **References** 10 *(pp 589, 593)*; 11 *(pp 134–138)*.

19. Answer B

The arrowheads in this transesophageal echocardiographic image show right atrial trabeculations or pectinate muscles. The right atrium is more trabeculated than the left atrium. (See also Question 18.) **References** 10 *(pp 589, 593)*; 11 *(pp 134–138)*.

20. Answer E

The Chiari network was first described by the anatomist Chiari in 1897. It is the fenestrated vestige of an embryonic structure (the right valve of the sinus venosus). Usually, this thin, weblike membrane with multiple fenestration extends from the inlet of the inferior vena cava to the interatrial septum. Although the Chiari network is generally associated with the orifice of the inferior vena cava, its primary origin may vary. **References** 10 *(pp 589, 592)*; 25 *(p 639)*; 26 *(pp 416, 418)*; 42 *(pp 849, 1169)*.

21. Answer D

The Chiari network is a prominent inferior vena cava valve with fibrous extensions that are fenestrated and lax, forming a network. The Chiari network is observed in about 2% of patients undergoing transesophageal echocardiography. During this examination, the Chiari network is seen as filamentous structures with rapid chaotic motion in the right atrium. The Chiari network has been reported to be a site of thrombus formation as well as a site of entrapment for a right heart catheter. However, it is not a frequent site of vegetation formation. **References** 10 *(pp 589, 592)*; 13 *(p 639)*; 26 *(pp 416, 418)*; 42 *(pp 849, 1169)*.

22. Answer E

23. Answer A

The preoperative transesophageal echocardiographic image shows a filamentous structure in the right atrium. This structure is the Chiari network. Generally, the Chiari network itself is nonpathologic and does not cause obstruction or embolization. However, there is a high likelihood of an associated atrial septal aneurysm or patent foramen ovale. **References** 10 *(pp 589, 592)*; 13 *(p 639)*; 26 *(pp 416, 418)*; 42 *(pp 849, 1169)*.

24. Answer C

In this transesophageal echocardiographic image, the arrowheads point to lipomatous hypertrophy of the atrial septum. The atrial septum surrounding the centrally located membrane of the fossa ovalis is fat laden. When excessively thick, it is referred to as lipomatous hypertrophy. A characteristic mass effect is observed. A dumbbell shape of the atrial septum is pathognomonic for the lipomatous hypertrophy of the atrial septum. Usually, the lipomatous atrial septum appears as an echo-dense mass of variable size and consistency. The amount of fatty infiltrate varies but can be impressive. Generally, this condition is considered benign but can easily be misinterpreted as a pathologic mass by an inexperienced examiner. **Reference** 11 *(pp 138–140)*.

25. Answer B

This left atrial pseudomass is the normal partition between the left atrial appendage and the left upper pulmonary vein. This partition is also called the "Coumadin ridge" or "warfarin ridge," because historically, it was frequently misdiagnosed as thrombus in the left atrium and many patients were treated with warfarin unnecessarily. The terminal portion of this partition can be fat laden and appears globular or bulbous. The proximal portion of this common wall is usually thin. Thus, the normal partition frequently has the appearance of a cotton-tipped applicator on the transesophageal echocardiographic image, hence the term "Q-tip sign." Sometimes, the distal globular end can be quite large and masslike, mimicking a left atrial tumor. Awareness of this common anatomic variant should prevent serious misinterpretation. **Reference** 11 *(pp 138–139)*.

26. Answer B

The accompanying transesophageal echocardiographic image (LA, left atrium; LAA, left atrial appendage) shows a large coronary sinus, which suggests that most likely this patient also has a persistent left superior vena cava. Frequently, the persistent left superior vena cava enters the right atrium through the coronary sinus. In such a situation, the patient has a severely dilated coronary sinus because of the blood flow from the persistent left superior vena cava. During transesophageal echocardiographic imaging in patients with persistent left superior vena cava, the partition between the left atrial appendage and the left upper pulmonary vein can appear as a space and then is confirmed as a persistent left superior vena cava after an agitated saline injection into a left arm vein. The dilated coronary sinus shows the contrast (arrow) as in the accompanying figure. **References** 10 *(pp 399–402)*; 11 *(pp 137–138)*; 23 *(p 235)*; 26 *(pp 355, 403, 415–416)*.

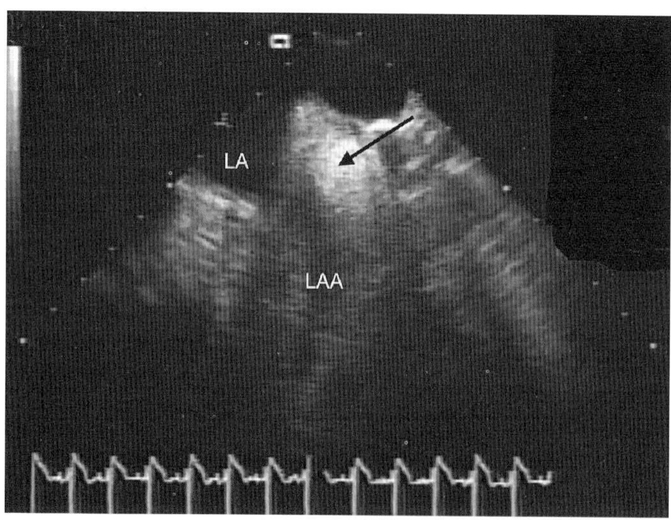

27. Answer E

This image shows a normal left atrial appendage with pectinate muscles. Generally, thrombus can be differentiated from pectinate muscles because it has different texture or echo density, although a highly trabeculated atrial appendage may be difficult to clearly differentiate from thrombus. In this case, the patient does not need to be treated with any anticoagulant before cardioversion because the left atrial appendage with pectinate muscles has a normal transesophageal echocardiographic appearance and the atrial fibrillation is of short duration. **References** 10 *(pp 589, 593)*; 11 *(pp 134–138, 367, 372)*.

28. Answer E

This transesophageal echocardiographic image shows a normal aortic valve. The pseudomass on the noncoronary cusp appears when the noncoronary cusp is cut obliquely in the short axis. This frequently observed mass effect of a coronary cusp is easily mistaken for an aortic valve vegetation or tumor. To eliminate this imaging pitfall, the aortic valve should be examined with a true orthogonal short axis plane and the analysis should be confirmed in other imaging planes. **Reference** 11 *(pp 140–141)*.

29. Answer A

A moderator band is a muscular ridge found only in the right ventricle. Anatomically, the moderator band is present in the majority of normal individuals and contains fibers of the right bundle branch, but it is often mistaken for a pathologic structure. Echocardiographically, the moderator band appears as a thick, echo-dense band extending from the lower interventricular septum across the right ventricular cavity to the base of the anterior papillary muscle. **References** 10 *(pp 85, 352–353, 589–590)*; 42 *(pp 987, 1170–1171)*.

30. Answer C

31. Answer A

In this transesophageal echocardiographic image, the large white arrow points to a pulmonary artery catheter in the right ventricular outflow tract. Because the pulmonary artery catheter has increased echo density and produces high attenuation, it results in reverberation or mirror imaging artifact behind it. The three smaller arrows in the image point to the artifact from the original pulmonary artery catheter. **References** 9 *(p 207)*; 10 *(pp 25–26)*.

32. Answer E

Left ventricular false tendons are filamentous, fibrous structures that traverse the left ventricular cavity. This structure is thought to represent false chordae tendineae and is of no pathologic importance. Unlike true chordae tendineae, which originate from papillary muscles and insert onto valve leaflets, false tendons pass between papillary muscles, from papillary muscle to the ventricular septum, from free wall to free wall, or from free wall to interventricular septum. They may be single or multiple. Echocardiographically, false tendons appear as linear, echo-dense structures that course through the left ventricular cavity. It is important to differentiate false tendons from thrombi, vegetation, pedunculated tumor, and other abnormalities of the mitral valve or septum. **References** 10 *(p 85)*; 42 *(p 1171)*.

33. Answer C

This transesophageal echocardiographic image is a scan of the atrial septum. The white arrow indicates the membrane of the fossa ovalis. If the valve of the fossa ovalis is patent, shunting from one atrium to the other can be observed within this space. **Reference** 11 *(pp 136, 141)*.

34. Answer D

The transverse sinus is a pericardial reflection between the left atrium and the great vessels (the ascending aorta and pulmonary artery). A posterior pericardial reflection between the pulmonary veins is the oblique sinus, which can appear as a fluid-filled space interposed between the left atrium and the esophagus. **References** 11 *(pp 135–136, 143–144)*; 23 *(pp 34, 213)*.

35. Answer E

In this transesophageal echocardiographic image, the arrows indicate a pseudomass in the pericardial reflection between the left atrium and the great vessels. This pericardial reflection is the transverse sinus, and the pseudomass may be epicardial fat or part of the left atrial appendage. Normally, there is epicardial fat within the transverse sinus. When the transverse sinus contains fluid, the epicardial fat or part of the left atrial appendage may appear masslike during transesophageal echocardiographic imaging. It could be misdiagnosed as a thrombus or tumor mass. **References** 11 *(pp 135–136, 143–144)*; 23 *(pp 34, 213)*.

36. Answer D

The arrows in the accompanying transesophageal echocardiographic images indicate linear reverberation. Frequently, it occurs within the upper ascending aorta and mid descending aorta. There is air-filled lung in the immediate far-field image. This is a common cause of linear echoes within the aorta that mimic dissections. Linear artifacts often lie in nonanatomic planes, cross normal anatomy, have artifactual motion, do not alter Doppler-depicted blood flow, and may disappear with change in imaging orientation. It is important to distinguish reverberation artifact from true aortic dissection. Reverberation does not require surgery. **Reference** 11 *(pp 145, 147–148)*.

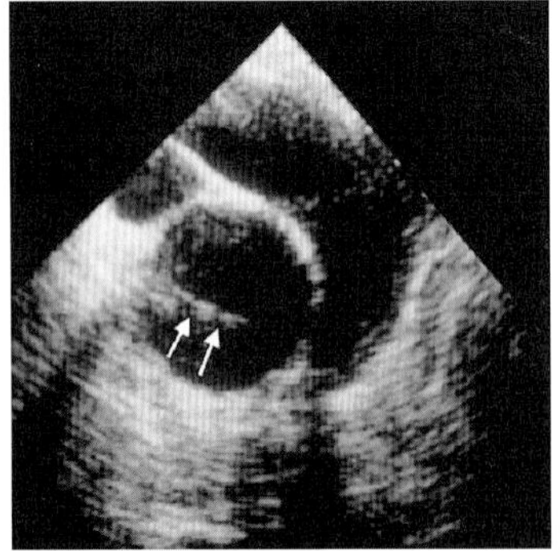

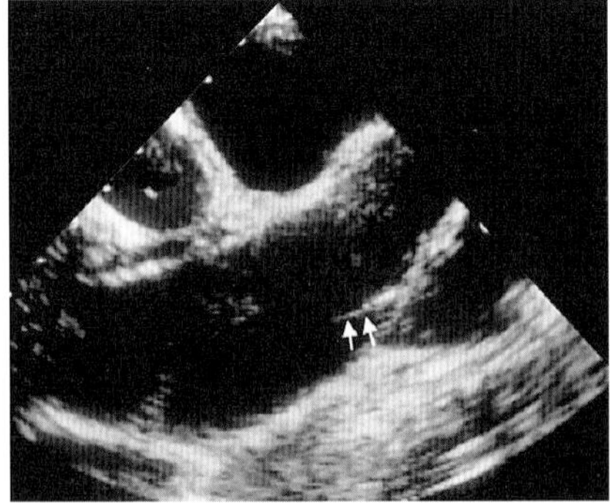

Figure from Seward et al. (35). Used with permission.

37. Answer D

The arrow in this transesophageal echocardiographic image indicates the stomach. In patients with hiatal hernia, the stomach can herniate into the thorax and become interposed between the normal esophagus and the heart. Rugal folds within the stomach can be mistaken for a tumor or mass. The heart can be obscured from visualization. When filled with fluid, the herniated stomach can appear as a thick-walled cystic mass posterior to the left atrium. When filled with gas, it produces the expected problem of interference with ultrasound transmission resulting in a technically difficult examination. **Reference** 11 *(p 144)*.

38. Answer E

The eustachian valve is also called the valve of the inferior vena cava. It has its origin from the margin of the inferior vena cava. During fetal development, the eustachian valve has its course across the right atrium to become continuous with the border of the fossa ovalis. Thus, it directs blood returning from the inferior vena cava across the fossa ovalis in the fetus. During transesophageal echocardiographic imaging, the eustachian valve often appears as a mobile, undulating membrane encircling the orifice of the inferior vena cava as it enters the floor of the right atrium. When it is large and mobile, it may simulate vegetation, thrombus, or tumor. **References** 10 *(pp 85–86, 354, 589–591)*; 11 *(p 143)*; 42 *(p 1169)*.

39. Answer D

This is a pseudomass of the tricuspid valve anulus. The tricuspid anulus normally contains fat. The amount of fatty tissue varies. When the fatty tissue is increased, it can produce a mass effect in the tricuspid atrioventricular groove. This common observation should not be misinterpreted as a tumor or ring abscess. **Reference** 11 *(p 140)*.

Chapter 4

Quantitative Echocardiography

Questions

Multiple choice (choose the *one* best answer):

1. The American Society of Echocardiography recommends that all M-mode measurements be made from
   A. leading edge to leading edge.
   B. trailing edge to trailing edge.
   C. leading edge to trailing edge.
   D. trailing edge to leading edge.
   E. any of the above.
2. During two-dimensional imaging, the aortic diameter should be measured from
   A. leading edge to leading edge.
   B. trailing edge to trailing edge.
   C. leading edge to trailing edge.
   D. trailing edge to leading edge.
   E. any of the above.
3. According to the American Society of Echocardiography recommendation, the end of diastole is indicated by
   A. the peak of the R wave on the electrocardiogram.
   B. the Q wave on the electrocardiogram.
   C. the S wave on the electrocardiogram.
   D. the QRS complex on the electrocardiogram.
   E. the PR interval on the electrocardiogram.
4. Which one of the following best describes what the centerline method is used for?
   A. Regional wall motion analysis.
   B. Estimation of left ventricular volume.
   C. Assessment of left ventricular symmetry.
   D. Measurement of left ventricular diameter.
   E. Evaluation of both left ventricular systolic and diastolic functions.
5. The referencing centroid method
   A. may use a fixed center.
   B. may use a floating center.

C. uses the center area as an internal reference point to measure the endocardial excursion quantitatively.
D. uses all of the above.
E. uses none of the above.

6. Which one of the following is used most commonly to evaluate left ventricular systolic function in the operating room?
A. Referencing centroids with a fixed axis.
B. Referencing centroids with a floating axis.
C. Visual assessment.
D. The centerline method.
E. Left ventricular movement.

7. Which one of the following is the method recommended by the American Society of Echocardiography for left ventricular volume calculation?
A. Simplified Simpson's method.
B. Prolate ellipse.
C. Simpson's method.
D. Modified Simpson's rule technique with two-chamber and four-chamber views.
E. Single-plane area length.

8. Generally, cardiac volume determined by the two-dimensional method is
A. greater than that measured by angiography.
B. less than that measured by angiography.
C. equal to that measured by angiography.
D. as accurate as that measured by angiography.
E. more accurate than that measured by angiography.

9. Fractional area change (FAC) is
A. a three-dimensional systolic index.
B. measured at the base of the left ventricle in the short axis.
C. calculated as the difference between left ventricular end-diastolic volume (LVEDV) and left ventricular end-systolic volume (LVESV) divided by the former (FAC = [LVEDV – LVESV]/LVEDV).
D. a truly global assessment, even in the presence of regional wall motion abnormality.
E. none of the above.

10. Circumferential shortening is used for evaluation of
A. left ventricular diameter.
B. left ventricular area.
C. left ventricular volume.
D. left ventricular systolic function.
E. left ventricular global systolic and diastolic functions.

11. Left ventricular ejection fraction, where left ventricular end-diastolic and end-systolic areas are denoted by LVEDV and LVESV, respectively, is calculated as

A. (LVEDV – LVESV) × 100.
B. [(LVESV – LVEDV)/LVESV] × 100.
C. [(LVEDV – LVESV)/LVEDV] × 100.
D. [(LVEDV – LVESV)/LVESV] × 100.
E. [(LVESV – LVEDV)/LVEDV] × 100.

12. Which one of the following is preload and afterload dependent?

A. Circumferential shortening.
B. Fractional area change.
C. Ejection fraction.
D. Cardiac output.
E. All of the above.

13. Which statement about measuring wall thickness and chamber dimension is true?

A. Two-dimensional approach is less accurate than M-mode measurement.
B. M-mode measurement always reflects the true dimension.
C. Measuring left ventricular volume using a single M-mode dimension is always reliable.
D. M-mode measurement is always accurate without being guided by a two-dimensional echocardiogram.
E. None of the above.

14. Which one of the following is recommended by the American Society of Echocardiography for measuring left ventricular mass?

A. M-mode technique.
B. Area length technique.
C. Truncated ellipsoid approach.
D. B and C.
E. All of the above.

15. When analyzing Doppler recordings, which one of the following parameters should be taken into consideration?

A. Timing of Doppler velocity.
B. Direction of blood flow.
C. Flow configuration.
D. Peak velocity.
E. All of the above.

16. Doppler echocardiography can be used to determine

A. intracardiac pressures.
B. transvalvular gradient.
C. valve area.
D. diastolic function.
E. all of the above.

17. Transmitral pressure gradients measured by Doppler
   A. are higher than those simultaneously measured by cardiac catheterization.
   B. are lower than those simultaneously measured by cardiac catheterization.
   C. correlate well with those simultaneously measured by cardiac catheterization.
   D. do not correlate well with those measured by cardiac catheterization in patients with mitral stenosis.
   E. do not correlate well with those measured by cardiac catheterization in the presence of prosthetic valves.

18. The time velocity integral
   A. is the sum of the velocities.
   B. is the stroke distance.
   C. equals the area enclosed by the baseline and the Doppler spectrum.
   D. is all of the above.
   E. is none of the above.

19. The simplified Bernoulli equation ignores
   A. flow acceleration.
   B. viscous friction.
   C. proximal flow velocity.
   D. all of the above.
   E. none of the above.

20. Which one of the following about the peak-to-peak gradient and the maximum instantaneous gradient is true?
   A. The maximum instantaneous gradient measured by Doppler is always higher than the peak-to-peak gradient measured in the cardiac catheterization laboratory.
   B. The peak-to-peak gradient is the pressure difference between the peak left ventricular and peak aortic pressures.
   C. The peak-to-peak gradient is a nonphysiologic measurement.
   D. The maximum Doppler velocity is converted to the maximum instantaneous gradient by the simplified Bernoulli equation.
   E. All of the above.

21. Atrial fibrillation creates problems in quantitation of Doppler echocardiographic information because Doppler velocities vary on the basis of R-R intervals. Therefore, for patients with atrial fibrillation, which one of the following is true?
   A. Doppler information can never be quantitated.
   B. Doppler information can be quantitated in the same way as for any other patients without atrial fibrillation.
   C. Three cycles should be averaged when Doppler velocity is measured.
   D. Seven to ten cycles should be averaged.
   E. None of the above.

22. Pressure half-time is the same as the interval for a peak velocity to decline to a velocity equal to
A. 0.5 × maximum velocity.
B. 1.4 × maximum velocity.
C. maximum velocity/1.4.
D. 4 × maximum velocity.
E. 4 × maximum velocity^2.

23. The empiric formula using pressure half-time to estimate the area of a stenotic native mitral valve is
A. 220 × pressure half-time.
B. 220/pressure half-time.
C. pressure half-time/220.
D. pressure half-time + 220.
E. 220 – pressure half-time.

24. The empiric formula in Question 23 should not be used in patients
A. with a prosthetic valve.
B. with atrial fibrillation.
C. with diastolic dysfunction.
D. immediately after balloon valvuloplasty.
E. with all of the above.

25. Which one of the following statements best describes the relationship between pressure half-time and deceleration time?
A. Pressure half-time is always proportionally related to deceleration time.
B. Pressure half-time is inversely related to deceleration time.
C. Pressure half-time is not proportionally related to deceleration time.
D. Pressure half-time is equal to approximately 60% of deceleration time.
E. Pressure half-time is equal to deceleration time.

26. The pressure half-time of aortic regurgitation Doppler velocity is
A. shortened in severe aortic regurgitation.
B. increased in severe aortic regurgitation.
C. dramatically shortened even in mild aortic regurgitation.
D. dramatically increased even in mild aortic regurgitation.
E. not influenced by the severity of aortic regurgitation.

27. Blood volume across a fixed orifice is equal to
A. the product of cross-sectional area and time velocity integral.
B. 0.785 × diameter^2 × time velocity integral.
C. π × (0.5 × diameter)^2 × time velocity integral.
D. all of the above.
E. none of the above.

28. The continuity equation uses the concept of conservation of
A. red blood cell number.
B. red blood cell mass.
C. red blood cell volume.
D. flow mass.
E. pressure.

29. The continuity equation can be used to calculate
A. peak pressure gradient.
B. mean pressure gradient.
C. valve area.
D. peak-to-peak gradient.
E. maximum instantaneous gradient.

30. Which one of the following represents the continuity equation?
A. Pressure 1 × time velocity integral 1 = pressure 2 × time velocity integral 2.
B. Mean pressure 1 × time velocity integral 2 = mean pressure 2 × time velocity integral 1.
C. Maximum instantaneous gradient 1 × time velocity integral 1 = maximum instantaneous gradient 2× time velocity integral 2.
D. Cross-sectional area 1 × time velocity integral 1 = cross-sectional area 2 × time velocity integral 2.
E. Cross-sectional area 1 × velocity 2 = cross-sectional area 2 × velocity 1.

31. During preoperative transesophageal echocardiography, a 56-year-old patient has a left ventricular outflow tract diameter of 2.1 cm and a time velocity integral of 16 cm. If this patient's heart rate is 72 beats per minute and his blood pressure is 120/60 mm Hg, his cardiac output is approximately
A. 2 L/min.
B. 3 L/min.
C. 4 L/min.
D. 5 L/min.
E. 6 L/min.

32. If the patient in Question 31 has body surface area of 1.88 m^2, his cardiac index is
A. 1.6 L/m^2.
B. 2.1 L/m^2.
C. 2.6 L/m^2.
D. 3.1 L/m^2.
E. 3.6 L/m^2.

33. Flow rate across a fixed orifice
A. equals the product of pressure gradient and flow velocity.
B. equals the product of the cross-sectional area and the flow velocity.
C. equals 0.785 × diameter^2 × the time velocity integral.

D. equals $\pi \times \text{diameter}^2 \times$ the time velocity integral.
E. can only be determined qualitatively, not quantitatively.

34. In patients with both mitral and aortic regurgitation, the mitral regurgitant volume
A. should be estimated by a volumetric method only.
B. should not be estimated by the proximal isovelocity surface area method.
C. is underestimated by the volumetric method.
D. is overestimated by the volumetric method.
E. is accurately estimated by the volumetric method.

35. The mitral inflow volume is calculated as a product of mitral valve area and mitral inflow time velocity integral. The mitral inflow time velocity integral is obtained by
A. placing a sample volume between the tips of mitral leaflets.
B. placing a sample volume below the tips of mitral leaflets.
C. placing a sample volume beyond the tips of mitral leaflets.
D. placing a sample volume at the center of the mitral anulus.
E. continuous wave Doppler without sample volume.

36. The proximal isovelocity surface area method
A. can only be used to calculate mitral regurgitant volume.
B. can only be used to calculate mitral valve area in patients with mitral stenosis.
C. can only be used to calculate the effective regurgitant orifice in patients with mitral regurgitation.
D. can be used to calculate the mitral regurgitant volume and effective regurgitant orifice, but not the mitral valve area in patients with mitral stenosis.
E. may be used to calculate the mitral regurgitant volume, effective regurgitant orifice, and mitral valve area in patients with mitral stenosis.

37. The proximal isovelocity surface area is calculated as
A. $2\pi \times \text{radius}^2$.
B. $\pi \times (2 \times \text{radius})^2$.
C. $\pi \times \text{radius}^2$.
D. $\pi \times 0.5 \times \text{diameter}^2$.
E. $\pi \times 0.25 \times \text{diameter}^2$.

38. The flow rate across the proximal isovelocity surface area
A. equals the product of the hemispheric area and the aliasing velocity.
B. equals the product of the hemispheric area and the regurgitant flow time velocity integral.
C. is greater than the flow rate across the effective regurgitant orifice.
D. is less than the flow rate across the effective regurgitant orifice.
E. is not equal to the flow rate across the effective regurgitant orifice.

39. If the peak velocity of the mitral regurgitant flow and the distance from the aliasing velocity to the mitral regurgitant orifice are known, which one of the following measurements should be obtained to calculate the effective regurgitant orifice?

A. The aliasing velocity.
B. The mean velocity of the mitral regurgitant flow.
C. The time velocity integral of the mitral regurgitant flow.
D. The time velocity integral of the mitral inflow.
E. The mitral annular diameter.

40. To calculate mitral regurgitant volume by the proximal isovelocity surface area method, all the following should be obtained ***except***

A. mitral inflow time velocity integral.
B. aliasing velocity.
C. proximal isovelocity surface area.
D. time velocity integral of mitral regurgitant flow.
E. peak velocity of mitral regurgitant flow.

41. The following measurements were obtained intraoperatively from a 72-year-old patient with mitral regurgitation: aliasing velocity of 44 cm/s, mitral regurgitant proximal isovelocity surface area (MR PISA) radius of 0.6 cm; at aliasing velocity of 39 cm/s, MR PISA radius of 0.8 cm. The MR peak velocity of 5 m/s and time velocity integral of 160 cm were measured by continuous wave Doppler. The effective regurgitant orifice in this patient is

A. 0.1 cm^2.
B. 0.2 cm^2.
C. 0.3 cm^2.
D. 0.4 cm^2.
E. 0.5 cm^2.

42. This patient's mitral regurgitant volume is

A. 28 mL.
B. 32 mL.
C. 38 mL.
D. 42 mL.
E. 48 mL.

43. If the patient described in Question 41 has a mitral annular diameter of 3 cm and a mitral inflow time velocity integral of 18 cm, the patient's regurgitant fraction is

A. 10%.
B. 22%.
C. 30%.
D. 38%.
E. 45%.

44. When the proximal isovelocity surface area method is used to calculate mitral valve area in patients with mitral stenosis, angle correction may be necessary. The angle α represents

A. the angle between the ultrasound beam and the mitral valve leaflets.
B. the angle between the ultrasound beam and the mitral anulus.
C. the angle between two mitral leaflets on the atrial side.
D. the angle between two mitral leaflets on the ventricular side.
E. the angle of the multiplane transesophageal echocardiographic probe orientation.

45. A 65-year-old patient had thickened mitral leaflets with diastolic doming. A proximal isovelocity surface area with a radius of 1.3 cm at an aliasing velocity of 32 cm/s was detected on the atrial side during diastole. The angle α was 120°. The peak mitral inflow velocity was 220 cm/s as measured by Doppler echocardiography. This patient's mitral valve area is

A. 0.5 cm^2.
B. 1.0 cm^2.
C. 1.5 cm^2.
D. 2.0 cm^2.
E. 2.5 cm^2.

46. Which one of the following statements about Qp/Qs is true?

A. It indicates the magnitude of intracardiac shunt.
B. Pulmonary flow is calculated from the right ventricular outflow tract.
C. Systemic flow is calculated from the left ventricular outflow tract.
D. All of the above.
E. None of the above.

47. Which one of the following statements about dp/dt is true?

A. It is the rate of left ventricular pressure change during the isovolumic contraction period.
B. It is an index of left ventricular relaxation.
C. Doppler-derived dp/dt does not correlate well with catheter-derived dp/dt.
D. A dp/dt of 1,200 mm Hg/s is abnormal.
E. It is used to evaluate both systolic and diastolic functions.

48. A 68-year-old patient has preoperative echocardiography, which reveals a dp/dt of 880 mm Hg/s. This patient has

A. decreased left ventricular diastolic function.
B. decreased left ventricular systolic function.
C. increased left ventricular diastolic function.
D. increased left ventricular systolic function.
E. normal left ventricular systolic function.

49. To calculate dp/dt, which one of the following should be measured?

A. Mitral inflow duration.
B. Aortic outflow duration.

C. Time interval for mitral regurgitant velocity to change from 1 m/s to 3 m/s.
D. Time interval of aortic regurgitant flow.
E. Left ventricular systolic duration.

50. The Doppler-derived index of myocardial performance reflects
A. systolic function only.
B. diastolic function only.
C. both systolic and diastolic myocardial function.
D. left atrial function.
E. right atrial function.

51. A 78-year-old patient has a left ventricular ejection time of 320 ms. To calculate the Doppler-derived index of myocardial performance, which one of the following should be obtained?
A. Isovolumic contraction and relaxation time.
B. Peak velocity of mitral inflow.
C. Left ventricular outflow tract maximum flow velocity.
D. Mitral valve closing to opening time.
E. A or D.

52. Which one of the following about the index of myocardial performance is true?
A. The index of myocardial performance is useful only for the left ventricle.
B. It provides prognostic information for patients with primary pulmonary hypertension.
C. The index of myocardial performance is decreased in dilated cardiomyopathy.
D. Systolic dysfunction results in a shortened isovolumic contraction time and ejection time.
E. Both systolic and diastolic dysfunction result in decreased isovolumic relaxation time.

53. In patients without pulmonary stenosis and right ventricular outflow tract obstruction, the tricuspid regurgitant velocity can be used to estimate
A. left atrial pressure.
B. right ventricular end-diastolic pressure.
C. pulmonary arterial end-diastolic pressure.
D. pulmonary arterial mean pressure.
E. none of the above.

54. A patient has tricuspid regurgitation with peak gradient 14 mm Hg. The mean velocity of the tricuspid regurgitant flow is 1.5 m/s. The patient's central venous pressure is 8 mm Hg. The estimated pulmonary arterial systolic pressure is
A. 12 mm Hg.
B. 22 mm Hg.
C. 30 mm Hg.
D. 45 mm Hg.
E. undetermined.

55. During an intraoperative transesophageal echocardiographic study, a 58-year-old patient has mitral regurgitation with a peak velocity of 5 m/s. His left ventricular outflow tract and aortic valve are normal. The vital signs are heart rate of 78 beats per minute and blood pressure of 115/60 mm Hg. This patient's left atrial pressure is
A. 10 mm Hg.
B. 15 mm Hg.
C. 20 mm Hg.
D. 25 mm Hg.
E. undetermined.

56. A 62-year-old patient with pulmonary regurgitation has preoperative transesophageal echocardiography. Doppler echocardiography reveals a pulmonary regurgitation signal with peak velocity of 1.8 m/s and end-diastolic velocity of 1.2 m/s. Other than the pulmonary regurgitation, the patient's physical examination findings are within normal limits. No jugular venous distention is found. This patient's pulmonary arterial end-diastolic pressure is about
A. 16 mm Hg.
B. 26 mm Hg.
C. 36 mm Hg.
D. 46 mm Hg.
E. undetermined.

57. An 80-year-old patient has aortic regurgitation with end-diastolic velocity of 2.5 m/s. The patient's blood pressure is 148/52 mm Hg. His left ventricular end-diastolic pressure is
A. 9 mm Hg.
B. 18 mm Hg.
C. 27 mm Hg.
D. 36 mm Hg.
E. undetermined.

58. Doppler interrogation of the flow across a ventricular septal defect reveals a peak velocity of 4.0 m/s at a systemic blood pressure 103/58 mm Hg. The patient has normal mitral and aortic valves without left ventricular outflow tract obstruction. The right ventricular systolic pressure is approximately
A. 20 mm Hg.
B. 30 mm Hg.
C. 40 mm Hg.
D. 50 mm Hg.
E. undetermined.

59. A 58-year-old patient has intraoperative transesophageal echocardiography which shows a normal right atrium and the presence of tricuspid regurgitation with peak velocity of 2 m/s. His systemic blood pressure is 110/58 mm Hg. The estimated right ventricular systolic pressure in this patient is
A. 16 mm Hg.
B. 26 mm Hg.

C. 36 mm Hg.
D. 49 mm Hg.
E. undetermined.

60. During intraoperative transesophageal echocardiography, a 32-year-old patient is found to have a patent foramen ovale with a left-to-right flow. The patent foramen ovale flow velocity is 1 m/s. The patient's central venous pressure is 6 mm Hg. This patient's left atrial pressure is
A. 5 mm Hg.
B. 7.5 mm Hg.
C. 10 mm Hg.
D. 12.5 mm Hg.
E. 15 mm Hg.

61. A 78-year-old patient has left ventricular outflow tract diameter of 2.0 cm measured by transesophageal echocardiography. To calculate this patient's stroke volume, one should measure
A. left ventricular outflow tract peak velocity by pulsed wave Doppler.
B. left ventricular outflow tract peak velocity by continuous wave Doppler.
C. left ventricular outflow tract time velocity integral by pulsed wave Doppler.
D. left ventricular outflow tract time velocity integral by continuous wave Doppler.
E. left ventricular outflow tract mean velocity by pulsed wave Doppler.

62. If the patient in Question 61 has left ventricular outflow tract peak velocity of 0.9 m/s, mean velocity of 100 cm/s, and left ventricular outflow tract time velocity integral of 22 cm, his stroke volume is
A. 59 mL.
B. 69 mL.
C. 79 mL.
D. 89 mL.
E. unable to be determined.

63. A 50-year-old patient with hypertrophic obstructive cardiomyopathy has a left ventricular outflow tract peak velocity of 4 m/s measured by continuous wave Doppler. His left ventricular outflow tract pressure gradient is
A. 4 mm Hg.
B. 16 mm Hg.
C. 32 mm Hg.
D. 64 mm Hg.
E. 72 mm Hg.

64. The area of a stenotic mitral valve may be estimated by
A. planimetry.
B. the pressure half-time method.
C. the continuity equation.
D. the proximal isovelocity surface area method.
E. all of the above.

65. A 66-year-old patient has mitral inflow deceleration time of 520 ms. The patient's mitral valve area is approximately
A. 1.5 cm^2.
B. 2.5 cm^2.
C. 3.5 cm^2.
D. 4.5 cm^2.
E. unable to be determined.

66. An 88-year-old patient has mitral regurgitation with a proximal isovelocity surface area radius of 7 mm at an aliasing velocity of 38 cm/s. His mitral regurgitant flow has a peak velocity of 3 m/s. To calculate the mitral regurgitant volume, which one of the following parameters should be measured?
A. The mitral regurgitant time velocity integral.
B. The mean velocity of mitral regurgitant flow.
C. The peak velocity of mitral inflow.
D. The mean velocity of mitral inflow.
E. The mitral annular diameter.

67. The peak velocity of mitral regurgitation is
A. higher than that of aortic stenosis.
B. lower than that of aortic stenosis.
C. usually lower but occasionally higher than that of aortic stenosis.
D. usually variable when compared with aortic stenosis.
E. never higher than that of aortic stenosis.

68. Severe aortic stenosis is indicated by a transaortic peak velocity greater than 4.5 m/s. If a patient with aortic stenosis has coexisting low cardiac output,
A. the continuity equation is less accurate than the Doppler velocity to estimate the severity of aortic stenosis.
B. the continuity equation is more accurate than the peak Doppler velocity to estimate the severity of aortic stenosis.
C. the Doppler-derived pressure gradient is more accurate than the continuity method to estimate the severity of aortic stenosis.
D. the peak velocity is more accurate than the continuity equation to estimate the severity of aortic stenosis.
E. the peak velocity is unchanged because the aortic valve area is unchanged.

Answers & Discussion

1. Answer A

When echocardiography is used to examine any structure or reflector with a finite width, the edge of the echo closest to the transducer is called the "leading edge" and that away from the transducer is called the "trailing edge." For optimal measurement accuracy, the American Society of Echocardiography recommends that all M-mode measurements be made from leading edge to leading edge of each interface of interest because the width of the M-mode echoes may vary from one instrument to another and at times even with gain. **Reference** 10 *(p 123–124)*.

2. Answer D

Although M-mode measurements are taken from leading edge to leading edge, two-dimensional measurements are taken from trailing edge to leading edge. Therefore, the aortic diameter should be measured from trailing edge to leading edge during two-dimensional imaging. **Reference** 10 *(p 123–124)*.

3. Answer B

The American Society of Echocardiography recommends that the end of diastole is best indicated by the Q wave of the electrocardiogram rather than by the R wave. This recommendation is based on the fact that the electrocardiogram frequently is not of the highest quality, and the R wave may vary. **Reference** 10 *(p 134)*.

4. Answer A

The centerline method is used for regional wall motion analysis. In this method, a centerline is drawn midway between the end-diastolic (ED) and end-systolic (ES) contours. Motion is measured along 100 equidistant chords perpendicular to the centerline. The motion at each chord is normalized by the ED perimeter to yield fractional shortening of a dimensionless chord. **Reference** 25 *(pp 29, 33)*.

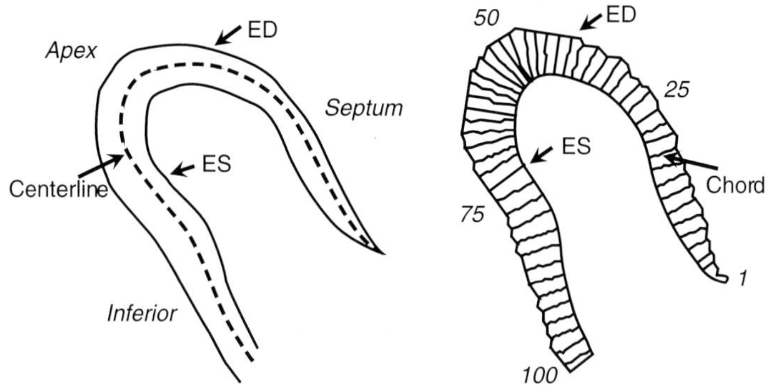

Figure from Wohlgelernter D, Cleman M, Highman HA, Fetterman RC, Duncan JS, Zaret BL, et al. Regional myocardial dysfunction during coronary angioplasty: evaluation by two-dimensional echocardiography and 12 lead electrocardiography. J Am Coll Cardiol 1986;7:1245–1254. Used with permission.

5. Answer D

A centroid is the center of a mass or area, which serves as an internal reference point to measure the endocardial excursion quantitatively. There are two types of referencing centroids: 1) the fixed center or fixed axis method and 2) the floating center or floating axis method. A fixed reference system uses a diastolic frame and traces the endocardial contour from which a centroid is computed. Cardiac contraction is assessed by tracking each point on the endocardial contour as it moves toward or away from the original diastolic center. The centroid of the left ventricle may have different spatial coordinates in systole compared with diastole, especially in patients with translation or regional wall motion abnormalities. A floating centroid entails computing a new center of mass for each time frame. Therefore, in the floating axis system, the end-diastolic and end-systolic centroids are superimposed to compensate for translation. Dyskinesis may produce false exaggeration or underestimation of contraction when using a referencing centroid with a floating axis. In general, a referencing centroid with a fixed axis is more accurate when assessing dyskinetic myocardial contraction if translation is minimal. Conversely, in the presence of translation or rotation, a referencing centroid with a floating axis is preferred because recalibration of the centroid with each time frame compensates for movement discrepancies. **Reference** 42 *(pp 631–633)*.

6. Answer C

Visual assessment of the left ventricular ejection fraction is the most commonly used method to evaluate left ventricular systolic function. Typically, ejection fraction is visually assessed in the interval of 5% to 10%, and an estimated ejection fraction range is reported (eg, 35%–40%). According to the ejection fraction, left ventricular systolic function can be classified as follows: >50%, normal systolic function; 40%–49%, mild systolic dysfunction; 30%–39%, moderate systolic dysfunction; and <30%, severe systolic dysfunction. The major limitation of visual assessment is that the accuracy of the estimated ejection fraction depends on the skill and experience of the observer. Because visual assessment is relatively subjective, the results may vary from observer to observer. However, a well-trained eye can accurately estimate ejection fraction and, hence, left ventricular systolic function. **References** 10 *(pp 143–144)*; 25 *(pp 31–33)*; 26 *(p 103)*; 42 *(pp 605–607, 629)*.

7. Answer D

Although all the methods listed in response to this question are used to calculate left ventricular volume, the American Society of Echocardiography's recommended method is the modified Simpson's rule technique. The principle for measuring volume with Simpson's rule is to divide the object into slices of known thickness. The volume of the object is then equal to the sum of the volumes of the slices. Although Simpson's method is accurate, it is clinically inapplicable because of the limitation in obtaining multiple short axis examinations. The modified Simpson's rule technique is a biplane method based on nearly orthogonal planes from two- and four-chamber views. Calculation of volume results from summation of volumes of 20 disks of equal height. This method is less sensitive to geometric distortions. Since it treats the ventricle as a stack of disks or slices, it is also called the method of disks or the disk summation method.

The modified Simpson's method is recommended by the American Society of Echocardiography because it is independent of preconceived ventricular shape and can be performed as rapidly as any other method. When only one view is of adequate quality for assessment, it is acceptable but less accurate to use a single-plane area length method. A different technique describes the left ventricle as a prolate ellipse. The long axis of the prolate ellipse is directly measured. The two minor axes can be either directly measured or calculated by measuring the area of the cavity in various planes. Then, the volume of a prolate ellipse is calculated according to the mathematic formula. The principal difficulty with using the prolate ellipse model for the left ventricle is that the chamber frequently does not resemble a prolate ellipse. With any significant dilation, the geometric model is distorted. Even a normal ventricle does not resemble a prolate ellipse in systole. This method is not recommended by the American Society of Echocardiography for calculation of left ventricular volume. **References** 10 *(pp 137–142)*; 33 *(pp 362–364)*.

8. Answer B

Generally, cardiac volume measured by a two-dimensional technique is less than that determined by angiography. One explanation is that echocardiography obtains tomographic views that are not necessarily the maximum dimensions. The angiographic technique relies on data from the silhouette of the angiographic dye, which visualizes the maximum distances between opposing walls. Another explanation for differences in volumes is that all the two-dimensional echocardiographic techniques require an accurate measurement of chamber length. Unfortunately, because it is easy to foreshorten the ventricular length, the measurement may be artifactually small and the volume may be underestimated. In addition, a two-dimensional echocardiographic calculation of left ventricular volumes requires identification of the endocardium. The two- and four-chamber views may have endocardial dropout because of the lateral resolution. Therefore, the two-dimensional echocardiographic method usually gives volumes that are smaller than those determined by angiography. **Reference** 10 *(pp 141–142)*.

9. Answer E

Fractional area change (FAC) is a two-dimensional area ejection fraction from a planar image. It is a systolic index used to assess global function. The systolic and diastolic areas are measured at the level of midpapillary muscle in the short-axis view of the left ventricle. The FAC is calculated by the following formula: FAC (%) = [(LVEDA − LVESA)/LVEDA] × 100, where LVEDA and LVESA denote left ventricular end-diastolic and end-systolic areas, respectively. The normal FAC is approximately 60% or more. The advantage of the FAC is that the measurements are not squared, and thus, the FAC reduces the magnification of any measurement error. The limitation of this method is that it is based only on a single cross-section of the left ventricle. Therefore, FAC is not truly global if the ventricle has regional wall motion abnormalities and is not contracting symmetrically. **References** 10 *(pp 143–144)*; 11 *(p 156)*; 33 *(p 364)*.

10. Answer D

Circumferential shortening is used to evaluate left ventricular systolic function. It is a way of converting the diameter into circumference and obtaining a systolic index. Circumferential shortening can be calculated by the following formula: Circumferential shortening = (diastolic circumference-systolic circumference)/diastolic circumference. **Reference** 10 *(p 144)*.

11. Answer C

Left ventricular ejection fraction (LVEF) reflects left ventricular systolic function. It can be calculated by the following formula: LVEF = [(LVEDV − LVESV)/LVEDV] × 100, where LVEDV and LVESV denote left ventricular end-diastolic and left ventricular end-systolic volumes, respectively. During intraoperative transesophageal echocardiography, the left ventricular ejection fraction usually is estimated using the short axis of left ventricular transgastric view at the midpapillary muscle level. (See also Question 6.) **References** 10 *(pp 143–144)*; 23 *(pp 40–41)*; 26 *(p 103)*; 33 *(pp 364–365)*; 42 *(p 605)*.

12. Answer E

Left ventricular global systolic function is evaluated by systolic indices such as ejection fraction, cardiac output, circumferential shortening, and fractional area change. All the systolic indices are preload and afterload dependent. **References** 10 *(pp 143–147)*; 23 *(pp 40–41)*; 26 *(pp 100–120)*; 42 *(pp 605–611)*.

13. Answer E

Although both M-mode and two-dimensional echocardiograms can be used to measure left ventricular wall thickness and chamber dimension, the two-dimensional approach is more accurate than M-mode in some ways. When measuring left ventricular wall thickness, the M-mode beam does not always cut across the walls perpendicularly. This inherent limitation of M-mode is improved if the M-mode measurement is guided by a two-dimensional echocardiogram. When a patient has regional wall motion abnormalities, the M-mode dimension may not reflect the true left ventricular dimension because it only reflects a slice where the ultrasound beam cuts across, which may or may not include the abnormal segment. Therefore, the M-mode dimensions are limited in evaluating global left ventricular function in patients with regional wall motion abnormalities. For the same reason, measuring left ventricular volumes by a single M-mode dimension is usually unreliable. **Reference** 10 *(pp 136–137)*.

14. Answer D

Left ventricular mass is the total weight of the myocardium, which equals the product of the volume of myocardium and the specific density of cardiac muscle. The area length and truncated ellipsoid techniques are the methods recommended by the American Society of Echocardiography to measure left ventricular mass. Both methods use two-dimensional mode. The M-mode technique can also be used to measure left ventricular wall volume and, hence, to calculate left ventricular mass. Then, the specific gravity of cardiac muscle is used to convert the left ventricular wall volume into left ventricular mass. The principal limitation of the M-mode technique is the inaccuracy of a single dimension to measure volumes. The M-mode technique is not the method recommended by the American Society of Echocardiography for measuring left ventricular mass. **References** 10 *(pp 155–158)*; 33 *(p 365)*.

15. Answer E

When analyzing Doppler recordings, several parameters need to be taken into consideration: timing of Doppler velocity, direction of blood flow, peak velocity, flow duration, flow configuration, and other accompanying signals. To identify whether the blood flow is normal or abnormal (eg, regurgitant), one needs to know when the flow occurs and which direction it goes. Peak velocity of the flow through an abnormal valvular orifice may indicate the degree of valvular stenosis or regurgitation. Flow duration is helpful to differentiate left ventricular outflow tract or transaortic forward flow from mitral regurgitant flow. Because there is no flow across the aortic valve during isovolumic contraction periods, the flow duration of transaortic forward flow is shorter than mitral regurgitant flow. Flow configuration helps recognition of flows at different valvular sites as well as differential diagnosis of certain cardiac diseases. A dagger-shaped systolic velocity is characteristic for dynamic left ventricular outflow tract obstruction. **References** 10 *(pp 26–42)*; 23 *(pp 16–19)*; 26 *(pp 50, 51–54)*.

16. Answer E

Doppler echocardiography can be used to determine transvalvular pressure gradients, intracardiac pressures, valve areas, flow volume, and diastolic function. On the basis of the Doppler shift, Doppler echocardiography measures blood flow velocities in cardiac chambers as well as in the greater vessels. Pressure gradient is converted from Doppler velocity according to the Bernoulli equation, and then intracardiac pressures can be calculated. Valve areas and flow volume can be calculated using various Doppler hemodynamic methods, including the continuity equation and the proximal isovelocity surface area. Diastolic function can be evaluated by Doppler flow velocities of mitral inflow and pulmonary vein for the left ventricle and those of tricuspid inflow and hepatic vein for the right ventricle. **References** 10 *(pp 35–36)*; 23 *(pp 59–70)*.

17. Answer C

Transmitral pressure gradients can be estimated by Doppler echocardiography using the simplified Bernoulli equation. Several studies have shown that Doppler-derived pressure gradients are highly accurate, with an excellent correlation with transseptal catheter–derived pressure gradients, even in patients with mitral stenosis and various prosthetic valves. Therefore, Doppler echocardiography is an optimal noninvasive method to estimate transmitral pressure gradients. **Reference** 23 *(pp 64–66)*.

18. Answer D

The time velocity integral is also called the velocity time integral. It is the sum of velocities and represents the distance blood travels with each heartbeat, ie, the stroke distance. The time velocity integral is calculated as the area enclosed by the baseline and the Doppler spectrum and can be measured readily with the built-in calculation package in the ultrasound system by tracing the Doppler velocity signal. **References** 8 *(p 191)*; 11 *(p 158)*; 23 *(pp 59, 61)*.

19. Answer D

Using the Bernoulli equation, we can calculate a pressure gradient across an orifice from blood flow velocity. The Bernoulli equation has three components: convective acceleration, flow acceleration, and viscous friction. In a clinical setting, the viscous friction factor can be ignored because the velocity profile in the center of the lumen is usually flat. The flow acceleration can also be ignored with reasonable accurate estimation of the pressure gradient. When blood flow passes through a narrowed orifice, the proximal velocity is much less than the distal velocity ($V_1 \ll V_2$). Therefore, the proximal velocity V_1 can be ignored in the calculation of the pressure gradient. After ignoring flow acceleration, viscous friction, and proximal flow velocity, we have the following simplified Bernoulli equation: $\Delta P = (2V)^2$ and thus $\Delta P = 4V^2$, where ΔP stands for pressure gradient and V is the distal flow velocity. **References** 8 *(pp 194–196)*; 10 *(pp 195–196)*; 23 *(pp 64–65)*; 26 *(pp 49, 230–231)*.

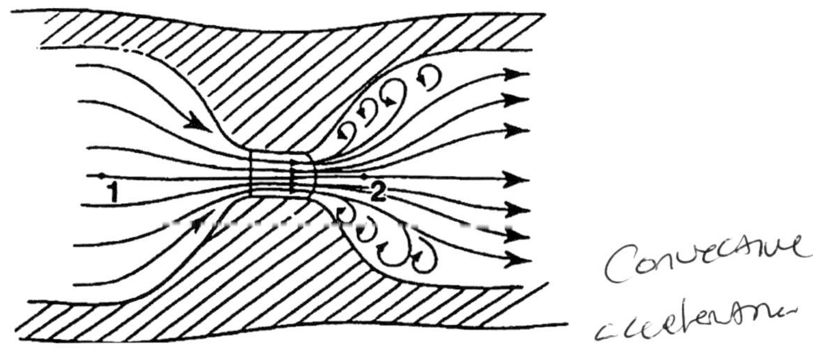

Bernoulli Equation

$$P_1 - P_2 = \underbrace{\tfrac{1}{2}\rho(V_2^2 - V_1^1)}_{\text{Convective acceleration}} + \underbrace{\rho \int_1^2 \frac{d\vec{V}}{dt}\, d\vec{s}}_{\text{Flow acceleration}} + \underbrace{R(\vec{V})}_{\text{Viscous friction}}$$

P_1 = pressure at location 1
P_2 = pressure at location 2
ρ = mass density of the blood 1.06 x 103 kg/m^3
V_1 = velocity at location 1
V_2 = velocity at location 2

Figure from Oh et al. (23). Used with permission of Mayo Foundation for Medical Education and Research.

20. Answer E

It is important to understand how the different pressure gradients are derived. The maximum instantaneous gradient is derived from the peak velocity using the simplified Bernoulli equation. The peak-to-peak gradient is the pressure difference between the peak left ventricular (LV) and peak aortic (Ao) pressures. Because the peak LV pressure occurs before the peak Ao pressure, the peak-to-peak gradient is a nonphysiologic measurement. From the accompanying diagram, it is obvious that the maximum instantaneous gradient measured by Doppler is always higher than the peak-to-peak gradient measured in the cardiac catheterization laboratory. **References** 23 *(pp 64–65)*; 26 *(pp 236–238)*.

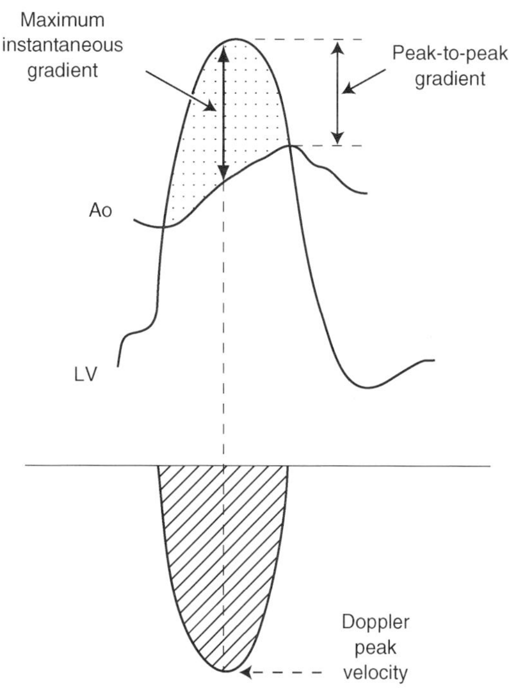

From Oh et al. (23). Used with permission of Mayo Foundation for Medical Education and Research.

21. Answer D

Atrial fibrillation creates problems in quantitation of Doppler echocardiographic information because Doppler velocities vary, depending on R-R intervals. In normal subjects, three to five cycles are usually averaged when quantitating Doppler information. For patients with atrial fibrillation, quantitative Doppler echocardiography still can be done, but seven to ten cycles should be averaged. **References** 10 *(pp 229, 233)*; 11 *(p 159)*; 23 *(p 118)*.

22. Answer C

Pressure half-time is the time interval for the maximum or peak pressure gradient to reach its half level. It is the same as the interval for the peak velocity to decline to a velocity equal to the peak velocity divided by 1.4. **References** 10 *(pp 244, 246)*; 23 *(pp 67–68)*; 26 *(pp 251–253)*.

23. Answer B

24. Answer E

The empiric formula using pressure half-time to estimate the amount of a stenotic native mitral valve is the constant 220 divided by the pressure half-time. This empiric formula overestimates the area of a normal prosthetic mitral valve. It is also not valid in patients with atrial fibrillation or diastolic dysfunction and immediately after balloon valvuloplasty. **References** 10 *(pp 244, 246)*; 23 *(pp 67–68)*; 26 *(pp 251–253)*.

25. Answer A

Pressure half-time is always proportionally related to deceleration time, equaling 29% of deceleration time. **Reference** 23 *(pp 67–68)*.

26. Answer A

An important clinical application of pressure half-time is to evaluate the severity of aortic regurgitation. In patients with severe aortic regurgitation, left ventricular pressure increases rapidly and aortic pressure decreases during diastole. Because of this decrease in the pressure gradient between the aorta and the left ventricle during diastole, the pressure half-time of aortic regurgitation Doppler velocity becomes much shorter (<250 ms) in severe aortic regurgitation. **Reference** 23 *(pp 120, 122)*.

27. Answer D

A certain amount of blood in a blood vessel can be considered a cylinder. Mathematically, the volume of a cylinder equals the product of the cross-sectional area (CSA) times the height of the cylinder. Therefore, the blood volume across a fixed orifice can be calculated as the following: Blood volume $=$ CSA $\times$ TVI, where TVI denotes time velocity integral. Because the radius is half the diameter, the CSA is calculated as CSA $= \pi r^2 = \pi \times (\text{diameter}/2)^2 = 0.785 \times \text{diameter}^2$. **Reference** 23 *(pp 59, 61–62)*.

28. Answer D

The continuity equation uses the concept of conservation of flow mass. It states that "what comes in must go out." The continuity equation expresses the continuity of flow mass at sequential points along the flow stream. According to the continuity equation, the flow mass through the mitral orifice is equal to the flow mass across the aortic orifice if the mitral and aortic valves are normal. **References** 10 *(pp 246–247)*; 23 *(p 65)*; 26 *(pp 237–239)*.

29. Answer C

30. Answer D

The continuity equation can be used to calculate valve area. After obtaining the time velocity integral (TVI) by tracing the Doppler velocity signal, the flow volume can be calculated by multiplying the TVI times the cross-sectional area (CSA).

According to the continuity equation, the flow volume across orifice 1 is equal to that across orifice 2. Thus, CSA 1 $\times$ TVI 1 $=$ CSA 2 $\times$ TVI 2. **References** 10 *(pp 246–247)*; 11 *(p 272)*; 23 *(p 65)*; 26 *(pp 237–239)*.

31. Answer C

32. Answer B

Cardiac output is calculated as the product of stroke volume (SV) and heart rate (HR). The SV is calculated as the product of the area of the left ventricular outflow tract (LVOT) and the distance the blood flow travels per stroke, which is the LVOT time velocity integral (TVI). The LVOT area is calculated as πr^2 or $0.785 \times$ LVOT diameter^2. Therefore, SV $= 0.785 \times$ LVOT diameter$^2 \times$ LVOT TVI $= 0.785 \times 2.1\ \text{cm}^2 \times 16\ \text{cm} = 55.4$ mL. Because the patient's SV is 55.4 mL and HR is 72 beats per minute, his cardiac output is SV $\times$ HR $= 55.4$ mL $\times$ 72 beats per minute $= 3988.8$ mL/min. So the patient's cardiac output is approximately 4 L/min. The cardiac index is the cardiac output per unit body surface area. This patient's body surface area is 1.88 m^2, and hence, his cardiac index is 4 L/1.88 $m^2 = 2.1$ L/m^2. Therefore, the patient's cardiac output and cardiac index are 4 L/min and 2.1 L/m^2, respectively. (See also Question 27.) **References** 11 *(pp 158–159)*; 23 *(pp 59, 61–62)*.

33. Answer B

In quantitative Doppler echocardiography, the flow rate across a fixed orifice can be calculated as the product of the cross-sectional area and the flow velocity. During mitral regurgitation, the regurgitant flow rate is equal to the product of the effective regurgitant orifice and the peak velocity of regurgitant flow. **References** 11 *(pp 210–214)*; 23 *(pp 59, 62–64)*.

34. Answer C

Regurgitant volume can be estimated by two different echocardiographic methods, ie, the volumetric and the proximal isovelocity surface area methods. With the volumetric method, the mitral valve regurgitant volume is estimated as the mitral inflow volume minus the left ventricular outflow tract stroke volume. In patients with aortic regurgitation, the left ventricular outflow tract stroke volume equals the sum of the aortic forward stroke volume and the aortic regurgitant volume. Therefore, the mitral regurgitant volume is underestimated by the volumetric method in patients with coexisting aortic regurgitation. In such a situation, the proximal isovelocity surface area method is more accurate to estimate the mitral regurgitant volume. **References** 11 *(pp 210–214)*; 23 *(pp 62–63)*.

35. Answer D

The mitral inflow volume equals the mitral valve area times the mitral inflow time velocity integral. The mitral inflow time velocity index should be measured by pulsed wave Doppler with the sample volume placed at the center of the mitral anulus.

36. Answer E

The proximal isovelocity surface area method is well known for calculation of the mitral regurgitant volume and effective regurgitant orifice. The principle of conservation of mass is applied in the region proximal to the orifice to measure the regurgitant orifice and volume. The concept of proximal isovelocity surface area can also be applied for calculating the area of a stenotic orifice. This method has been validated for mitral valve area in patients with mitral stenosis. **References** 11 *(pp 210–214)*; 23 *(pp 62–64)*.

37. Answer A

38. Answer A

The proximal isovelocity surface area (PISA) method can be used to calculate the volume of valvular regurgitation. As blood flow converges toward the regurgitant orifice, blood flow velocity increases with the formation of multiple shells of isovelocity of hemispheric shape. The flow rate at the surface of a hemispheric shell is equal to the flow rate across the regurgitant orifice because of the conservation of flow. By adjusting the Nyquist limit of the color flow map, the hemisphere can be maximized and the flow velocity at the hemispheric surface can be determined. The radius of the hemisphere is measured as the distance from the aliasing velocity to the regurgitant orifice, and the PISA is calculated as $2\pi r^2$, PISA $= 2\pi r^2$. Because the flow rate equals the cross-sectional area multiplied by the velocity, the flow rate by the PISA method equals the product of the hemispheric area and the aliasing velocity. **References** 11 *(pp 210–214)*; 23 *(pp 62–64)*.

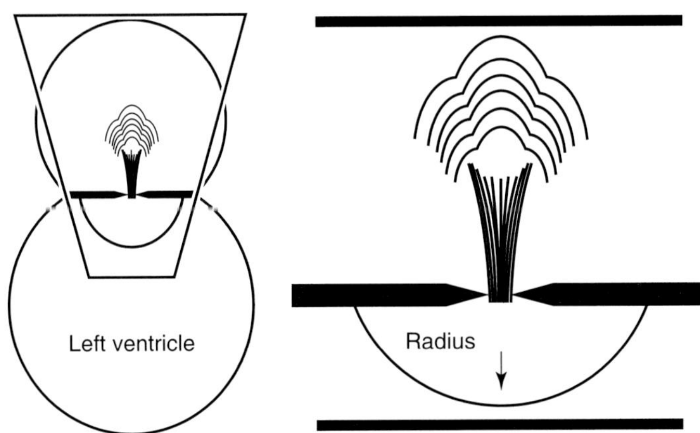

39. Answer A

As mentioned in Answer 38, flow rate equals the cross-sectional area multiplied by velocity. Hence, the flow rate across the effective regurgitant orifice (ERO) equals the effective regurgitant orifice multiplied by the aliasing velocity. The proximal isovelocity surface area method is an application of continuity equation. Because of the conservation of flow, the flow rate across the proximal isovelocity surface area should equal that across the ERO: $2\pi r^2 \times$ aliasing velocity $=$ ERO $\times$ peak regurgitant velocity. Rearranging the above equation, the ERO can be calculated as follows: ERO $= 2\pi r^2 \times$ aliasing velocity/peak regurgitant velocity. Therefore, if the peak velocity of mitral regurgitation and the distance from the aliasing velocity to the mitral regurgitant orifice are known, the aliasing velocity should be obtained to calculate the mitral ERO. **References** 11 *(pp 210–214)*; 23 *(pp 62–64)*.

40. Answer A

The proximal isovelocity surface area (PISA) method can be used to calculate mitral regurgitant volume. Because volume is calculated as the product of the area and the time velocity integral (TVI), the mitral regurgitant (MR) volume equals the product of the effective regurgitant orifice (ERO) and the TVI of the MR flow: RV = ERO × MR TVI. As mentioned in Answer 39, the mitral ERO is calculated according to the following equation: ERO = $2\pi r^2$ × aliasing velocity/peak regurgitant velocity. Thus, by combining these two equations, we obtain the following equation for calculation of MR volume: Regurgitant volume = $2\pi r^2$ × aliasing velocity × MR TVI/peak MR velocity, where $2\pi r^2$ is the PISA. Hence, to calculate MR volume by the PISA method, one needs to know the PISA, aliasing velocity, peak MR velocity, and MR TVI. **References** 11 *(pp 210–214)*; 23 *(pp 62–64)*.

41. Answer C

42. Answer E

43. Answer D

The effective regurgitant orifice (ERO) of mitral regurgitation can be calculated using the proximal isovelocity surface area (PISA) method. Because the hemisphere size changes as the aliasing velocity changes, the aliasing velocity should be adjusted so that the largest hemisphere is measured for calculation. When two sets of measurements are made for PISA, the measurement of the larger hemisphere should be used. In Question 41, the PISA radius of 0.8 cm and aliasing velocity of 39 cm/s should be used for calculation of the ERO. The mitral regurgitant (MR) peak velocity of 5 m/s should be converted to 500 cm/s to calculate the ERO or regurgitant volume (RV) by the PISA method. Thus, ERO = ($2\pi r^2$ × aliasing velocity)/MR peak velocity = $(2\pi \times 0.8^2 \times 39)/500 = 0.3\ \text{cm}^2$.

In Doppler hemodynamic study, flow volume is calculated as the product of the cross-sectional area (CSA) and the flow time velocity integral (TVI). Thus, the MR volume equals the product of the ERO and the TVI of the MR flow: RV = ERO × MR TVI = $0.3\ \text{cm}^2 \times 160\ \text{cm} = 48$ mL.

Regurgitant fraction (RF) is simply the percentage of regurgitant volume compared with the total flow volume across the regurgitant valve. This patient's mitral RF can be calculated as RF = MR volume × 100% mitral inflow volume, where mitral inflow volume equals the product of the mitral valve area and the mitral inflow TVI. This patient has mitral annular diameter of 3 cm and mitral inflow TVI of 18 cm. His mitral inflow volume is calculated as follows: Mitral inflow volume = MVA × mitral TVI = πr^2 × TVI = $\pi \times (1.5\ \text{cm})^2 \times 18\ \text{cm} = 127$ mL. Therefore, the patient's mitral RF is calculated as follows: Mitral RF = MR volume/mitral inflow volume = 48 mL/127 mL = 38%. **References** 11 *(pp 210–214)*; 23 *(pp 62–64)*.

44. Answer C

When the concept of the proximal isovelocity surface area is applied to calculate mitral valve area (MVA) in patients with mitral stenosis, it should be considered that the proximal isovelocity surface area proximal to a stenotic mitral orifice may not be a complete hemisphere but rather a portion of a hemisphere because of the geometry of mitral leaflets on the atrial side. Therefore, an angle correction factor may be necessary. Thus, MVA = $2\pi r^2$ × (aliasing volume/peak mitral stenosis velocity) × ($\alpha/180$), where α is the angle between two mitral leaflets on the atrial side. **References** 11 *(pp 210–214)*; 23 *(pp 62–64)*.

45. Answer B

This patient had a proximal isovelocity surface area radius of 1.3 cm, aliasing velocity of 32 cm/s, angle α of 120°, and peak mitral inflow velocity 220 cm/s. Entering these values into the equation used in Answer 44, we can calculate the mitral valve area (MVA) as follows: MVA $= 2\pi r^2 \times$ (aliasing velocity/peak mitral inflow velocity) $\times$ $(\alpha/180) = 2\pi \times 1.3^2 \times (32/220) \times (120/180) = 1.01$ cm^2. Therefore, this patient's MVA is approximately 1.0 cm^2 using the proximal isovelocity surface area method. **References** 11 *(pp 210–214)*; 23 *(pp 62–64)*.

46. Answer D

Qp/Qs is the flow ratio between the pulmonary and the systemic circulations. In the presence of an intracardiac shunt, this flow ratio indicates the magnitude of the intracardiac shunt. Pulmonary flow (Qp) is calculated from the right ventricular outflow tract (RVOT), and systemic flow (Qs) is calculated from the left ventricular outflow tract (LVOT). Thus, Qp = RVOT CSA × RVOT TVI and Qs = LVOT CSA × LVOT TVI, where CSA is the cross-sectional area, and TVI is the time velocity integral. Therefore, Qp/Qs can be calculated as the following: Qp/Qs = (RVOT CSA × RVOT TVI)/(LVOT CSA × LVOT TVI). **Reference** 23 *(p 64)*.

47. Answer A

48. Answer B

The dp/dt represents the rate of ventricular pressure rise during the isovolumic contraction period. It is an index of left ventricular contractility and provides information about left ventricular systolic function. There is good correlation between noninvasive Doppler-derived and catheter-derived dp/dt. Normal dp/dt is 1,200 mm Hg/s or higher. A dp/dt less than 1,000 mm Hg/s indicates decreased left ventricular systolic function. Because the patient has a dp/dt of 880 mm Hg/s, his left ventricular function is decreased. **References** 23 *(p 70)*; 25 *(p 51)*.

49. Answer C

The dp/dt can be estimated from a mitral regurgitation jet by continuous wave Doppler. The rate of pressure rise in the left ventricle is calculated from the time interval (dt) required to achieve mitral regurgitant velocity from 1 m/s to 3 m/s. Since there is no significant change in left atrial pressure during the isovolumic contraction period, mitral regurgitant velocity changes during this period reflect dp/dt. According to the simplified Bernoulli equation, pressure $= 4 \times$ velocity^2. Therefore, the pressures at mitral regurgitant velocities of 1 m/s and 3 m/s can be calculated as follows: Pressure at 1 m/s $= 4 \times 1^2 = 4$ mm Hg and Pressure at 3 m/s $= 4 \times 3^2 = 36$ mm Hg.

When mitral regurgitant velocity rises from 1 m/s to 3 m/s, the pressure change (dp) is calculated as follows: dp = pressure at 3 m/s − pressure at 1 m/s $= 36 - 4 = 32$ mm Hg. That is, there is a 32 mm Hg pressure rise. Therefore, to calculate dp/dt, one needs to measure the time interval (dt) for mitral regurgitant velocity to change from 1 m/s to 3 m/s: dp/dt = pressure at 3 m/s − pressure at 1 m/s/time interval dt (in seconds) = 32/dt (mm Hg/s). **Reference** 23 *(p 70)*.

50. Answer C

51. Answer E

The Doppler-derived index of myocardial performance combines systolic and diastolic parameters and reflects global myocardial function independent of ventricular geometry. The normal value of the index of myocardial performance is 0.39 ± 0.05. Left ventricular (LV) systolic and diastolic dysfunction frequently coexists in heart failure. Two-dimensional echocardiography (ECG) is excellent for diagnosing systolic dysfunction, and Doppler echocardiography is reliable for evaluating diastolic function. However, the two-dimensional echocardiographic assessment of LV systolic function may be difficult because of poorly defined ventricular endocardial borders. Doppler analysis of diastolic function may be limited because of fusion of the early and late mitral inflow waves during tachycardia, and a normal inflow pattern may be difficult to separate from pseudonormalization. Under these conditions, the Doppler-derived index of myocardial performance, defined as the sum of isovolumic contraction time (ICT) and isovolumic relaxation time (IRT) divided by ejection time (ET), can be used to obtain a combined measure of systolic and diastolic myocardial function. If the patient's ET is known, the ICT and IRT should be obtained to calculate the index of myocardial performance. Since the sum of the ICT and IRT equal the interval between cessation and onset of the mitral inflow minus the ET, one can calculate the index of myocardial performance if the ET and the mitral valve closing to opening (MCO) time are known. **Reference** 23 *(pp 55–56)*.

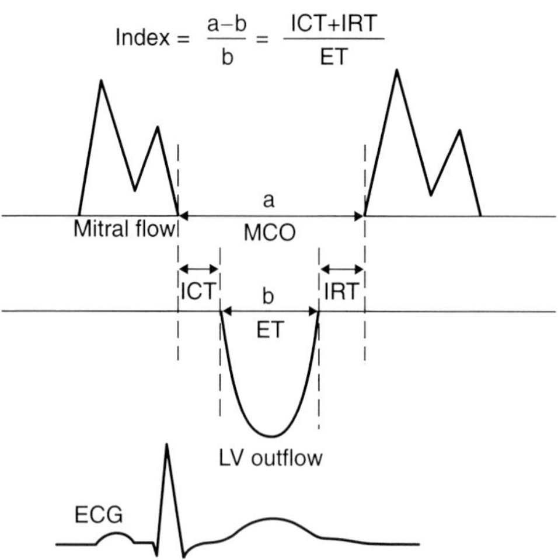

From Oh et al. (23). Used with permission of Mayo Foundation for Medical Education and Research.

52. Answer B

The index of myocardial performance is related to morbidity and mortality in cardiac diseases. Systolic dysfunction results in a prolonged isovolumic contraction time and a shortened ejection time. Abnormal myocardial relaxation prolongs isovolumic relaxation time. The index of myocardial performance is increased in patients with dilated cardiomyopathy.

The index of myocardial performance was evaluated for the right ventricle, especially in patients with primary pulmonary hypertension. In these patients, the right index of myocardial performance (RIMP) correlates with symptoms and survival and is the single most powerful variable for discriminating patients with primary pulmonary hypertension from normal subjects. The RIMP is calculated as follows: RIMP = (TVCO − PVET)/PVET, where TVCO denotes tricuspid valve closing and opening time, and PVET is the pulmonary valve ejection time (ie, the ejection time of flow across the pulmonary valve). A normal RIMP value is 0.28 ± 0.04. A value of 0.89 ± 0.25 indicates a poor prognosis in patients with primary pulmonary hypertension. **Reference** 23 *(pp 55–56)*.

53. Answer E

Regurgitant velocities can be used to determine intracardiac and pulmonary arterial (PA) pressures because the velocity of the regurgitant flow is directly related to the pressure difference across the orifice or valve. The tricuspid regurgitant (TR) velocity reflects the systolic pressure difference between the right ventricle (RV) and the right atrium (RA). According to the simplified Bernoulli equation, the RV systolic pressure, the RA pressure, and the TR flow velocity have the following relationship: RV systolic pressure − estimated RA pressure = 4 × TR velocity^2. Rearranging the equation, we can calculate the RV pressure as follows: RV systolic pressure = 4 × TR velocity^2 + estimated RA pressure. The RA pressure is roughly estimated by inspecting the jugular venous pressure at the bedside. An empiric value of 10 mm Hg is used for a normal RA; an empiric value of 14 or 20 mm Hg is used for patients with increased RA pressure. In the absence of pulmonary stenosis and RV outflow tract obstruction, the PA systolic pressure is practically the same as the calculated RV systolic pressure, that is, PA systolic pressure = RV systolic pressure and PA systolic pressure = estimated RA pressure + (4 × TR velocity^2). Therefore, TR flow velocity can be used to calculate RV systolic pressure or PA systolic pressure in patients without pulmonary stenosis or RV outflow tract obstruction. **Reference** 23 *(p 68)*.

54. Answer B

As mentioned in Answer 53, tricuspid regurgitant flow velocity or pressure gradient reflects right ventricular (RV) systolic pressure and, therefore, pulmonary arterial systolic pressure in patients without pulmonary stenosis or RV outflow tract obstruction. Here, the patient has central venous pressure (CVP) of 8 mm Hg and tricuspid regurgitation with peak gradient of 14 mm Hg: Tricuspid regurgitant peak gradient = RV systolic pressure − CVP. Rearranging the equation, we can calculate the RV systolic pressure as follows: RV systolic pressure = tricuspid regurgitant peak gradient + CVP = 14 mm Hg + 8 mm Hg = 22 mm Hg. Because the pulmonary arterial systolic pressure is practically the same as the RV systolic pressure, the estimated pulmonary arterial systolic pressure for this patient is approximately 22 mm Hg. Mean velocity of tricuspid regurgitant flow is not used for calculation of RV systolic pressure or pulmonary arterial systolic pressure. **Reference** 23 *(p 68)*.

55. Answer B

The flow velocity (V) of mitral regurgitation (MR) can be used to calculate the left atrial (LA) pressure. According to the simplified Bernoulli equation, the pressure difference (ΔP) between the left ventricle (LV) and the LA is calculated as follows: LV systolic pressure − LA pressure = 4 × MR velocity^2. In patients without LV outflow tract obstruction, systolic blood pressure (SBP) is practically the same as LV systolic pressure. Rearranging this equation, we can calculate the LA pressure as follows: LA pressure = LV systolic pressure − 4 × MR velocity^2 LA pressure = SBP − 4 × MR velocity^2 = 115 − 4 × 5^2 = 115 mm Hg−100 mm Hg = 15 mm Hg. Therefore, the patient's LA pressure was 15 mm Hg. **Reference** 23 *(pp 68–69)*.

56. Answer A

Pulmonary regurgitant (PR) end-diastolic velocity (EDV) reflects the pressure difference between the pulmonary artery (PA) and the right ventricle (RV) at the end of diastole. According to the simplified Bernoulli equation, we have the following equation: PA EDP − RV EDP = 4 × PR EDV^2, where EDP stands for end-diastolic pressure. Rearranging the equation, we have the following equation to calculate PA EDP: PA EDP = 4 × PR EDV^2 + RV EDP. Because the RV EDP is practically the same as RA pressure, the PA EDP can be calculated as follows: PA EDP = 4 × PR EDV^2 + RA pressure. In a patient with normal RA pressure, an empiric value of 10 is used for RA pressure. Therefore, PA EDP = 4 × 1.2^2 + 10 mm Hg = 16 mm Hg + 10 mm Hg = 26 mm Hg. Thus, the patient's PA EDP is 16 mm Hg. **Reference** 23 *(p 68)*.

57. Answer C

Aortic regurgitation (AR) velocity reflects the diastolic pressure difference between the aorta and the left ventricle. According to the simplified Bernoulli equation, the end-diastolic pressure gradient between the aorta and the left ventricle is calculated as follows: DBP − LVEDP = 4 × AR EDV^2, where DBP, LVEDP, and EDV stand for diastolic blood pressure, left ventricular end-diastolic pressure, and end-diastolic velocity, respectively. Rearranging the above equation, we can calculate the LVEDP as follows: LVEDP = DBP − 4 × AR EDV^2. The patient in Question 57 has DBP of 52 mm Hg and AR EDV 2.5 m/s. Entering these values into the equation yields the following: LVEDP = 52 − (4 × 2.5^2) = 27 mm Hg. Therefore, this patient's LVEDP is 27 mm Hg. **Reference** 23 *(pp 68–69)*.

58. Answer C

The pressure difference between the left ventricle (LV) and the right ventricle (RV) produces the gradient across a ventricular septal defect (VSD). Knowing the VSD flow velocity, this pressure gradient can be calculated using the simplified Bernoulli equation: LV systolic pressure − RV systolic pressure = 4 × VSD velocity^2. In a patient with a normal aortic valve without LV outflow tract obstruction, the LV systolic pressure is practically the same as the systolic blood pressure (SBP). If we rearrange the equation using SBP instead of LV systolic pressure, the following equation is obtained for calculation of RV systolic pressure: RV systolic pressure = SBP − 4 × VSD velocity^2. Because the patient has SBP of 103 mm Hg and VSD velocity of 4.0 m/s, his RV systolic pressure can be calculated as follows: RV systolic pressure = 103 − 4 × 4^2 = 103 mm Hg − 64 mm Hg = 39 mm Hg. Therefore, the patient's RV systolic pressure is 39 mm Hg, or approximately 40 mm Hg.

59. Answer B

Tricuspid regurgitant (TR) velocity can be used to estimate the right ventricular (RV) systolic pressure. According to the simplified Bernoulli equation, the pressure gradient between the RV and the right atrium (RA) can be calculated from the TR velocity: Pressure gradient = 4 × TR velocity^2. Because this pressure gradient is the systolic pressure difference between the RV and the RA, we have the following equation: RV systolic pressure − RA pressure = 4 × TR velocity^2. Because the patient's RA is normal, an empiric value of 10 mm Hg can be used for the RA pressure. Rearranging the preceding equation, we can calculate the RV systolic pressure as follows: RV systolic pressure = 4 × TR velocity^2 + RA pressure = 4 × 2^2 + 10 = 16 mm Hg + 10 mm Hg = 26 mm Hg. Therefore, the patient's RV systolic pressure is 26 mm Hg. **Reference** 23 *(p 68)*.

60. Answer C

Left atrial (LA) pressure can be estimated from velocity of flow across the patent foramen ovale or atrial septal defect. Using the Bernoulli equation, we have the following equation: LA pressure − RA pressure = 4 × PFO velocity^2. The left atrial pressure can be calculated by rearranging the equation and using central venous pressure (CVP) for right atrial (RA) pressure: LA pressure = 4 × PFO velocity^2 + CVP = 4 × 1^2 + 6 = 4 mm Hg + 6 mm Hg = 10 mm Hg. Therefore, the patient's LA pressure was 10 mm Hg. **Reference** 23 *(pp 69–70)*.

61. Answer C

62. Answer B

Because flow volume equals the product of area and time velocity integral (TVI), the patient's stroke volume (SV) can be calculated as the product of the left ventricular outflow tract (LVOT) area and the LVOT TVI. The LVOT TVI is measured by pulsed wave Doppler with the sample volume placed at the level of aortic anulus. Because the patient's LVOT diameter (D) is 2 cm, his LVOT area is calculated as follows: LVOT area = 0.785 × D^2 = 0.785 × 2^2 = 3.14 cm^2. Knowing the patient's LVOT area, one needs to measure the LVOT TVI by pulsed wave Doppler to calculate his SV. If the patient's LVOT TVI is 22 cm, his SV can be calculated as follows: SV = LVOT area × LVOT TVI = 3.14 mL × 22 mL = 69 mL. (See also Questions 27 and 31.) **References** 8 *(p 191)*; 11 *(pp 158–159)*; 23 *(pp 59, 61–62)*.

63. Answer D

The simplified Bernoulli equation is used to calculate the pressure gradient from the flow velocity. Knowing the patient's left ventricular outflow tract (LVOT) peak velocity is 4 m/s, one can calculate the gradient as follows: Pressure gradient = 4 × LVOT velocity^2 = 4 × 4^2 = 4 mm Hg × 16 mm Hg = 64 mm Hg. Therefore, this patient's LVOT pressure gradient is 64 mm Hg. **References** 8 *(pp 194–196)*; 10 *(pp 195–196)*; 23 *(pp 64–65)*; 26 *(pp 49, 230–231)*.

64. Answer E

The area of a stenotic mitral valve can be estimated by planimetry, continuity equation, pressure half-time, and proximal isovelocity surface area methods. Each method has its pros and cons. When the valve is severely calcified, its surface area is difficult to estimate accurately by planimetry. In the presence of a mitral prosthesis or immediately after valvuloplasty, the pressure half-time method is not accurate and should not be used. Also, the pressure half-time method may be inaccurate in the presence of aortic regurgitation or abnormal relaxation. The continuity equation is not accurate if multivalvular regurgitant lesions or significant shunts are present. It is also difficult to calculate mitral valve area accurately in the presence of dense annular calcification. Although the proximal isovelocity surface area method can be used to calculate mitral valve area in the presence of aortic regurgitation, the pitfall of the proximal isovelocity surface area method is the inability to accurately measure the radius in some patients. In addition, the assumption of hemispherical flow convergence area may not be accurate in a noncircular regurgitant orifice. Therefore, it is important to be aware of limitations of each method when we estimate mitral valve area. **References** 10 *(pp 244, 246–247)*; 11 *(pp 210–214, 272)*; 23 *(pp 62–64, 67–68, 113–115)*; 26 *(pp 237–239, 250–253)*.

65. Answer A

Pressure half-time is the time interval for the peak pressure gradient to reach its half level. Deceleration time (DT) is the time interval from the peak velocity to zero baseline. Pressure half-time is 29% of the deceleration time. If this patient's deceleration time is 520 ms, the pressure half-time can be calculated as follows: Pressure half-time $= 0.29 \times 520 = 150$ ms. The patient's mitral valve area (MVA) can be estimated by the pressure half-time method using the following empiric formula: MVA = 220 ms/pressure half-time = 220 ms/150 ms = 1.47 cm^2. Therefore, the patient's mitral valve area is approximately 1.5 cm^2. **References** 10 *(pp 244, 246)*; 23 *(pp 67–68)*; 26 *(pp 251–253)*.

66. Answer A

Using the proximal isovelocity surface area method, we can calculate the mitral regurgitant (MR) volume according to the following equation: MR volume = ($2\pi r^2 \times$ aliasing velocity/MR peak velocity) × MR TVI, where TVI is the time velocity integral. Because the radius of the hemisphere, the aliasing velocity, and MR peak velocity are known, the MR TVI should be measured to calculate the MR volume. **References** 10 *(pp 255, 257–258)*; 11 *(pp 210–214)*; 23 *(pp 62–64, 125–127)*.

67. Answer A

Normal left ventricular systolic pressure is 100 to 140 mm Hg, and normal left atrial pressure is 5 to 15 mm Hg, so the pressure difference between the left ventricle and the left atrium in systole is 85 to 135 mm Hg. In patients with an incompetent mitral valve, this high-pressure gradient between the left ventricle and the left atrium produces mitral regurgitation during systole. Because the pressure gradient between the left ventricle and the left atrium is higher than that between the left ventricle and the aorta, the peak velocity of mitral regurgitation is usually higher than that of aortic stenosis. Typically, the mitral regurgitant velocity curve has a maximum velocity of 5 to 6 m/s. **Reference** 26 *(p 271)*.

68. Answer B

When cardiac output is normal, severe aortic stenosis is usually present if the peak velocity is greater than 4.5 m/s. However, when the cardiac output is decreased, the peak velocity may be less than that. Therefore, in patients with aortic stenosis and low cardiac output, the continuity equation is more accurate than the peak Doppler velocity to estimate the severity of aortic stenosis. **Reference** 23 *(pp 106, 111)*.

Chapter 5

Diastolic Function

Questions

Multiple choice (choose the *one* best answer):

1. Which one of the following disease(s) may cause abnormal diastolic relaxation?
A. Left ventricular hypertrophy.
B. Hypertrophic cardiomyopathy.
C. Coronary artery disease.
D. Dilated cardiomyopathy without mitral regurgitation.
E. All of the above.

2. Commonly, which one of the following is the earliest change during acute myocardial ischemia?
A. Systolic wall motion abnormalities.
B. Impaired relaxation.
C. Restrictive filling pattern.
D. Tachycardia.
E. Elevated ST segment on electrocardiography.

3. On the Doppler recording of pulmonary vein velocities, the pulmonary venous flow velocity in early ventricular systole is related to
A. left atrial relaxation.
B. left atrial contraction.
C. left ventricular relaxation.
D. left ventricular contraction.
E. diastasis.

4. The pulmonary venous flow velocity in late ventricular systole is produced by
A. atrial relaxation.
B. atrial contraction.
C. ventricular relaxation.
D. mitral anulus displacement.
E. decreased pulmonary venous pressure.

5. The pulmonary venous diastolic forward flow velocity
A. is produced by atrial relaxation.
B. is produced by atrial contraction.

C. is produced by left ventricular contraction.
D. is determined by the gradient between the pulmonary veins and the left ventricle.
E. occurs after mitral valve opening.

6. The pulmonary venous reverse flow velocity is due to
A. left atrial relaxation.
B. left atrial contraction.
C. left ventricular diastole.
D. left ventricular systole.
E. increased pulmonary venous pressure.

7. Deceleration time is
A. the interval from the peak velocity of the early mitral inflow diastolic wave (E) to zero velocity.
B. prolonged in abnormal relaxation.
C. shortened in patients with increased left atrial pressure.
D. shortened in normal young subjects.
E. all of the above.

8. Isovolumic relaxation time
A. is the interval from aortic valve closure to mitral valve opening.
B. generally parallels deceleration time.
C. is prolonged with abnormal relaxation.
D. is shortened with rapid relaxation.
E. is all of the above.

9. With aging,
A. the late mitral inflow diastolic velocity decreases.
B. the early mitral inflow diastolic (E) velocity decreases.
C. the E-wave duration increases.
D. the isovolumic relaxation time shortens.
E. the deceleration time shortens.

10. In normal subjects older than 70 years,
A. the ratio of early to late mitral inflow diastolic velocity changes but is not less than 1.0.
B. the peak pulmonary venous systolic forward flow velocity is unchanged.
C. the pulmonary venous diastolic forward flow velocity is unchanged.
D. the peak pulmonary venous systolic forward flow velocity becomes more prominent.
E. the pulmonary venous diastolic forward flow velocity becomes more prominent.

11. When the sample volume moves from the tips of the mitral leaflets toward the left atrium, the early mitral inflow diastolic wave has
A. increased velocity.
B. decreased velocity.

C. the same velocity.
D. increased duration.
E. decreased duration.

12. Fusion of the early (E) and late (A) mitral inflow diastolic velocities
A. occurs with tachycardia.
B. occurs with first-degree atrioventricular block.
C. increases A-wave velocity relatively.
D. affects the E/A ratio.
E. includes all of the above.

13. Which one of the following is found in a patient with normal diastolic filling?
A. Deceleration time of 180 ms.
B. Isovolumic relaxation time of 180 ms.
C. Deceleration time of 100 ms.
D. Isovolumic relaxation time of 100 ms.
E. Ratio of early to late diastolic velocity of 0.8.

14. The accompanying mitral inflow pattern is obtained during preoperative transesophageal echocardiography. With the Valsalva maneuver, the early (E) and late (A) mitral inflow diastolic velocities decrease proportionally, and the E/A ratio is unchanged. Most likely, the patient has
A. impaired relaxation.
B. restrictive physiology.
C. pseudonormalized filling pattern.
D. normal left ventricular diastolic function.
E. a condition that cannot be determined.

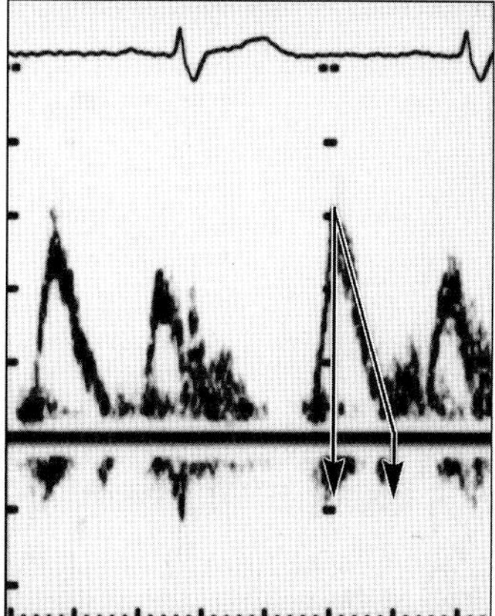

Figure from Oh et al. (23). Used with permission of Mayo Foundation for Medical Education and Research.

15. When the early (E) mitral inflow diastolic velocity is less than the late (A) diastolic velocity, impaired relaxation is usually present. Based only on the E and A waves, when the E velocity is greater than the A velocity,
   A. impaired relaxation is never present.
   B. impaired relaxation is usually present.
   C. impaired relaxation is always present.
   D. diastolic function is always normal.
   E. diastolic function cannot be determined.

16. Which one of the following can be used to distinguish a pseudonormal pattern from a true normal pattern?
   A. The patient has abnormal left ventricular size.
   B. The peak pulmonary venous reverse flow velocity at atrial contraction duration exceeds the duration of late diastole.
   C. Sitting up decreases the ratio of early to late diastole (E/A ratio).
   D. Sublingual nitroglycerine decreases the E/A ratio.
   E. All of the above.

17. When left ventricular relaxation is impaired,
   A. the pulmonary venous diastolic forward flow velocity (PVd) is decreased.
   B. pulmonary peak systolic forward flow velocity is decreased.
   C. PVd is increased.
   D. the pulmonary venous reverse flow velocity at atrial contraction (PVa) is decreased.
   E. the PVa duration is decreased.

18. When left atrial pressure is increased,
   A. the pulmonary venous reverse flow velocity at atrial contraction (PVa) is decreased.
   B. the PVa duration is decreased.
   C. the pulmonary venous systolic forward flow velocity (PVs) is decreased.
   D. the PVs is increased.
   E. the pulmonary venous diastolic forward flow velocity is decreased.

19. In patients with high left ventricular end-diastolic pressure,
   A. the pulmonary venous reverse flow velocity at atrial contraction PVa is decreased.
   B. the PVa is increased.
   C. the pulmonary venous systolic forward flow velocity PVs is increased.
   D. the pulmonary venous diastolic forward flow velocity is increased.
   E. the PVs duration is increased.

20. All of the following may occur in patients with impaired relaxation ***except***

A. a ratio of early to late diastolic velocity of less than 1.

B. peak pulmonary venous systolic forward flow velocity much greater than pulmonary venous diastolic forward flow velocity.

C. isovolumic relaxation time of 100 ms.

D. deceleration time of 120 ms.

E. normal or increased duration of peak pulmonary venous reverse flow velocity at atrial contraction.

21. A 77-year-old patient with a history of hypertensive heart disease has preoperative two-dimensional echocardiography with Doppler to evaluate left ventricular function. The accompanying mitral inflow pattern suggests

A. normal diastolic function.

B. impaired relaxation.

C. restrictive filling pattern

D. pseudonormalized filling pattern.

E. undetermined left ventricular diastolic function.

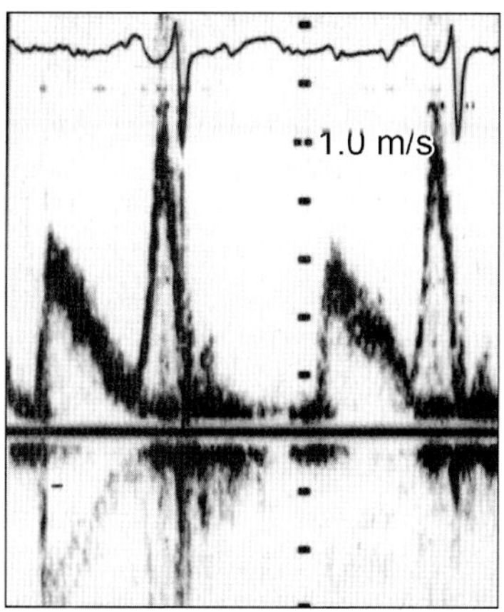

Figure from Oh et al. (23). Used with permission of Mayo Foundation for Medical Education and Research.

22. With restrictive diastolic filling, transmitral flow velocities are characterized by

A. a ratio of early to late diastole greater than 2.0.

B. a shortened isovolumic relaxation time.

C. shortened deceleration time.

D. shortened late mitral inflow diastolic duration.

E. all of the above.

23. A 88-year-old patient has the accompanying mitral inflow Doppler spectrum. Your diagnosis is

A. a normal filling pattern for all age groups.
B. a normal filling pattern for an elderly patient.
C. a restrictive filling pattern.
D. a pseudonormalized filling pattern.
E. impaired relaxation.

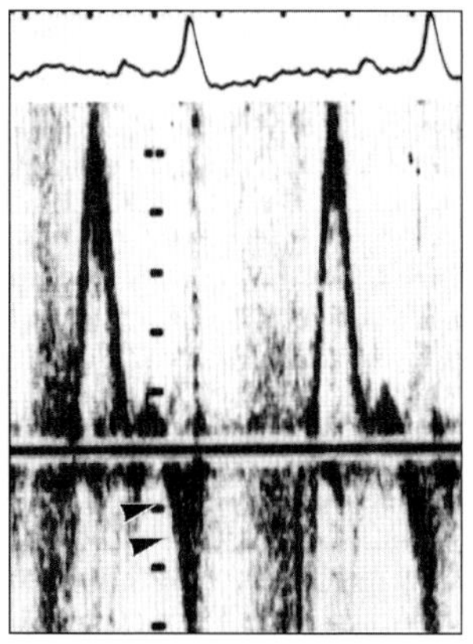

Figure from Oh et al. (23). Used with permission of Mayo Foundation for Medical Education and Research.

24. In patients with restrictive physiology, the Doppler spectrum of the pulmonary vein velocities is characterized by

A. increased pulmonary venous systolic forward flow velocity (PVs).
B. shortened pulmonary venous reverse flow velocity at atrial contraction (PVa) duration.
C. PVs much greater than pulmonary venous diastolic forward flow velocity.
D. PVa duration greater than the late mitral inflow diastolic duration.
E. normal PVa velocity.

25. A 48-year-old patient has preoperative transesophageal echocardiography. The accompanying Doppler spectra are obtained from mitral inflow and the pulmonary vein. Which one of the following is your diagnosis?

A. Normal diastolic function.

B. Impaired relaxation.

C. Pseudonormalized filling pattern.

D. Restrictive physiology.

E. Undetermined.

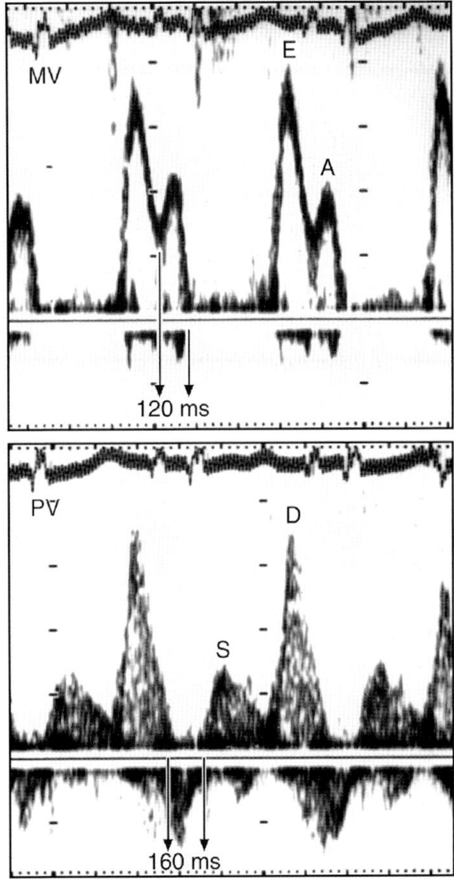

Figure from Oh et al. (23). Used with permission of Mayo Foundation for Medical Education and Research.

26. A 78-year-old patient has preoperative transesophageal echocardiography. His mitral inflow Doppler spectrum shows a single large wave (fusion of early and late diastolic velocities) with decreased deceleration time. The patient's heart rate is 130 to 140 beats per minute. Which one of the following best describes this patient's diastolic function?

A. Normal diastolic function.

B. Impaired relaxation.

C. Pseudonormalized filling pattern.

D. Restrictive physiology.

E. None of the above.

27. Which one of the following is consistent with restrictive physiology?

A. Ratio of early to late mitral inflow diastolic velocity of 1.2.

B. Isovolumic relaxation time of 80 ms.

C. Deceleration time of 272 ms.

D. Peak pulmonary venous reverse flow velocity at atrial contraction of 45 cm/s.

E. Age greater than 70 years.

28. In patients with acute myocardial ischemia, the initial change in the early mitral diastolic (E) wave is

A. increased E velocity with shortened deceleration time.

B. increased E velocity with prolonged deceleration time.

C. decreased E velocity with prolonged deceleration time.

D. decreased E velocity with shortened deceleration time.

E. dramatically increased E velocity.

29. Which one of the following about the grading of diastolic dysfunction is true?

A. Grade 1, normal diastolic function.

B. Grade 2, impaired diastolic relaxation.

C. Grade 3, reversible restrictive physiology.

D. Grade 4, pseudonormalized filling pattern.

E. Grade 5, irreversible restrictive filling pattern.

30. Which one of the following statements about tissue Doppler is correct?

A. Mitral anulus velocities are not useful in differentiating a pseudonormalized filling pattern from normal diastolic function.

B. In a pseudonormalized filling pattern, both early and late diastolic anulus velocities (E′ and A′) appear normal because of increased left atrial pressure.

C. In a restrictive pattern, early diastolic anulus velocity E′ is much greater than late diastolic anulus velocity A′ (E′/A′ ratio greater than 2).

D. All of the above.

E. None of the above.

31. In patients with a pseudonormalized filling pattern, which one of the following increases early diastolic anulus velocity E′?

A. Valsalva maneuver.

B. Sitting up.

C. Nitroglycerine.

D. All of the above.

E. None of the above.

32. Color M-mode Doppler

A. records pulmonary venous flow in order to evaluate diastolic function.

B. shows slow flow propagation in normal subjects.

C. shows flow reaches the apex immediately in diastolic dysfunction.

D. has a pseudonormal pattern in grade 2 diastolic dysfunction.

E. is none of the above.

Answers & Discussion

1. Answer E

Many cardiac diseases cause impaired diastolic relaxation. Typical examples of cardiac lesions that produce impaired relaxation include left ventricular hypertrophy, hypertrophic cardiomyopathy, myocardial ischemia, myocardial infarction, and dilated cardiomyopathy. In patients with left ventricular hypertrophy or hypertrophic cardiomyopathy, impaired relaxation is due to the inability of the hypertrophied left ventricle to relax quickly and develop a negative pressure gradient or "suction" after mitral opening. In patients with coronary artery disease, acute coronary occlusion can lead to diastolic dysfunction, with impaired relaxation as the most common diastolic filling pattern. Patients with dilated cardiomyopathy may present with any of the patterns in the spectrum of diastolic abnormalities. Dilated cardiomyopathy patients without mitral regurgitation typically may have a pattern of abnormal relaxation, and patients with mitral regurgitation may have a pseudonormalized filling pattern because of increased left atrial pressure. Therefore, all the cardiac diseases listed in this question may cause impaired relaxation. **References** 23 *(pp 45–57)*; 42 *(pp 765–775)*.

2. Answer B

Generally, impaired relaxation is the earliest change during acute myocardial ischemia. During coronary artery occlusion with a balloon, the earliest change was diastolic dysfunction with impaired relaxation as the most often exhibited pattern, which occurred within 15 seconds of balloon inflation, preceding electrocardiographic changes, chest pain, or systolic wall motion abnormalities.

In most cardiac diseases, including acute myocardial ischemia, the initial diastolic dysfunction is impaired relaxation. With time, the left atrial pressure increases, and impaired relaxation progresses to a pseudonormalized filling pattern; that is, the Doppler velocity pattern of mitral inflow appears similar to a normal filling pattern. Eventually, the diastolic filling pattern becomes restrictive because of a further decrease in left ventricular compliance and an increase in left atrial pressure.

Tachycardia may cause myocardial ischemia, and reflex tachycardia occurs secondary to systemic hypotension. However, tachycardia is not the earliest change during acute myocardial ischemia. **References** 23 *(pp 45–57, 85)*; 42 *(p 770)*.

3. Answer A

4. Answer D

5. Answer E

6. Answer B

Pulmonary vein Doppler recordings have four distinct velocity components: two systolic velocities (PVs1 and PVs2), diastolic velocity (PVd), and atrial flow reversal (PVa). The accompanying Doppler spectrum demonstrates the four velocity components of normal pulmonary venous flow.

PVs1 occurs in early systole and is related to atrial relaxation, which decreases left atrial pressure. The pressure gradient between the pulmonary vein and the left atrium drives pulmonary venous flow into the left atrium.

PVs2 is the second systolic forward flow of the pulmonary vein. It occurs in late systole and is produced by the mitral anulus displacement, that is, the apical systolic motion of the mitral anulus. The mitral anulus displacement causes an increase in atrial volume and a decrease in pressure with a corresponding increase in flow from the pulmonary veins into the left atrium. With normal atrioventricular conduction, the systolic components are closely connected and a distinct PVs1 peak velocity may not be seen in 70% of patients.

PVd occurs after mitral valve opening and is produced by left ventricular diastole. Initial mitral valve opening causes a decrease in left atrial pressure and an increase in the pressure gradient between the pulmonary vein and the left atrium. This pressure gradient causes blood flow from the pulmonary veins to enter the left atrium. Since the left atrium is open to the left ventricle during diastole, the pulmonary veins essentially "see" left ventricular pressure. Therefore, the PVd is determined by the pressure gradient between the pulmonary vein and the left ventricle. Generally, the diastolic component of pulmonary vein velocities reflects left ventricular early filling, and the systolic component reflects left atrial pressure.

PVa is the atrial flow reversal (blood pushed back into the pulmonary vein) caused by atrial contraction. Atrial contraction causes an increase in the left atrial pressure, resulting in both forward flow through the mitral valve and reversed flow into the pulmonary veins. Thus, the PVa wave is in the opposite direction as PVs and PVd waves on the pulmonary vein Doppler recording. **References** 23 *(pp 48–50)*; 42 *(pp 733–735)*.

7. Answer E

Deceleration time is the interval from the peak velocity of the early diastolic (E) wave to zero velocity, that is, to the point of intercept of the extrapolated slope with the baseline. The normal deceleration time for the E wave is 160 to 200 ms. This time reflects the speed with which the pressure between the left atrium and the left ventricle equalizes. Deceleration time is prolonged in patients with impaired relaxation because it takes longer for the left atrial and ventricular pressures to be equilibrated. Conversely, if there is a marked increase in the left atrial pressure or decrease in the left ventricular compliance, deceleration time is shortened because of rapid equilibration of left atrial and left ventricular pressures. In normal young subjects, filling is rapid because of vigorous left ventricular relaxation and elastic recoil. Therefore, the deceleration time is shortened. **Reference** 23 *(pp 48, 51–54)*.

8. Answer E

The isovolumic relaxation time (IVRT) is the interval from aortic valve closure to mitral valve opening. Its normal range is 70 to 90 ms. Generally, the IVRT parallels deceleration time. In normal young subjects, the IVRT is shortened because of rapid relaxation. As relaxation becomes impaired, the IVRT is prolonged. In patients with restrictive physiology, the IVRT is shortened because high left atrial pressure leads to earlier mitral opening. Conversely, volume depletion and low left atrial pressure have the opposite effect. It is important to remember that the IVRT is influenced not only by the relaxation rate but also by factors affecting left atrial pressure. Therefore, IVRT measurements are not used in isolation but rather to confirm other findings. **Reference** 23 *(pp 48, 51–54)*.

9. Answer B

The rates of myocardial relaxation and compliance vary in different age groups. With aging, the rate of myocardial relaxation as well as elastic recoil gradually decrease. In elderly patients, the pressure between the left ventricle and the left atrium occurs later, and the mitral valve opens later. Therefore, the isovolumic relaxation time is prolonged.

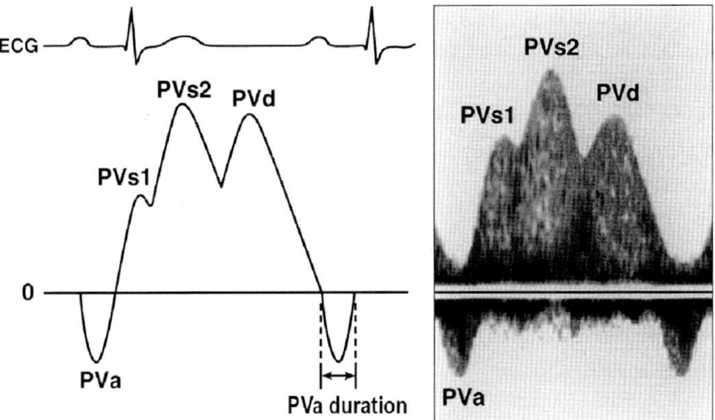

Figure from Oh et al. (23). Used with permission of Mayo Foundation for Medical Education and Research.

Because of the decreased early transmitral pressure gradient, early left ventricular filling is reduced, and the contribution of atrial contraction to left ventricular filling becomes more important. Hence, the early (E) diastolic velocity gradually decreases and the late diastolic velocity gradually increases with aging. Decreased filling in early diastole retards the equilibration of pressure between the left ventricle and the left atrium, resulting in a longer deceleration time. Generally, the E-wave duration is not measured for the evaluation of diastolic function. **Reference** 23 *(p 51)*.

10. Answer D

In normal subjects older than 70 years, the mitral inflow ratio of early to late diastolic velocity is usually less than 1.0. Pulmonary venous flow velocities show similar changes with aging: diastolic forward flow velocity decreases as more filling of the left ventricle occurs at atrial contraction, and systolic forward flow velocity becomes more prominent. **Reference** 23 *(p 51)*.

11. Answer B

When the sample volume moves from the tips of the mitral leaflets toward the left atrium, the early (E) mitral inflow diastolic velocity decreases. Recordings made between the mitral leaflet tips yield higher velocities of flow and a better assessment of the rapid filling phase. To measure mitral E velocity accurately, the sample volume should be placed between the tips of the mitral leaflets. If the sample volume is placed at the level of mitral anulus or further toward the left atrium, the E velocity will be underestimated. **References** 8 *(pp 199, 201)*; 42 *(pp 759–761)*.

12. Answer E

Both tachycardia and first-degree atrioventricular (AV) block may result in fusion of the early (E) and late (A) diastolic velocities. With increasing heart rates, there is a progressive merging of the E and A waves as the diastasis period shortens and then is obliterated. In patients with first-degree AV block, an increase in the AV interval delays the occurrence of ventricular contraction and hence the onset of the subsequent early diastolic filling (E wave). At a constant heart rate, an increase in the AV interval takes the E wave closer to the following A wave, and the waves may eventually fuse as the AV interval prolongs. When E-A fusion occurs, the A-wave velocity may be relatively increased because it starts before the E-wave velocity has reached zero. As a general rule, if the E-wave velocity is higher than 20 cm/s at the beginning of the A wave, both the A-wave velocity and E/A ratio are affected by the fusion of the E and A velocities. (See also Question 26.) **Reference** 23 *(pp 46, 50)*.

13. Answer A

Patients with normal diastolic function have a normal Doppler spectrum of mitral inflow velocities. A normal mitral inflow has an early (E) diastolic velocity greater than the late (A) diastolic velocity with the E/A ratio equal to 1.0 to 1.5. An E/A ratio of 0.8 is consistent with impaired relaxation, not normal diastolic function. The diastolic filling pattern is characterized further by measuring deceleration time and the isovolumic relaxation time (IVRT). The deceleration time is the interval from the peak of the E velocity to its extrapolation to the baseline, and its normal value is 160 to 200 ms. A deceleration time of 180 ms is consistent with normal diastolic function. The IVRT is the interval from aortic valve closure to mitral valve opening. The normal IVRT is approximately 70 to 90 ms. A prolonged IVRT (>90 ms) is frequently found in patients with impaired relaxation. **Reference** 23 *(pp 51–55)*.

14. Answer D

The Doppler spectrum of mitral inflow velocities is normal. The early (E) diastolic velocity is the peak mitral inflow velocity during the rapid filling phase in early diastole. The A velocity is defined as the peak velocity of the late filling wave due to atrial contraction. The two phases of forward flow in early diastole (E wave) and late diastole (A wave) are separated by a brief period of diastasis. Normally, the E velocity is in the range of 70 to 100 cm/s with peak A wave of 45 to 70 cm/s, resulting in an E/A ratio of 1.0 to 1.5. In normal young subjects, most filling is completed during early diastole with only a small contribution at atrial contraction because the left ventricular elastic recoil is vigorous and myocardial relaxation is swift. With reduction in preload (Valsalva maneuver), normal subjects have proportionally decreased E and A velocities, keeping the E/A ratio unchanged. In contrast, in patients with a pseudonormal pattern, a reduction in preload by the Valsalva maneuver unmasks the underlying impaired relaxation, decreasing the E/A ratio to less than 1.0.

Most likely, the patient in this question has a normal left ventricular diastolic function because the preoperative transesophageal echocardiographic study revealed an E/A ratio higher than 1.0 (but less than 2.0), which is unchanged by Valsalva maneuver. (See also Question 16.) **References** 23 *(pp 51–55)*; 25 *(pp 49–70)*.

15. Answer E

Whenever the early (E) mitral inflow diastolic velocity is less than the late (A) diastolic velocity (ie, the E/A ratio is less than 1.0), impaired relaxation is usually present. However, the reverse is not true. When the mitral inflow E velocity is greater than the A velocity, diastolic function is not always normal because a pseudonormal pattern may be present. The pseudonormal pattern is a transitional phase from impaired relaxation to restrictive filling as diastolic function deteriorates. During the pseudonormal pattern, the mitral inflow pattern goes through a phase resembling a normal diastolic filling, that is, an E/A ratio of 1.0 to 1.5 and a normal deceleration time. This is the result of moderately increased left atrial pressure superimposed on a relaxation abnormality. The pseudonormalized filling pattern can be distinguished from a true normal pattern by other factors. (See also Question 16.) Therefore, when the mitral inflow E/A ratio is greater than 1.0, diastolic function cannot be determined on the basis of only the mitral inflow E/A ratio. **Reference** 23 *(pp 52–54)*.

16. Answer E

A pseudonormalized filling pattern can be distinguished from a true normal pattern in several ways:

1. When patients have an abnormal left ventricular size, increased wall thickness, or systolic dysfunction, impaired relaxation is expected. In these patients, a normal ratio of early to late diastole suggests that the increased left atrial pressure is masking the abnormal relaxation.
2. Patients with a pseudonormal pattern usually have a duration of reverse flow velocity at atrial contraction greater than duration of late diastole.
3. A reduction in preload by sitting, Valsalva maneuver, or sublingual nitroglycerine may unmask the underlying impaired relaxation of the left ventricle and decrease the ratio of early to late diastole to less than 1.0.
4. The color M-mode of the mitral inflow shows slow flow propagation because of impaired myocardial relaxation.
5. The mitral anulus velocity by tissue Doppler shows decreased early diastolic anulus velocity E′, and the E/E′ ratio is greater than 15, indicating persistent underlying relaxation abnormality even though the mitral inflow pattern is pseudonormal. (See also Questions 30, 31, and 32.) **Reference** 23 *(pp 52–55)*.

17. Answer A

When left ventricular relaxation is impaired, the diastolic forward flow velocity (PVd) is decreased. During ventricular diastole, the pulmonary venous flow passes through the left atrium and enters the left ventricle because of the pressure gradient between the pulmonary veins and the left ventricle. This pulmonary venous flow produces PVd on the Doppler recording. In patients with impaired diastolic relaxation, the left ventricular pressure is elevated in early diastole, which leads to a decreased pressure gradient between the pulmonary veins and the left ventricle. Because the systolic forward flow velocity is determined by the gradient between the pulmonary veins and the left ventricle, the PVd decreases if the gradient is reduced secondary to impaired relaxation. (See also Question 6.) **Reference** 23 *(pp 48, 51–52)*.

18. Answer C

Antegrade systolic flow (PVs) is produced by the pressure gradient between the pulmonary veins and the left atrium. This pressure gradient is produced both by the decrease in atrial pressure during atrial relaxation and by the increase in atrial volume due to apical systolic motion of the mitral anulus. When left atrial pressure is increased, the pressure gradient between the pulmonary veins and the left atrium is decreased. Therefore, the PVs velocity decreases correspondingly. (See also Questions 3 and 4.) **Reference** 23 *(pp 48, 52)*.

19. Answer B

The atrial flow reversal (PVa) wave is defined as the reversal flow from the left atrium to the pulmonary veins, produced by left atrial contraction during late diastole. Atrial contraction causes both forward flow through the mitral valve and reversed flow into the pulmonary veins. The atrial systolic pressure and the amount of forward flow are influenced by the ventricular pressure against which the atrium must contract. For any given atrial systolic pressure, retrograde flow into the pulmonary veins increases in proportion to the resistance to forward flow into the left ventricle because pulmonary vein compliance is greater than ventricular compliance. When the left ventricular end-diastolic pressure is high, there is less forward flow through the mitral valve and more reverse flow from the left atrium into the pulmonary veins during atrial contraction. Therefore, the PVa wave is larger with both increased velocity and duration in patients with elevated left ventricular end-diastolic pressure. (See also Question 5.) **Reference** 23 *(pp 48, 52)*.

20. Answer D

In patients with impaired myocardial relaxation, early (E) diastolic velocity is decreased and late (A) diastolic velocity is increased, resulting in a mitral E/A ratio of less than 1.0. Both isovolumic relaxation time and deceleration time are prolonged. Pulmonary diastolic forward flow velocity (PVd) parallels mitral E velocity and is also decreased with compensatory increased flow in systole, leading to systolic forward flow velocity much greater than PVd. Usually, the duration and velocity of the atrial flow reversal (PVa) wave are normal. However, when the left ventricular end-diastolic pressure is elevated, both duration and velocity of PVa may be increased. Hence, PVa duration greater than mitral A duration occurs. All the answers characterize the impaired myocardial relaxation pattern except deceleration time of 120 ms. Generally, a decreased deceleration time is consistent with restrictive physiology but not impaired relaxation. **Reference** 23 *(pp 51–52, 54)*.

21. Answer B

The Doppler transmitral flow pattern from this patient exhibits features characteristic of impaired relaxation. The spectral profile shows a reduced early (E) diastolic velocity and a predominant late (A) diastolic velocity, leading to an E/A ratio of less than 1.0. Generally, whenever the E/A ratio is less than 1.0, impaired relaxation is present. The diminished early diastolic flow produces a decreased peak E-wave velocity. The increased peak A-wave velocity is likely the result of higher left atrial residual volume at the time of atrial contraction, secondary to reduced early diastolic flow. Therefore, these features are consistent with impaired relaxation. **Reference** 23 *(pp 51–52, 54)*.

22. Answer E

A restrictive filling pattern or restrictive physiology can be present in any cardiac abnormality that produces decreased left ventricular compliance and markedly increased left atrial pressure. The increase in left atrial pressure produces a greater initial transmitral gradient with a high early (E) diastolic velocity. High left atrial pressure also leads to earlier opening of mitral valve, which produces a shortened isovolumic relaxation time. Earlier diastolic filling into a noncompliant left ventricle causes a rapid increase in early left ventricular diastolic pressure with rapid equalization of left ventricular and left atrial pressures, resulting in a shortened deceleration time. Although atrial contraction increases left atrial pressure, both late (A) diastolic wave velocity and duration are shortened because left ventricular pressure increases even more rapidly. Therefore, with a restrictive diastolic filling pattern or restrictive physiology, the Doppler spectrum of mitral inflow is characterized by shortened isovolumic relaxation time, reduced deceleration time, decreased A-wave duration, and a mitral E/A ratio greater than 2.0 (increased mitral inflow E velocity and decreased A velocity). **Reference** 23 *(pp 52, 54)*.

23. Answer C

The spectral Doppler tracing is characterized by an increased early (E) diastolic wave and decreased late (A) diastolic wave velocities with an E/A ratio greater than 2.0. These findings are typical for the restrictive transmitral flow pattern. Other features of transmitral flow velocities in patients with restrictive physiology are decreased A-wave duration, shortened isovolumic relaxation time, and reduced deceleration time. Therefore, this patient's transmitral Doppler spectrum is a restrictive filling pattern. **Reference** 23 *(pp 52, 54)*.

24. Answer D

In patients with restrictive physiology, the features of pulmonary vein velocity waveforms are characterized by a small systolic forward flow wave (PVs) and a large diastolic forward flow wave (PVd). Because of increased left atrial pressure, the pressure gradient between the pulmonary veins and the left atrium is diminished, leading to decreased systolic forward flow velocity in the pulmonary vein with compensatory increased flow during diastole. Therefore, PVs velocity is much less than PVd velocity. The wave size and duration of reverse flow at atrial contraction (PVa) vary, depending on the state of left atrial function. Usually, the PVa wave is characterized by increased velocity and prolonged duration. However, if left atrial failure has occurred due to chronic dilation, the PVa wave may become diminutive. **Reference** 23 *(pp 48, 52)*.

25. Answer C

The Doppler spectra obtained from the mitral inflow and pulmonary vein indicate pseudonormalized filling pattern. The pseudonormal pattern represents an intermediate pattern between impaired relaxation and restrictive phases and may be viewed as a transition from one pattern to another. As the result from counterbalancing influences of both abnormal relaxation and restrictive forces, the pseudonormal pattern has characteristics of normal transmitral velocities, that is, nearly equal early (E) and late (A) diastolic wave velocities with an E/A ratio of 1.0 to 1.5. Because atrial compliance often becomes gradually reduced in this group of patients, the pulmonary venous flow during systole is reduced owing to decreased atrial relaxation and increased left atrial pressure. Thus, the diastolic wave becomes more predominant than the systolic wave. Another characteristic feature of this pattern is a larger wave during atrial contraction, reflecting reduced ventricular compliance. **Reference** 23 *(pp 52–53)*.

26. Answer E

Early (E) and late (A) mitral inflow diastolic fusion occurs in the presence of tachycardia, making measurements of E and A difficult. As the heart rate increases, the period of diastasis shortens progressively. Hence, the E and A mitral inflow waves become closer and eventually merge together. Generally, at heart rates higher than 100 beats per minute, the individual E and A waves often become fused. At higher heart rates (around 130 beats per minute), peak velocities may not be readily discriminated and appear as a single large wave. Therefore, the diastolic function cannot be determined based on mitral inflow pattern in the presence of mitral E-A fusion secondary to tachycardia. In such patients, one should slow down the heart rate first to determine the E/A ratio. Other useful methods to determine diastolic function in patients with tachycardia include pulmonary venous flow pattern and the ratio of early diastolic mitral inflow E velocity to early diastolic mitral anulus E′ velocity (E/E′ ratio). The E/E′ ratio is a useful index in the estimation of left ventricular filling pressure. Although the mitral anulus E′ and A′ waves may fuse in the presence of tachycardia, the E/E′ ratio remains a valid index to evaluate the left ventricular filling pressure. (See also Question 12.) **References** 23 *(pp 46–55)*; 42 *(pp 761–763)*.

27. Answer D

The flow velocity at atrial contraction (PVa) of 45 cm/s is consistent with restrictive physiology. As mentioned previously, PVa velocity is usually increased in restrictive filling pattern (>35 cm/s). A mitral early to late diastolic ratio (E/A ratio) of 1.2 and an isovolumic relaxation time of 80 ms are consistent with normal diastolic function. A prolonged deceleration time (272 ms) is seen in impaired relaxation. Age greater than 70 years may lead to decreased E velocity with E/A ratio less than 1.0. Aging does not result in restrictive filling pattern. (See also Questions 16 and 25.) **Reference** 23 *(pp 51–55)*.

28. Answer C

In patients with acute myocardial ischemia, the initial change of the early (E) mitral diastolic wave is decreased E-wave velocity with prolonged deceleration time because of impaired relaxation, which occurs before pseudonormal or restrictive filling pattern. (See also Questions 2, 20, and 21.) **References** 23 *(pp 45–57, 85)*; 42 *(p 770)*.

29. Answer C

According to the diastolic filling pattern, diastolic dysfunction can be graded as follows: grade 1, impaired relaxation; grade 2, pseudonormalized pattern; grade 3, reversible restrictive pattern; and grade 4, irreversible restrictive pattern.

The restrictive pattern is graded as "reversible" if it moves from a restrictive to a pseudonormalized filling pattern after volume unloading, such as Valsalva maneuver, sitting up, nitroglycerine, and diuretics.

The grading system provides important prognostic information for various cardiac diseases. Reversible restrictive filling has a worse prognosis than impaired relaxation, and an irreversible restrictive filling pattern indicates a poor prognosis. Generally, treatments are aimed at improving the diastolic filling pattern toward the lower grade. The Doppler echocardiographic evaluation of the diastolic filling pattern may be helpful in assessing the patient's response to the treatment. **Reference** 23 *(p 56)*.

30. Answer E

Doppler tissue imaging, or tissue Doppler, has been applied to evaluate diastolic function by measuring mitral anulus velocity during diastole. The mitral anulus velocity profile during diastole reflects the rate of change in the long axis dimension and in left ventricular volume. In a normal diastolic pattern, early diastolic anulus velocity (E′) is greater than late diastolic anulus velocity (A′), and the normal value of the ratio of early (E) mitral diastolic velocity to early diastolic anulus (E′) velocity (E/E′) ratio is 7.7 ± 3.0. In abnormal relaxation, the E′ and late diastolic anulus velocity (A′) parallel the E and A velocities of mitral inflow. In pseudonormalized and restrictive filling patterns, the E′ remains decreased (ie, persistent underlying relaxation abnormality), and mitral inflow E velocity increases due to increased left atrial pressure, leading to increased E/E′ ratio (>15). Because the E′ remains decreased with high left atrial pressure, mitral anulus velocity is useful in differentiating pseudonormal from normal mitral inflow velocity pattern. Shown in the accompanying figure are the patterns of mitral inflow and mitral anulus velocity from normal to restrictive physiology. **Reference** 23 *(pp 51–55)*.

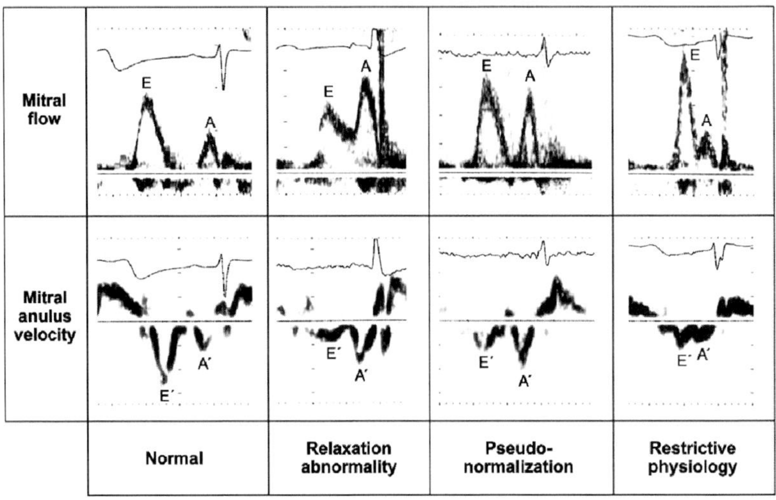

Figure from Oh et al. (23). Used with permission of Mayo Foundation for Medical Education and Research.

31. Answer E

In contrast to transmitral velocity, which is preload dependent, the mitral anulus velocity determined by Doppler tissue imaging is relatively preload-independent. In patients with grade 2 diastolic dysfunction (pseudonormalized filling pattern), the early diastolic anulus velocity remains decreased due to persistent underlying impaired relaxation and is not increased by volume unloading such as the Valsalva maneuver, sitting up, and nitroglycerine administration. **Reference** 23 *(pp 52–55)*.

32. Answer E

Color M-mode Doppler is a new method for relating mitral inflow velocities to left ventricular relaxation. It assesses the rate of diastolic flow propagation from base to apex. In normal subjects with intact elastic recoil and suction, mitral inflow reaches the apex immediately, which gives rise to a straight flow propagation on color M-mode recording. In patients with diastolic dysfunction, the color M-mode shows slow flow propagation because of impaired myocardial relaxation. The color M-mode method is a useful tool to differentiate pseudonormal from normal filling patterns because the slow flow propagation is not altered by increased left atrial pressure. **Reference** 23 *(pp 54–55)*.

Chapter 6

Equipment, Infection Control, and Safety

Questions

Multiple choice (choose the *one* best answer):

1. Which one of the following statements about dosimetric quantities is true?
A. Acoustic energy is the capacity to do work or to produce a biological effect.
B. Acoustic power is the amount of acoustic energy per unit time.
C. Pressure is force per area.
D. Intensity is the concentration of power within an area.
E. All of the above.

2. When the operator increases transmit gain,
A. the amplification function of the ultrasound machine is increased.
B. the ultrasound intensity is increased.
C. the electrical voltage from the pulser to the transducer does not change.
D. the power is not affected.
E. the pressure is decreased.

3. To optimize the image quality and minimize the acoustic exposure to the patient, the operator should
A. increase both the transmit gain and receiver gain.
B. decrease both the transmit gain and receiver gain.
C. increase the transmit gain and decrease the receiver gain.
D. increase the receiver gain and decrease the transmit gain.
E. increase the transmit gain and not change the receiver gain.

4. The mechanisms of the ultrasound bioeffects include
A. the thermal effect of cooling.
B. cavitation.
C. reflection.
D. refraction.
E. focusing.

5. All of the following increase the tissue temperature during ultrasound examination ***except***
A. high tissue density.
B. increased absorption.
C. increased tissue perfusion.
D. increased ultrasound intensity.
E. increased power output.

6. In comparison with transthoracic echocardiography, transesophageal echocardiography has
A. no problem with heat generation.
B. fewer problems with heat generation.
C. the same problem with heat generation.
D. more problems with heat generation.
E. none of the above.

7. A 70-year-old patient is undergoing coronary artery bypass graft surgery and mitral valve repair. The transesophageal echocardiographic image is frozen during cardiopulmonary bypass. Before coming off cardiopulmonary bypass, the perfusionist rewarms the patient to a nasopharyngeal temperature above 39°C. When the surgeon asks the cardiologist to look at the newly repaired mitral valve, the monitor screen says "Probe auto-cool imminent." Most likely, this is due to
A. an overused probe.
B. dysfunction of the transducer.
C. long bypass time with the probe in esophagus.
D. the patient's elevated temperature.
E. malfunction of the heat-sensing device.

8. Cavitation
A. is the creation of small fluid-filled bodies by the ultrasound beam.
B. tends to occur only with low intensity exposures.
C. occurs when large, macroscopic gas bubbles located in tissues vibrate as a result of interaction with ultrasound waves.
D. is all of the above.
E. is none of the above.

9. Stable cavitation occurs when the small bubbles
A. rhythmically grow and shrink but do not burst.
B. randomly change their size and stably enlarge.
C. change their size and burst constantly.
D. burst quickly but do not change their size.
E. never change their size with time.

10. Transient cavitation occurs when
A. the surrounding tissue cells transiently melt and then heal quickly.
B. the changing energy in an ultrasound beam causes transient heat to melt surrounding tissue cells.

C. the changing heat in an ultrasound beam causes transient microbubbles in the soft tissue.
D. the changing pressure in an ultrasound beam causes a microbubble to contract and expand violently and burst.
E. the small bubbles located in tissues transiently decrease in size but do not burst as an ultrasound wave strikes them.

11. In comparison with an unfocused ultrasound beam, a highly focused ultrasound beam is
A. less likely to dissipate heat by conduction.
B. more likely to dissipate heat by conduction.
C. less likely to lose heat through convection.
D. more likely to lose heat through convection.
E. more likely to cause higher tissue temperature because of decreased conduction.

12. Which one of the following statements about electrical and mechanical hazards during transesophageal echocardiography is true?
A. The ultrasound machine exposes the patient to electrical hazard, but the probe never exposes the patient to mechanical hazard.
B. The transducer has the greatest potential to expose the patient to electrical hazard.
C. The ultrasound machine is the component that has the greatest potential to expose the patient to electrical hazard, and the probe exposes the patient to mechanical hazard only.
D. If the transducer case is cracked, the operator may continue to use it for the scheduled case but should stop using it after finishing the scheduled examination.
E. A cracked transducer housing presents mechanical hazard but not electrical hazard to the patient.

13. Which one of the following statements about the safety of diagnostic ultrasound is true?
A. After many years of clinical use, several adverse effects from exposure to diagnostic ultrasound have been confirmed.
B. In a randomized study, many adverse effects such as low birth weight in humans have been identified as resulting from exposure to diagnostic ultrasound.
C. So far, no biological effects on patients or instrument operators have been confirmed as being caused by exposure to intensities typical of present diagnostic ultrasound instruments.
D. To minimize the patient's exposure to ultrasound, the American Institute of Ultrasound in Medicine has suggested using the maximum output power and maximum amplification to optimize image quality.
E. To minimize the patient's exposure to ultrasound, the American Institute of Ultrasound in Medicine has suggested using the maximum output power and minimum amplification to optimize image quality.

14. All of the following statements about the care of the transesophageal echocardiographic probe are true ***except***
A. After each examination, the probe should be inspected carefully for defects with the transducer tip in the neutral position and all flexed directions.

B. Transesophageal echocardiographic probe defects include cracks and sheath corrosion.
C. Visual inspection of the probe alone always guarantees that the outer insulating layer is intact.
D. Leakage current should be measured regularly by qualified technicians.
E. Sheath corrosion may expose the patient to leakage current.

15. Which one of the following may be used to clean the transesophageal echocardiographic probe?
A. Heat sterilization.
B. Enzymatic solution.
C. Glutaraldehyde disinfectant solution.
D. B and C.
E. All of the above.

16. According to current American Heart Association guidelines, antibiotic prophylaxis for subacute bacterial endocarditis is
A. recommended for all the patients with valvular diseases undergoing transesophageal echocardiography.
B. not recommended for patients undergoing transesophageal echocardiography.
C. recommended for all the patients with native valvular diseases or prosthetic valves, at least 30 minutes before insertion of the transesophageal echocardiographic probe.
D. recommended for patients with prosthetic valves but not for those with native valvular diseases.
E. recommended for patients undergoing transesophageal echocardiography, who had subacute bacterial endocarditis in the past.

17. Before transesophageal echocardiography,
A. the patient should be examined for loose teeth.
B. the patient's mouth should be examined for preexisting injuries.
C. the transesophageal echocardiographic probe should be inspected for cracks.
D. the control wheels should be checked and unlocked.
E. all of the above should be done.

18. A 37-year-old febrile patient is referred to the echocardiography laboratory for transesophageal echocardiography to rule out suspected infective endocarditis. On the way to the echo laboratory, the patient has a motor vehicle accident with multiple trauma. Urgent surgery is planned and preoperative transesophageal echocardiography is performed in the emergency department, which reveals a prolapsed mitral valve with vegetation. This patient should receive
A. antibiotics for subacute bacterial endocarditis prophylaxis at least 30 minutes before transesophageal echocardiography.
B. antibiotic prophylaxis for infective endocarditis at least 60 minutes before transesophageal echocardiography.

C. antibiotics for subacute bacterial endocarditis prophylaxis as soon as he arrives in the emergency department.
D. antibiotics for subacute bacterial endocarditis prophylaxis at the same time the transesophageal echocardiographic probe was inserted.
E. antibiotic treatment after the blood culture is obtained.

19. If intraoperative withdrawal of the transesophageal echocardiographic probe is difficult,
A. the probe should be removed surgically.
B. the tip should be anteflexed and the control wheel locked before withdrawing the probe.
C. the control wheel should be locked and the probe withdrawn.
D. the probe should be withdrawn forcefully to pass the resistance.
E. the probe should be advanced into the stomach.

20. A 58-year-old patient has a known history of moderate mitral regurgitation. Before this patient's preoperative transesophageal echocardiography, antibiotic prophylaxis for subacute bacterial endocarditis
A. is recommended by the American Heart Association.
B. is not recommended by the American Heart Association.
C. should be administered 30 minutes before scheduled transesophageal examination because transesophageal examination uses an endoscope placed in the upper gastrointestinal tract.
D. should be administered at least 60 minutes before the placement of the transesophageal echocardiographic probe.
E. is both A and C.

Answers & Discussion

1. Answer E

Dosimetry is the science of identifying and measuring the characteristics of an ultrasound field that are relevant to its potential for producing biological effects. Dosimetric quantities, such as pressure, intensity, and power, are important ultrasound characteristics that determine the patient's acoustic exposure during echocardiography. Acoustic energy is the capacity of the sound wave to do work or to produce a biological effect. The amount of acoustic energy per unit time is called acoustic power. Intensity is the concentration of power per area. It may also be called power intensity. Pressure is defined as force per area. **References** 9 *(pp 8, 15–17, 226)*; 10 *(p 59)*.

2. Answer B

When the operator increases the transmit gain, the pulser sends a stronger electrical voltage to the transducer, leading to an increase in pressure, intensity, and power delivered to the patient. At the intensity levels currently used, clinical imaging ultrasound appears to be a safe procedure. However, no current data prove ultrasound is absolutely safe. Although the benefits of an ultrasound examination outweigh the risks, it is important for the operator to minimize the pressure, intensity, and power delivered to the patient. The amplification function of the ultrasound machine is controlled by the receiver gain, but not the transmit gain. **References** 9 *(pp 8, 15–17, 226)*; 10 *(p 59)*.

3. Answer D

Acoustic exposure is the ultrasound dose given to the patient undergoing an ultrasound examination. To minimize acoustic exposure to the patient, the operator should decrease the examination time, decrease the transmit gain, and increase the receiver gain. Decreasing the examination time decreases the total dose of ultrasound delivered to the patient and hence decreases the acoustic exposure to the patient. The operator can use the transmit gain to control the output power that supplies electrical shock to the piezoelectric element. The stronger the electrical pulse delivered to the transducer, the greater the intensity of the ultrasound pulse to the patient. Thus, decreasing transmit gain reduces the power and intensity delivered to the patient, resulting in decreased acoustic exposure. The receiver gain controls the amplification function of the ultrasound machine. It determines the voltage of all returned signals. Receiver gain has no effect on the transmitted ultrasound intensity. To decrease the risk of bioeffects and reduce patient exposure to ultrasound intensity, the operator should decrease the transmit gain and increase the receiver gain to optimize image quality. **References** 10 *(pp 59–60)*; 31 *(p 370)*.

4. Answer B

The interaction of ultrasound waves with biological tissue forms the basis of ultrasound bioeffects that may have the potential to produce cell injury. Two proposed mechanisms of ultrasound bioeffects are postulated. These two mechanisms are cavitation and the thermal effect of heating. **References** 9 *(pp 227–231)*; 10 *(pp 59–60)*.

5. Answer C

Heat is produced whenever ultrasonic energy is absorbed by any biological material. During absorption, acoustic energy is converted into heat energy that remains in the soft tissue. This energy transformation may lead to an increase in tissue temperature. The rate of temperature elevation depends on the absorption coefficient of the tissue for a given frequency, the specific heat of the tissue, the density of the tissue, and the ultrasound intensity. Increased absorption converts more acoustic energy into heat energy. Tissues with high density heat more rapidly than those with low density. The amount of heat production is directly related to the ultrasound intensity, which is determined by the output power. Therefore, increased absorption, high tissue density, and increased power output and ultrasound intensity increase the tissue temperature during ultrasound examination.

Perfusion of tissue by blood has a cooling effect and may offset temperature elevation due to ultrasound exposure. The physical transport of heat from a tissue region by blood or fluid flow is called convection. Direct diffusion of heat to the neighboring region may dissipate heat, decreasing local temperature. This mechanism is called conduction. Therefore, the degree of tissue heating depends on multiple factors, including tissue perfusion and direct heat diffusion.

The actual elevation in temperature for a specific tissue is difficult to predict because of the complexity of the entire biologic system and because it is difficult to assess accurately the intensity of ultrasound exposure. Usually, tissue temperature elevation is less than 1.0°C at the intensities typical of diagnostic imaging instrumentation. Soft tissue can tolerate this temperature elevation without harmful effects. The American Institute of Ultrasound in Medicine stated the conclusions regarding the thermal bioeffect mechanism as follows: "Based solely on a thermal criterion, a diagnostic exposure that produces a maximum temperature rise of 1°C above normal physiological levels may be used in clinical examinations without reservation." **References** 9 *(pp 228–229)*; 10 *(p 60)*.

6. Answer D

7. Answer D

Compared with transthoracic echocardiography, transesophageal echocardiography has a unique problem with heat generation because of its proximity to the esophagus and the fact that the probe may be left in place for long periods when monitoring a patient during surgery. As a result, the manufacturers have inserted a heat-sensing device that automatically shuts off or cools the transducer when a certain temperature is reached. If the patient's temperature is high, the sensing device may shut off the probe. Because this patient is rewarmed to the nasopharyngeal temperature higher than 39°C, the esophageal temperature is also elevated. The transesophageal echocardiographic heat-sensing device detects the increased temperature and is about to start auto-cooling. If the transesophageal echocardiographic image is frozen during cardiopulmonary bypass, the probe does not produce heat. **Reference** 10 *(p 60)*.

8. Answer E

Cavitation is the creation of small gas-filled bodies by the ultrasound beam. It occurs when small, microscopic gas bubbles located in tissues vibrate as a result of interaction with ultrasound waves. Cavitation tends to occur only with exposure to high ultrasound intensity and is one of the mechanisms that may have the potential to cause bioeffects in tissues. Therefore, none of the statements about cavitation listed in this question is correct. **References** 9 *(pp 230–231)*; 10 *(p 60)*.

9. Answer A

10. Answer D

The two forms of cavitation are stable and transient cavitations. Stable cavitation occurs when the small bubbles located in tissues rhythmically grow and shrink as an ultrasound wave strikes them. Stable cavitation is like a pulsating microbubble that does not burst. The bubble rhythmically bounces against surrounding tissues and, theoretically, may cause cell injury. Stable cavitation is not believed to occur with pulsed wave Doppler, but it may occur with continuous wave Doppler. Also, two-dimensional imaging instruments have not been demonstrated to produce stable cavitation.

Transient cavitation is also called normal or inertial cavitation. It occurs when the changing pressure in an ultrasound beam causes a microbubble to expand and collapse violently, leading to burst or microscopic explosion. Transient cavitation is like an exploding microbomb. The bursting bubble causes shock waves that may result in cell injury. However, cavitation is not considered a clinically significant risk to patients; if harmful effects do occur, they are found only in a few cells. **References** 9 *(pp 230–231)*; 10 *(p 60)*.

11. Answer B

In comparison with nonfocused ultrasound beam, a highly focused ultrasound beam is more likely to dissipate heat to a neighboring region by conduction, that is, direct diffusion of heat to the neighboring region. This occurs because a highly focused ultrasound beam delivers heat only to a small area of the tissue, and the heat energy can be rapidly unloaded or transferred to neighboring regions that are cooler. This elimination of heat energy makes extreme temperature elevation unlikely. In contrast, with nonfocused ultrasound beams, the tissue area exposed to ultrasound energy is large. It is relatively difficult for tissue within the beam to transfer heat energy rapidly to neighboring regions. Hence, there is a greater likelihood for heat to build up, resulting in elevated tissue temperature. (See also Question 5.) **References** 9 *(pp 228–229, 233)*; 10 *(p 60)*.

12. Answer B

During transesophageal echocardiography, the patient's exposure to the electrical hazard is minimal under normal diagnostic condition. Ultrasound systems usually do not present special electrical hazards to the patient. Mechanically, the machine should be inspected regularly to assure proper physical status. Because the transducer is in direct contact with the patient, it is the component that has the greatest potential to expose the patient to electrical hazard. If a transducer case is cracked, it may cause current leakage and present a substantial electrical hazard to the patient. Therefore, the operator should check the transducer case before inserting the probe into the patient. If the transducer case is cracked, the operator should stop using it immediately to avoid the potential electrical hazard. **References** 9 *(p 236)*; 11 *(pp 19–20)*.

13. Answer C

The American Institute of Ultrasound in Medicine has developed and published official conclusions regarding the safety and bioeffects of diagnostic ultrasound.

The conclusion regarding epidemiology said that, after 25 years of clinical use, no adverse effects from exposure to diagnostic ultrasound have been indicated; in a randomized study, no adverse effects such as low birth weight in humans have been identified as a result of exposure to diagnostic ultrasound.

The conclusions regarding the overall clinical safety of ultrasound stated, "No confirmed biological effects on patients or instrument operators caused by exposure at intensities typical of present diagnostic ultrasound instruments have ever been reported. Although the possibility exists that such biological effects may be identified in the future, current data indicate that the benefits to patients of the prudent use of diagnostic ultrasound outweigh the risks, if any, that may be present."

To minimize a patient's exposure to ultrasound, the institute suggested using the minimum output power and maximum amplification to optimize image quality. (See also Question 3.) **References** 9 *(pp 232–234)*; 10 *(pp 59–60)*.

14. Answer C

It is important to maintain the integrity of the transesophageal echocardiographic probe. After each examination, the probe should be carefully inspected for defects with the transducer tip in the neutral position and in all flexed directions. The probe defects that may be seen include metallic protrusions, perforations, cracks, and sheath corrosion. These defects may cause mechanical trauma or expose the patient to infective, caustic, or electrical complications. Whenever a defect is suspected, the probe should not be used until additional safety inspections and necessary repairs have been made by qualified personnel. Visual inspection of the probe alone does not always guarantee that the outer insulating layer is intact. The electrical safety of the probe should be tested regularly by either a qualified technician or a commercially available meter to detect leakage current. **References** 9 *(p 236)*; 11 *(pp 19–20)*.

15. Answer D

After each procedure, the transesophageal echocardiographic probe must be cleaned and disinfected. The probe is first washed in an enzymatic solution to remove any adherent mucus or secretions. Then, the probe is rinsed with tap water and soaked in a glutaraldehyde disinfectant solution for 20 minutes. This period is sufficient to destroy any viral or bacterial contaminants acquired from patients, including those under strict isolation. Finally, the probe is rinsed thoroughly with tap water and then air dried for 20 minutes to allow any residual adherent glutaraldehyde to evaporate. The disinfectant solution should be changed according to package instructions or approximately every two weeks, and the enzymatic solution should be discarded after each use. Cleaning the probe with enzymatic solution is not mandatory but is routine in the echocardiography laboratory at Mayo Clinic.

Heat sterilization should never be used for these probes because high temperature depolarizes the piezoelectric crystal inside the probe and the transducer loses its piezoelectricity forever. **Reference** 11 *(pp 20–22)*.

16. Answer B

The important consideration regarding antibiotic prophylaxis for subacute bacterial endocarditis is the balance between the magnitude of the risk of bacteremia during transesophageal echocardiography and the well-known risks of widespread use of prophylactic antibiotics in both individual patients and the general population. Prospective studies showed that the incidence of transesophageal echocardiography–related bacteremia is extremely low, and a general recommendation for antibiotic prophylaxis during transesophageal echocardiography is not warranted. In 1997, the American Heart Association published its recommendations for prophylaxis of bacterial endocarditis. In this article, the procedures that may cause bacteremia and for which prophylaxis is recommended are clearly specified. Prophylaxis for bacterial endocarditis is not recommended by the American Heart Association for transesophageal echocardiography. **References** 7; 11 *(p 32)*.

17. Answer E

Before transesophageal echocardiography, the patient's mouth should be examined for preexisting injuries and loose teeth because oral or dental injuries may occur during transesophageal echocardiography, especially during insertion and removal of the probe. To prevent any mechanical, thermal, or electrical injuries to the patient, the transducer must be inspected for any damage to its outer surface, such as cracks or sheath corrosion, before its insertion into the patient. In addition, the control wheels should be checked to be sure they are working and unlocked. During insertion and removal of the probe, the steering wheels must never be locked. Also, lubricant gel should be applied to the tip of the transducer for easier probe insertion, which decreases the incidence of oral or esophageal injuries. **References** 11 *(pp 19–20, 28–29)*; 37.

18. Answer E

Apparently, this patient does not need antibiotic prophylaxis for subacute bacterial endocarditis anymore because he actually has infective endocarditis (fever and vegetation confirmed by transesophageal echocardiography). He should receive antibiotic treatment for his infective endocarditis after the blood culture is obtained. For patients with a referral diagnosis of infective endocarditis, antibiotics should not be administered until the blood culture specimens have been analyzed. **References** 7; 11 *(p 32)*.

19. Answer E

Once the transesophageal echocardiographic probe is in the esophagus, the transducer should never be forced through any resistance. If resistance is met, the tip of the transducer should be allowed to return to the neutral position before advancing or withdrawing the probe. At no time should excessive force be applied when moving the transducer in the esophagus or flexing the tip with the control wheels. Frequently, the resistance is caused by excessively anteflexing or retroflexing the tip of the probe. Further anteflexing or retroflexing the tip of the probe does not resolve the problem. By locking the control wheel, the tip of the transducer may be locked in the position that causes the resistance. The most serious mechanical problem is buckling of the tip while the probe is in the esophagus. Four such cases have been reported in the literature. In the course of the examination, the probe tip buckled over on itself, leading to difficulty in probe withdrawal. In these instances, the probe was safely removed after it was advanced into the stomach, where the buckled tip unfolded. **References** 11 *(p 50)*; 37.

20. Answer B

Although transesophageal echocardiography can be considered as an endoscopic procedure in the esophagus, the American Heart Association believes that the risk of endocarditis as a direct result of an endoscopic procedure in the gastrointestinal tract is small. Transient bacteremia may occur during or immediately after endoscopy; however, there are few reports of infective endocarditis attributable to endoscopy. For most gastrointestinal endoscopic procedures, the rate of bacteremia is 2% to 5%, and the organisms typically identified are unlikely to cause endocarditis. For transesophageal echocardiography, the reported incidence of bacteremia in most studies is 0% to 4%, and there is little direct evidence that patients experience clinical consequences. According to the current American Heart Association guidelines, antibiotic prophylaxis for subacute bacterial endocarditis is not recommended for transesophageal echocardiography. **References** 7; 11 *(p 32)*.

Chapter 7

Indications, Contraindications, and Complications of Transesophageal Echocardiography

Questions

Multiple choice (choose the *one* best answer):

1. A category II indication for perioperative transesophageal echocardiography means
   A. weaker evidence and expert consensus.
   B. strong evidence and expert consensus.
   C. strong scientific evidence but weak expert support.
   D. weak scientific evidence but strong expert support.
   E. no current scientific and expert support.

2. Which one of the following is a category II indication?
   A. Intraoperative transesophageal echocardiographic assessment of mitral valve replacement.
   B. Intraoperative use of transesophageal echocardiography in evaluating mitral valve repair.
   C. Intraoperative use of transesophageal echocardiography in evaluating aortic valve repair.
   D. B and C.
   E. All of the above.

3. A category I indication means
   A. the surgeon requested intraoperative transesophageal echocardiography.
   B. there is no scientific evidence although there is expert support.
   C. strongest evidence or expert support.
   D. weakest evidence or expert support.
   E. strong scientific evidence but no expert support.

4. Category I indications include intraoperative transesophageal echocardiographic evaluation of

A. pericardial window procedures.
B. pericardiectomy.
C. pericardial surgery.
D. all of the above.
E. none of the above.

5. A category III indication means

A. strongest evidence and expert support.
B. weak scientific evidence but strong expert support.
C. strong scientific evidence but weak expert support.
D. little current scientific and expert support.
E. no benefit and intervention may be harmful.

6. All of the following are category III indications ***except***

A. monitoring placement and function of left ventricular assist devices.
B. monitoring placement of intra-aortic balloon pumps.
C. monitoring placement of pulmonary artery catheters.
D. monitoring placement of automatic implantable cardiac defibrillators.
E. monitoring cardioplegia administration.

7. A 38-year-old patient has a motor vehicle accident. In the emergency department, he is hemodynamically stable but chest radiography shows a widened mediastinum. To rule out suspected thoracic aortic dissection, a transesophageal echocardiography is performed. This clinical setting is

A. a category I indication.
B. a category II indication.
C. a category III indication.
D. an indication for transesophageal echocardiography supported by strong evidence and expert opinion.
E. A and D.

8. Which one of the following statements about intraoperative use of transesophageal echocardiography in the case described in Question 7 is true?

A. Intraoperative use of transesophageal echocardiography in this case without suspected aortic valve involvement is a category III indication.
B. Intraoperative use of transesophageal echocardiography in this case with aortic valve involvement is a category II indication.
C. Intraoperative assessment of aortic valve function in this case with possible aortic valve involvement is a category I indication.
D. Intraoperative use of transesophageal echocardiography in this case without aortic valve involvement is a category I indication.

9. Contraindications to transesophageal echocardiography include

A. recent esophageal surgery.
B. recent gastric surgery.

C. esophageal tumor.
D. esophageal stricture.
E. all of the above.

10. For small children,
A. a pediatric transesophageal echocardiographic probe can be used only for patients who weigh more than 10 pounds.
B. a pediatric transesophageal echocardiographic probe can be used for patients at least 1 year old.
C. airway pressure is never a concern during intraoperative transesophageal echocardiography because the pediatric probe is small and safe.
D. airway pressure does not need to be monitored in pediatric patients undergoing transesophageal echocardiography because the probe is inserted into the esophagus, not the trachea.
E. airway pressure should be monitored before and after insertion of the transesophageal echocardiographic probe, as well as during transesophageal echocardiography even though the probe is inserted into the esophagus.

11. Minor complications from transesophageal echocardiography include
A. lip and dental injuries.
B. bradycardia.
C. dysphagia.
D. hoarseness.
E. all of the above.

12. During noncardiac surgery, a 90-year-old patient with a history of stable angina suddenly develops severe hypotension. Since no obvious cause explains the acute hypotension that does not respond to treatment, the anesthesiologist decides to perform intraoperative transesophageal echocardiography to evaluate the left ventricular function and determine the cause of the acute hypotension. This is
A. a category I indication.
B. a category II indication.
C. a category III indication.
D. a weak indication for intraoperative transesophageal echocardiography.
E. an indication with weak evidence and expert consensus because it was noncardiac surgery.

13. A 65-year-old patient with a history of mild coronary artery disease, hypertension, smoking, and hypercholesterolemia is scheduled for descending thoracic aortic aneurysm repair. The vascular surgeon requests intraoperative transesophageal echocardiography to monitor the left ventricular function and hemodynamic disturbance during aortic cross-clamp. According to the American Society of Anesthesiologists/Society of Cardiovascular Anesthesiologists practice guidelines for transesophageal echocardiography, this scenario is
A. a category I indication.
B. a category II indication.
C. a category III indication.

D. not indicated.
E. absolutely contraindicated.

14. Intraoperative transesophageal echocardiography for congenital heart surgery is
A. a category III indication for all types of the lesions.
B. a category III indication for most lesions requiring cardiopulmonary bypass.
C. a category II indication for all types of the lesions.
D. a category II indication for most lesions requiring cardiopulmonary bypass.
E. a category I indication for most lesions requiring cardiopulmonary bypass.

15. A 28-year-old patient with the accompanying intraoperative transesophageal echocardiographic image (Ao, aorta; LA, left atrium; RA, right atrium) is scheduled for surgery. The cardiac surgeon asks about intraoperative use of transesophageal echocardiography in this case. Intraoperative transesophageal echocardiography in evaluation in this case is
A. supported by the strongest evidence or expert opinion.
B. never indicated because it is not useful in improving clinical outcomes.
C. supported by weaker evidence and expert consensus.
D. very useful in improving clinical outcomes and is always a category I indication.
E. A and D.

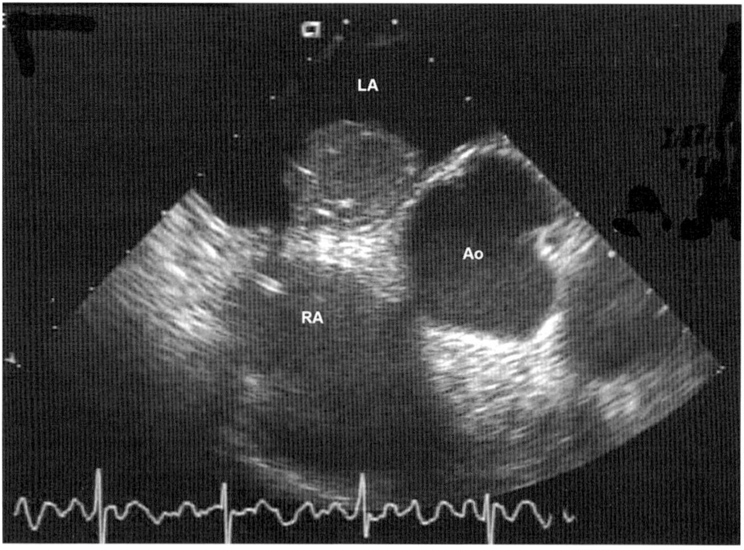

16. A 26-year-old patient has a motor vehicle accident with multiple trauma, including anterior chest injury. Intraoperatively, the patient is hemodynamically stable. The trauma surgeon requests intraoperative transesophageal echocardiography for suspected traumatic cardiac injury. This is
A. supported by the strongest evidence or expert opinion.
B. a strong indication for intraoperative transesophageal echocardiography because the surgeon requested it.

C. a category I indication.
D. a category II indication.
E. a category III indication.

17. A 32-year-old patient is currently taking antibiotics for his uncomplicated endocarditis. He is brought to the operating room for emergency open reduction and internal fixation of the left tibia. Considering his endocarditis, the surgeon asks the consulting cardiologist if intraoperative transesophageal echocardiography is indicated. In this case, the cardiologist advises that transesophageal echocardiography for uncomplicated endocarditis during noncardiac surgery is
A. a category II indication for intraoperative transesophageal echocardiography.
B. not an indication for intraoperative transesophageal echocardiography according to the American Society of Anesthesiologists/Society of Cardiovascular Anesthesiologists practice guidelines.
C. a category III indication.
D. a relative contraindication for intraoperative transesophageal echocardiography because of the risk of subacute bacterial endocarditis.
E. an indication strongly supported by expert opinion.

18. Serious complications during transesophageal echocardiography include all of the following ***except***
A. dysrhythmias.
B. phrenic nerve paralysis.
C. vocal cord paralysis.
D. esophageal bleeding or injury.
E. cardiac arrest.

19. Which one of the following is not a relative contraindication for transesophageal echocardiography?
A. Esophageal varices.
B. Barrett's esophagus.
C. Poorly maintained teeth with a loose front upper tooth.
D. Previous radiotherapy to the esophageal area.
E. Zenker's diverticulum.

20. During total hip replacement, the patient suddenly develops severe hypotension, which does not respond to treatment. Intraoperative transesophageal echocardiography reveals a large fat embolus in the right atrium. This is an example of
A. a category I indication.
B. a category II indication.
C. a category III indication.
D. a transesophageal echocardiographic indication that is not included in the American Society of Anesthesiologists/Society of Cardiovascular Anesthesiologists practice guidelines.
E. intraoperative transesophageal echocardiography with weak evidence and expert consensus.

21. Because of the experience described in Question 20, the surgeon asks the consulting cardiologist if intraoperative transesophageal echocardiography should be done in all patients undergoing total hip replacement. The cardiologist tells the surgeon that intraoperative monitoring for emboli during orthopedic procedures is

A. a category I indication.

B. a category II indication.

C. a category III indication.

D. an appropriate indication only if requested by the surgeon.

E. supported by strong evidence and expert opinion.

22. According to the American Society of Anesthesiologists/Society of Cardiovascular Anesthesiologists practice guidelines, which one of the following statements about intraoperative use of transesophageal echocardiography in patients with cardiomyopathies is true?

A. All cardiomyopathies are category I indications for intraoperative transesophageal echocardiography.

B. All cardiomyopathies are category II indications for intraoperative transesophageal echocardiography.

C. Dilated cardiomyopathy is a category I indication, and all the other types of cardiomyopathies are category III indications for intraoperative transesophageal echocardiography.

D. Hypertrophic cardiomyopathy is a category I indication, and the others are category III indications for intraoperative transesophageal echocardiography.

E. Restrictive cardiomyopathy is a category I indication, and the others are category II indications for intraoperative transesophageal echocardiography.

23. A 78-year-old patient with a Zenker's diverticulum is scheduled for coronary artery bypass graft surgery. The surgeon asks the cardiologist's opinion about the use of intraoperative transesophageal echocardiography to evaluate myocardial perfusion, coronary artery anatomy, and graft patency. The cardiologist should tell the surgeon that

A. intraoperative transesophageal echocardiography is strongly indicated if it is requested by the surgeon.

B. intraoperative transesophageal echocardiography is absolutely indicated but not contraindicated in this case.

C. if resistance is met, the transesophageal echocardiographic probe should be forced to advance it beyond the resistance.

D. intraoperative transesophageal echocardiography is not appropriate in this case.

E. intraoperative transesophageal echocardiography is a category I indication but is relatively contraindicated in this patient.

24. Detection of air emboli during cardiotomy, heart transplantation, and upright neurosurgical procedures is

A. a category I indication for intraoperative transesophageal echocardiography.

B. a category II indication for intraoperative transesophageal echocardiography.

C. a category III indication for intraoperative transesophageal echocardiography.

D. always requested by the cardiac surgeon or neurosurgeon.
E. A and D.

25. A 42-year-old patient is scheduled for pulmonary embolectomy. The surgeon requests intraoperative transesophageal echocardiography to detect any residual pulmonary emboli. The intraoperative use of transesophageal echocardiography to detect pulmonary emboli and to evaluate their surgical treatment is
A. indicated only if requested by the surgeon.
B. always indicated because there is very strong evidence that intraoperative transesophageal echocardiography improves clinical outcomes.
C. a category I indication.
D. a category II indication.
E. a category III indication.

26. A 70-year-old patient with a left ventricular aneurysm undergoes aneurysmectomy. Intraoperative transesophageal echocardiography is used to evaluate the surgical repair. According to the American Society of Anesthesiologists/Society of Cardiovascular Anesthesiologists practice guidelines for transesophageal echocardiography, assessing surgical repair of cardiac aneurysms
A. has strong evidence and expert support.
B. is supported by weak evidence and expert consensus.
C. is a category II indication.
D. is a category III indication.
E. is B and C.

Answers & Discussion

1. Answer A

According to the "Practice Guidelines for Perioperative Transesophageal Echocardiography" by the American Society of Anesthesiologists/Society of Cardiovascular Anesthesiologists task force on transesophageal echocardiography, the indications for transesophageal echocardiography are classified into three categories on the basis of the strength of supporting evidence or expert opinion that transesophageal echocardiography improves clinical outcomes. Category II indications are supported by weaker evidence and expert consensus. In the settings of category II indications, transesophageal echocardiography may be useful in improving clinical outcomes, but appropriate indications are less certain. **Reference** 41.

2. Answer A

In patients undergoing valve surgery, intraoperative transesophageal echocardiography is helpful in many ways. Preoperative transesophageal echocardiography may provide new information, resulting in prompt changes in the surgical plan. Postoperative transesophageal echocardiography is helpful in identifying severe valve dysfunction that may necessitate returning to bypass to rerepair or replace the valve. Thus, intraoperative transesophageal echocardiography makes it possible to recognize the need for further surgery in the operating room, which decreases postoperative complications and avoids a second operation. Other potential benefits of transesophageal echocardiography during valve surgery include detection of entrapped air and assessment of hemodynamic function, which is especially helpful in weaning the patient from cardiopulmonary bypass. The American Society of Anesthesiologists/Society of Cardiovascular Anesthesiologists practice guidelines for perioperative transesophageal echocardiography recommend that valve repair is a category I indication and valve replacement is a category II indication for the use of intraoperative transesophageal echocardiography. **Reference** 41.

3. Answer C

The indications for transesophageal echocardiography are classified on the basis of the strength of supporting evidence and expert opinion, not the surgeon's request. According to the American Society of Anesthesiologists/Society of Cardiovascular Anesthesiologists practice guidelines for transesophageal echocardiography, category I indications are supported by the strongest evidence or expert opinion. In this category of indications, transesophageal echocardiography frequently is useful in improving clinical outcomes and often is indicated, depending on individual circumstances. **Reference** 41.

4. Answer A

In patients undergoing pericardial window procedures, intraoperative use of transesophageal echocardiography to evaluate the adequacy of treatment is a category I indication as recommended by the American Society of Anesthesiologists/Society of Cardiovascular Anesthesiologists practice guidelines for transesophageal echocardiography. During pericardial window procedures, posterior or loculated pericardial effusions are easily missed by the surgeon. Intraoperative transesophageal echocardiography is helpful in detecting pericardial effusions missed by the surgeon, leading to decreased postoperative morbidity.

Perioperative transesophageal echocardiography may be more sensitive than transthoracic echocardiography in detecting pericardial effusions. Although supporting scientific evidence is limited, expert opinion believes that perioperative transesophageal echocardiography is clinically beneficial if it detects pericardial tamponade and avoids serious hemodynamic sequelae. In addition, intraoperative transesophageal echocardiography may be helpful in evaluating constrictive pericarditis and pericardiectomy procedures. The American Society of Anesthesiologists/Society of Cardiovascular Anesthesiologists practice guidelines for transesophageal echocardiography recommend that intraoperative evaluation of pericardiectomy or pericardial effusions and evaluation of pericardial surgery are category II indications for transesophageal echocardiography. **Reference** 41.

5. Answer D

In the American Society of Anesthesiologists/Society of Cardiovascular Anesthesiologists practice guidelines for transesophageal echocardiography, category III indications have little current scientific and expert support. In the clinical settings of category III indications, transesophageal echocardiography infrequently is useful in improving clinical outcomes, and appropriate indications are uncertain. The lack of supporting evidence for category III indications is often owing to the absence of relevant studies rather than to existing evidence of ineffectiveness. **Reference** 41.

6. Answer A

Although intraoperative transesophageal echocardiography can be used to aid placement and monitor function of ventricular assist devices, intra-aortic balloon pumps, automatic implantable cardiac defibrillators, and pulmonary artery catheters, there is little direct evidence that transesophageal echocardiography is necessary to insert and operate these devices safely or that its use results in improved clinical outcomes. However, expert opinion believes that intraoperative transesophageal echocardiography is beneficial in patients receiving mechanical circulatory assist devices because these patients usually are experiencing hemodynamic disturbances for which transesophageal echocardiography is considered beneficial. In addition, using intraoperative transesophageal echocardiography to confirm placement of such devices reduces the need for intraoperative radiography, thereby decreasing radiation exposure and operating room time. The American Society of Anesthesiologists/Society of Cardiovascular Anesthesiologists task force recommend that monitoring placement and function of ventricular assist devices is a category II indication, while monitoring placement of intra-aortic balloon pumps, automatic implantable cardiac defibrillators, or pulmonary artery catheters is a category III indication for transesophageal echocardiography.

The use of intraoperative transesophageal echocardiography to evaluate the distribution of cardioplegia solution and to aid placement of cannulas for cardioplegia infusions has been described. However, there is little direct evidence that using transesophageal echocardiography to monitor cardioplegia administration improved clinical outcomes. The American Society of Anesthesiologists/Society of Cardiovascular Anesthesiologists practice guidelines recommend that monitoring cardioplegia administration is a category III indication for intraoperative transesophageal echocardiography. **Reference** 41.

7. Answer B

The mortality rate in the first 48 hours of aortic dissection is about 1% per hour, necessitating prompt diagnosis and surgical intervention. In patients with acute aortic dissection or disruption, rapidly worsening hemodynamic instability and hemodynamic shock often preclude the performance of diagnostic tests before the patient is taken to surgery. In these clinical settings, angiography and other imaging studies are often impractical because of the above-mentioned reasons. Therefore, preoperative or intraoperative transesophageal echocardiography can play an important role in the early detection of acute aortic dissection or disruption. Expert opinion believes that any method enhancing prompt detection of acute aortic dissection or disruption is potentially beneficial, and early detection of aortic dissection or disruption improves clinical outcomes due to the life-threatening nature of the diseases. For preoperative use of transesophageal echocardiography in patients with suspected thoracic aortic aneurysm, dissection, or disruption, the American Society of Anesthesiologists/Society of Cardiovascular Anesthesiologists practice guidelines for transesophageal echocardiography recommend the following:

1. Preoperative use in unstable patients with suspected thoracic aortic aneurysm, dissection, or disruption is a category I indication.
2. Preoperative assessment of stable patients with suspected acute thoracic aortic dissections, aneurysm, or disruption is a category II indication.

The patient in this question has suspected aortic dissection or disruption because of widened mediastinum. Because this patient is hemodynamically stable, preoperative transesophageal echocardiography examination in this clinical setting is a category II indication according to the American Society of Anesthesiologists/Society of Cardiovascular Anesthesiologists practice guidelines for transesophageal echocardiography. **Reference** 41.

8. Answer C

In the setting of thoracic aortic disease, the American Society of Anesthesiologists/Society of Cardiovascular Anesthesiologists practice guidelines recommend the following:

1. Intraoperative use of transesophageal echocardiography for assessing aortic valve function in repair of aortic dissections with possible aortic valve involvement is a category I indication.
2. Intraoperative use of transesophageal echocardiography during repair of thoracic aortic dissections without suspected aortic valve involvement is a category II indication.

In patients with aortic dissection undergoing aortic reconstruction, the principle benefits of intraoperative transesophageal echocardiography are to assess hemodynamic status, document entry and exit sites, and confirm decompression of the false lumen. In patients with suspected aortic valve involvement, intraoperative transesophageal echocardiography is also used to determine whether aortic valve surgery is needed. **Reference** 41.

9. Answer E

Perioperative transesophageal echocardiography is safe when it is performed properly. Occasionally, serious complications may occur. One should always examine the patient and detect preexisting esophageal or gastric problems before performing transesophageal echocardiography. Avoiding transesophageal echocardiography in patients with extensive esophageal or gastric disease can minimize the risk of esophageal or gastric injury. According to the American Society of Anesthesiologists/Society of Cardiovascular Anesthesiologists practice guidelines for performing comprehensive intraoperative multiplane transesophageal echocardiography, contraindications to transesophageal echocardiography include esophageal stricture, diverticulum, tumor, and recent esophageal or gastric surgery. **References** 11 *(pp 47, 49)*; 41.

10. Answer E

At present, the smallest pediatric transesophageal echocardiographic probes available measure 5.9 mm in diameter and enable examination of children as small as 2,400 g. In addition to selecting an appropriate probe size for small children, airway pressure should be carefully monitored during perioperative transesophageal echocardiography. Generally, small children have a membranous trachea that is more easily compressed by the probe. For small children who are intubated under general anesthesia, the airway pressure should always be monitored during intraoperative transesophageal echocardiography, especially before and after inserting the probe, because it may compress on the relatively small endotracheal tube and hence impair ventilation. **References** 11 *(p 50)*; 22; 30.

11. Answer E

Minor complications from transesophageal echocardiography include lip injuries, dental injuries, hoarseness, dysphagia, and bradycardia. Among these minor complications, lip injuries occur most frequently and have an incidence of 13%. It is important to examine the patient's mouth for any preexisting lip damage or dental injuries. The incidence of hoarseness and dysphagia is 12% and 1.8%, respectively. Bradycardia occurs rarely (0.2%) and most likely secondary to vagal stimulation caused by the insertion or manipulation of the probe during transesophageal echocardiography. **References** 11 *(pp 49–51)*; 41.

12. Answer A

Transesophageal echocardiography is very helpful in assessing hemodynamic and global ventricular function. In the operating room or intensive care settings, transesophageal echocardiography can be used to diagnose the hemodynamic problems such as myocardial depression or hypovolemia. Hence, appropriate therapy can be administered to improve and stabilize the patient's hemodynamic status. In comparison with the pulmonary artery catheter, transesophageal echocardiography may be more expedient because it can be inserted more quickly and without sterile technique; transesophageal echocardiography is also safer because it does not enter the great vessels and heart. While a pulmonary artery catheter provides pressure measurements only, transesophageal echocardiography provides global hemodynamic information about the structure and function of the heart. Failing to take action to correct or prevent hemodynamic disturbances increases the risk of end-organ damage as well as perioperative morbidity and mortality. The American Society of Anesthesiologists/Society of Cardiovascular Anesthesiologists task force on transesophageal echocardiography believes that detecting acute hemodynamic disturbances during surgery improves clinical outcomes. The practice guidelines for transesophageal echocardiography recommend that the emergent use of perioperative transesophageal echocardiography to determine the cause of acute, persistent, and life-threatening hemodynamic disturbances in which ventricular function and its determinants are uncertain and have not responded to treatment is a category I indication.

This 90-year-old patient with a history of coronary artery disease has acute hypotension of unclear etiology, which has not responded to treatment. The emergent use of intraoperative transesophageal echocardiography to determine the etiology of this acute hemodynamic disturbance in this patient is a category I indication according to the American Society of Anesthesiologists/Society of Cardiovascular Anesthesiologists practice guidelines for transesophageal echocardiography. **References** 11 *(pp 33–34)*; 41.

13. Answer B

This patient has multiple risk factors for coronary artery disease and perioperative myocardial ischemia. He is scheduled for thoracic aortic aneurysm repair, which is a major vascular procedure associated with increased risk of myocardial ischemia and infarction. Traditional methods for monitoring myocardial ischemia during surgery, such as continuous electrocardiography, have limited sensitivity in the early detection of myocardial ischemia and tissue injury. Generally, regional wall motion abnormalities detected by transesophageal echocardiography precede electrocardiographic changes during myocardial ischemia. The development of regional ventricular dysfunction during surgery increases the patient's risk of perioperative myocardial infarction and sudden death. Since early treatment of myocardial ischemia and myocardial infarction improves survival, intraoperative transesophageal echocardiography is beneficial for patients with increased risk of myocardial ischemia undergoing high-risk procedures such as operations on major vessels or that involve aortic cross-clamping. Clinically, intraoperative transesophageal echocardiographic detection of myocardial ischemia permits corrective interventions, including alterations in surgery and anesthetic management. The American Society of Anesthesiologists/Society of Cardiovascular Anesthesiologists practice guidelines for transesophageal echocardiography recommend that the increased risks of hemodynamic disturbances and myocardial ischemia or infarction during the perioperative period are category II indications for perioperative transesophageal echocardiography. **Reference** 41.

14. Answer E

Transesophageal echocardiography has a special application in evaluating the adequacy of surgical repair of congenital heart lesions. When performed with biplane pediatric probes, intraoperative transesophageal echocardiography can detect lesions not seen on preoperative transthoracic echocardiography in as many as 30% of patients. In patients undergoing congenital heart surgery, findings before cardiopulmonary bypass result in new findings or altered medical therapy in 3% to 45% of cases, and postoperative transesophageal echocardiography detects information not available by transthoracic echocardiography in 15% to 48% of patients. The American Society of Anesthesiologists/Society of Cardiovascular Anesthesiologists task force on transesophageal echocardiography believes that the detection of residual defects improves clinical outcomes by reducing the residual hemodynamic burden of these lesions and by decreasing the patient's risk of pulmonary hypertension and endocarditis. The American Society of Anesthesiologists/Society of Cardiovascular Anesthesiologists practice guidelines for transesophageal echocardiography recommend that congenital heart surgery for most lesions requiring cardiopulmonary bypass is a category I indication for intraoperative transesophageal echocardiography, both before and after cardiopulmonary bypass. **References** 11 *(pp 33–34)*; 41.

15. Answer C

The image shows a left atrial myxoma. There is some evidence that intraoperative transesophageal echocardiography may be more accurate than preoperative testing in characterizing the anatomy of some cardiac tumors and intracardiac extensions of pulmonary or renal tumors, but there is little evidence beyond case reports that this information or the use of transesophageal echocardiography during resection of cardiac tumors results in improved clinical outcomes. Nevertheless, intraoperative transesophageal echocardiography may determine whether a cardiac mass has embolized or detect the new location of the mass, even if preoperative echocardiography is adequate. These new findings about the cardiac mass may lead to a change in surgical planning. According to the American Society of Anesthesiologists/Society of Cardiovascular Anesthesiologists practice guidelines, intraoperative use of transesophageal echocardiography in evaluation of removal of cardiac tumors is classified as a category II indication, which is supported by weaker evidence and expert consensus.

This 28-year-old patient is scheduled for surgical resection of myxoma. The use of intraoperative transesophageal echocardiography to evaluate the removal of myxoma is a category II indication. **References** 11 *(pp 33–34)*; 41.

16. Answer D

Intraoperative transesophageal echocardiography performed during trauma surgery may disclose unrecognized traumatic injuries to the heart. Therefore, the need to return for further surgery and the risk of complications may be reduced by intraoperative transesophageal echocardiography. Case reports describe the role of intraoperative transesophageal echocardiography in detecting unrecognized traumatic injuries to the heart and the role of postoperative transesophageal echocardiography in detecting injuries not seen on transthoracic echocardiography. However, there is little evidence that transesophageal echocardiography improves the clinical outcome of cardiac trauma patients. The American Society of Anesthesiologists/Society of Cardiovascular Anesthesiologists practice guidelines for transesophageal echocardiography recommend that suspected cardiac trauma is a category II indication for perioperative transesophageal echocardiography. **Reference** 41.

17. Answer C

Although the role of transesophageal echocardiography in detecting endocarditis is well established, there is little role for transesophageal echocardiography in evaluating endocarditis during noncardiac surgery, unless the preoperative examination is inadequate or the patient requires urgent surgery. Studies suggest that transesophageal echocardiographic evidence of vegetations may persist long after bacteriologic cure. However, negative transesophageal echocardiography does not rule out endocarditis. So far, little evidence beyond case reports supports the use of transesophageal echocardiography during noncardiac surgery as accurate in detecting endocarditis and achieving improved clinical outcomes. The American Society of Anesthesiologists/Society of Cardiovascular Anesthesiologists practice guidelines for transesophageal echocardiography recommend that noncardiac surgery involving patients with uncomplicated endocarditis is a category III indication for intraoperative transesophageal echocardiography. **Reference** 41.

18. Answer B

Serious complications of transesophageal echocardiography include esophageal injury or bleeding, vocal cord paralysis, dysrhythmias, hypotension, seizures, and cardiac arrest. These complications occur in less than 3% of transesophageal echocardiographic examinations, according to the American Society of Anesthesiologists/Society of Cardiovascular Anesthesiologists practice guidelines for transesophageal echocardiography. The reported mortality rate associated with transesophageal echocardiography is 0.01% to 0.03%, but in most cases, a causal link with transesophageal echocardiography has not been established. Generally, phrenic nerve paralysis does not occur during transesophageal echocardiography. **References** 11 *(pp 49–51)*; 41.

19. Answer C

Poorly maintained teeth with a loose front upper tooth is not a contraindication to transesophageal echocardiography. Patients with poorly maintained teeth or loose teeth are more susceptible to dental injury during transesophageal echocardiography examination, especially during the insertion or removal of the transesophageal echocardiographic probe. One should always examine the patient's mouth for any preexisting oral or dental injuries. If the patient has preexisting dental injury or loose teeth, one should pay special attention to avoid further damage to the patient's teeth. Esophageal varices, Zenker's diverticulum, Barrett's esophagus, and radiotherapy of the esophageal area are relative contraindications to transesophageal echocardiography according to the American Society of Anesthesiologists/Society of Cardiovascular Anesthesiologists practice guidelines. **References** 11 *(pp 47–51)*; 41.

20. Answer A

In this clinical setting, intraoperative transesophageal echocardiography is performed emergently during the orthopedic surgery to detect the cause of the acute hemodynamic disturbance that has not responded to any treatment. A large fat embolus in the right atrium is found, and the appropriate management is possible because of intraoperative transesophageal echocardiography. Failure to detect the large fat embolus in the right atrium leads to increased perioperative morbidity and mortality and hence poor clinical outcome. According to the American Society of Anesthesiologists/Society of Cardiovascular Anesthesiologists practice guidelines for transesophageal echocardiography, the emergent use of perioperative transesophageal echocardiography to determine the cause of acute, persistent, and life-threatening hemodynamic disturbances in which ventricular function and its determinants are uncertain and have not responded to treatment is a category I indication. **Reference** 41.

21. Answer C

The American Society of Anesthesiologists/Society of Cardiovascular Anesthesiologists practice guidelines for transesophageal echocardiography recommend that monitoring for emboli during orthopedic procedures is a category III indication for intraoperative transesophageal echocardiography. Although intraoperative transesophageal echocardiography can detect embolized air or medullary contents in patients undergoing total hip replacement or total knee replacement, there is little evidence that this information results in improved clinical outcomes unless the patient has acute hemodynamic disturbance secondary to the emboli. The task force on transesophageal echocardiography believes that in clinical practice, the ultimate benefit of intraoperative transesophageal echocardiography to the hemodynamically stable patient undergoing orthopedic surgery is uncertain. Therefore, intraoperative transesophageal echocardiography used routinely to monitor emboli during orthopedic procedures has little current scientific or expert support and is classified as a category III indication in the practice guidelines for transesophageal echocardiography. **Reference** 41.

22. Answer D

Although hypertrophic, dilated, and restrictive cardiomyopathies are diagnosed accurately by echocardiography, the use of intraoperative transesophageal echocardiography in patients with cardiomyopathies has centered on hypertrophic obstructive cardiomyopathy. It has been reported that the detection of persistent outflow tract gradients aided surgical revision in 20% of patients undergoing myectomy for hypertrophic obstructive cardiomyopathy. In addition, intraoperative transesophageal echocardiography enables the detection of systolic anterior motion or iatrogenic septal defects resulting from the surgical repair. However, there is little evidence that intraoperative transesophageal echocardiography alters therapy or improves outcomes in patients with dilated or restrictive cardiomyopathies. The American Society of Anesthesiologists/Society of Cardiovascular Anesthesiologists task force on transesophageal echocardiography recommends that use of intraoperative transesophageal echocardiography is a category I indication for hypertrophic obstructive cardiomyopathy repair and a category III indication for other cardiomyopathies. **Reference** 41.

23. Answer D

Transesophageal echocardiography is contraindicated in patients with Zenker's diverticulum. The use of perioperative transesophageal echocardiography to evaluate myocardial perfusion, coronary artery anatomy, or graft patency are category III indications that have little current scientific and expert support in improving clinical outcomes. Although intraoperative transesophageal echocardiography is capable of evaluating the myocardial perfusion pattern, coronary artery anatomy, and graft patency, few studies have examined whether this information improves clinical outcomes. Studies of cardiac surgery patients report the transesophageal echocardiographic findings were "valuable or essential" or resulted in a change in therapy such as graft revision and hemodynamic support, but there is no direct evidence that patients experience better outcomes as a result of these changes.

For this patient with Zenker's diverticulum undergoing coronary artery bypass graft surgery, the risk of transesophageal echocardiography outweighs its benefit. Therefore, intraoperative transesophageal echocardiography may not be appropriate in this case. **References** 11 *(pp 47, 49)*; 41.

24. Answer B

Transesophageal echocardiography is an extremely sensitive test in detecting air emboli. Usually, air emboli as small as 2 μm can be detected. However, the clinical importance of such very small air bubbles is unclear. Although animal studies suggest that air entrainment greater than 1 cm^3/kg increase the risk of neurologic complications, the threshold value for safe air volumes in humans is uncertain. Current evidence is inadequate to determine whether intraoperative transesophageal echocardiographic monitoring for small air emboli improves clinical outcomes.

The American Society of Anesthesiologists/Society of Cardiovascular Anesthesiologists task force on transesophageal echocardiography believes that patients benefit when transesophageal echocardiography detects air during cardiotomy and neurosurgical procedures. During cardiotomy, venting procedures before coming off cardiopulmonary bypass can eliminate retained air, which may decrease the patient's risk of embolic neurological events. In addition, the right coronary artery is anatomically susceptible to air embolism because of its position. Detection and removal of air before coming off cardiopulmonary bypass may decrease the risk of right coronary artery air embolism and, hence, myocardial infarction. Transesophageal echocardiographic monitoring offers similar benefits for patients undergoing sitting craniotomies, especially if the patient is not screened preoperatively for patent foramen ovale. In such a subpopulation, paradoxical emboli increase the risk of stroke and neurologic deficit. The task force on transesophageal echocardiography recommends that the detection of air emboli during cardiotomy, heart transplant operations, and upright neurosurgical procedures is a category II indication for intraoperative transesophageal echocardiography. **Reference** 41.

25. Answer D

The American Society of Anesthesiologists/Society of Cardiovascular Anesthesiologists task force believes that intraoperative transesophageal echocardiography is useful during pulmonary embolectomy to evaluate hemodynamic status and to detect residual emboli, although there is little evidence regarding the impact of intraoperative transesophageal echocardiography on clinical outcomes. Because about 30% of embolectomy procedures fail to completely remove all emboli and the residual emboli are potentially harmful to the patient, it would be beneficial for the patient to have an intraoperative transesophageal echocardiography in order to detect residual pulmonary emboli during the surgery, before the patient leaves the operating room.

According to the American Society of Anesthesiologists/Society of Cardiovascular Anesthesiologists practice guidelines on transesophageal echocardiography, pulmonary embolectomy is a category II indication for intraoperative transesophageal echocardiography, which is supported by weaker evidence and expert consensus. **Reference** 41.

26. Answer E

Although there is little evidence that intraoperative transesophageal echocardiography results in improved clinical outcomes for patients undergoing aneurysmectomy, the American Society of Anesthesiologists/Society of Cardiovascular Anesthesiologists task force believes that intraoperative transesophageal echocardiography can play an important role in evaluating the adequacy of surgical repair and, occasionally, in detecting previously unsuspected abnormalities such as pseudoaneurysms. In addition, patients with cardiac aneurysms typically have advanced ischemic heart disease and associated hemodynamic complications. Intraoperative transesophageal echocardiography is useful in evaluating regional wall motion abnormalities and assessing hemodynamic disturbances. Frequently, coming off cardiopulmonary bypass is difficult in patients undergoing aneurysmectomy. Intraoperative transesophageal echocardiography may monitor the patient's hemodynamic function and is helpful in weaning from cardiopulmonary bypass. The American Society of Anesthesiologists/Society of Cardiovascular Anesthesiologists practice guidelines recommend that assessing surgical repair of cardiac aneurysms is a category II indication for intraoperative transesophageal echocardiography, which is supported by weak evidence and expert consensus. **Reference** 41.

Chapter 8

Normal Anatomy and Flow During the Complete Examination

Questions

Multiple choice (choose the *one* best answer):

1. When the four-chamber view is used to evaluate the left ventricular apex,
   A. the tip of the transesophageal echocardiographic probe should always be in the neutral position to visualize the apex.
   B. the tip of the transesophageal echocardiographic probe needs to be anteflexed to see the left ventricular apex.
   C. the tip of the transesophageal echocardiographic probe may require retroflexion.
   D. the tip of the transesophageal echocardiographic probe should be locked.
   E. foreshortening is never a problem.

2. Transesophageal echocardiography may not visualize
   A. the distal aortic arch.
   B. the proximal descending aorta.
   C. the proximal ascending aorta.
   D. the distal aortic arch and the proximal descending aorta.
   E. the proximal aortic arch and the distal ascending aorta.

3. The accompanying transgastric image is
   A. a short axis view at the apical and midpapillary level.
   B. a short axis view at the basal and midpapillary level.
   C. an apical short axis view.
   D. a mid short axis view.
   E. a basal short axis view.

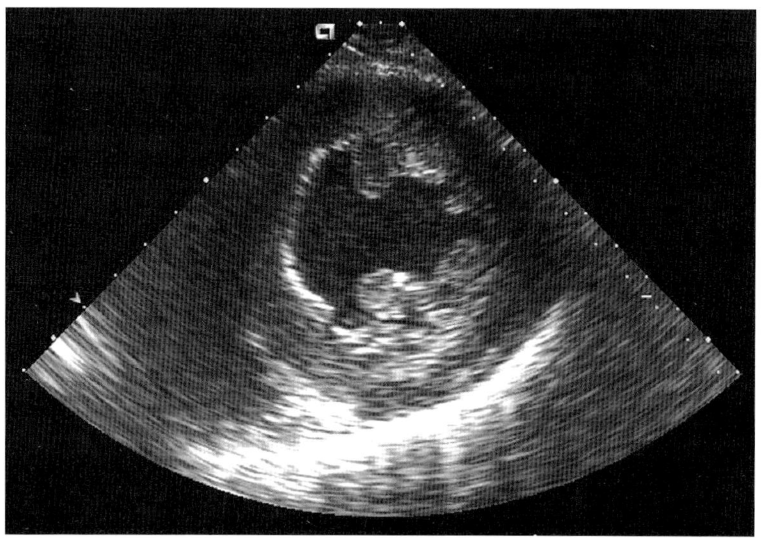

4. In the mid-esophageal four-chamber view,
   A. the anterior mitral leaflet is never longer than the posterior mitral leaflet.
   B. the anterior mitral leaflet and posterior mitral leaflet always have the same length.
   C. the posterior mitral leaflet is always longer than the anterior mitral leaflet.
   D. the anterior mitral leaflet is on the right of the image display and the posterior mitral leaflet is on the left.
   E. none of the above is correct.

5. In the accompanying image (Arch, mid aortic arch; MPA, main pulmonary artery; PV, pulmonic valve; RVOT, right ventricular outflow tract), the arrow points to

A. the false lumen of the dissected aortic arch.

B. the false lumen of the dissected ascending aorta.

C. the false lumen of the dissected descending aorta.

D. the superior vena cava.

E. the innominate vein.

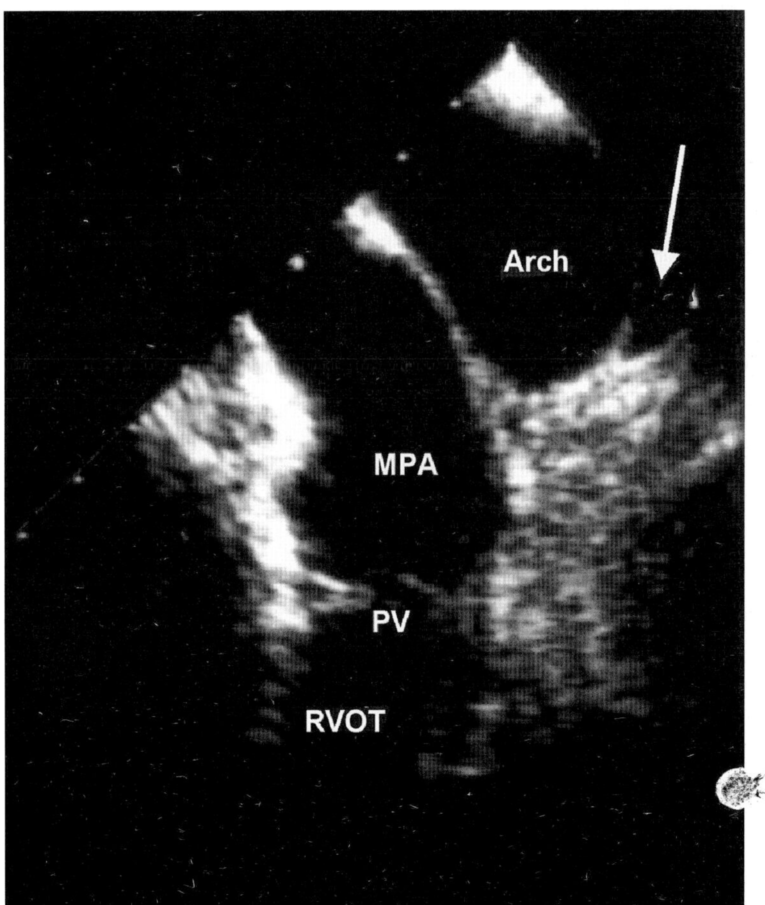

6. To obtain the image shown in Question 5, the transducer should be placed in

A. the upper esophagus.

B. the mid esophagus.

C. the lower esophagus.

D. the stomach.

E. the deep stomach.

7. The image shown in Question 5 is especially useful to evaluate

A. the dissected aortic arch.

B. aortic dissection.

C. aortic stenosis.

D. the superior vena cava.

E. Doppler flow velocity through the pulmonic valve.

8. In the accompanying mid-esophageal aortic valve short axis view, the structure indicated by the arrow is best described as

A. the ascending aorta.

B. the noncoronary cusp.

C. the left coronary cusp.

D. the right coronary cusp.

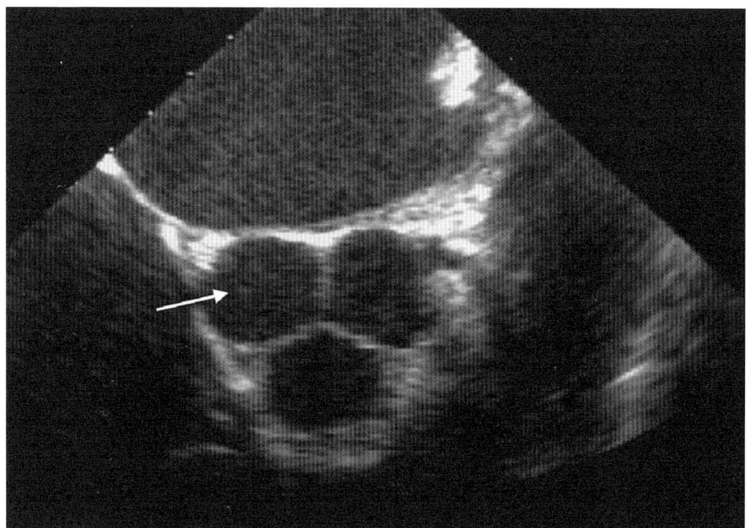

9. The arrow in the accompanying image points to
   A. the eustachian valve.
   B. the Chiari network.
   C. the cor triatrium.
   D. the tricuspid valve.
   E. the pulmonic valve.

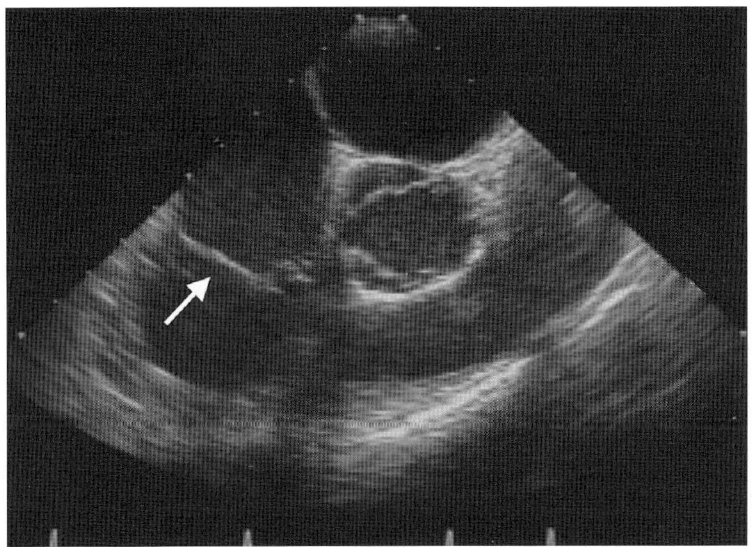

10. Which one of the following transesophageal echocardiographic views of the left atrium has good correlation with the transthoracic echocardiographically derived left atrial size?
   A. The mid-esophageal short axis view at the level of the aortic valve with the transducer rotated 30° to 60°.
   B. The mid-esophageal four-chamber view with 0° rotation.
   C. The mid-esophageal longitudinal two-chamber view with the transducer rotated to 90°.
   D. The mid-esophageal long axis view with the transducer rotated 120° to 150°.
   E. The transgastric long axis view.

11. The accompanying transesophageal echocardiographic images are obtained with the transducer placed

A. at the level of the aortic arch.
B. in the upper esophagus.
C. in the mid esophagus.
D. in the lower esophagus.
E. in the stomach.

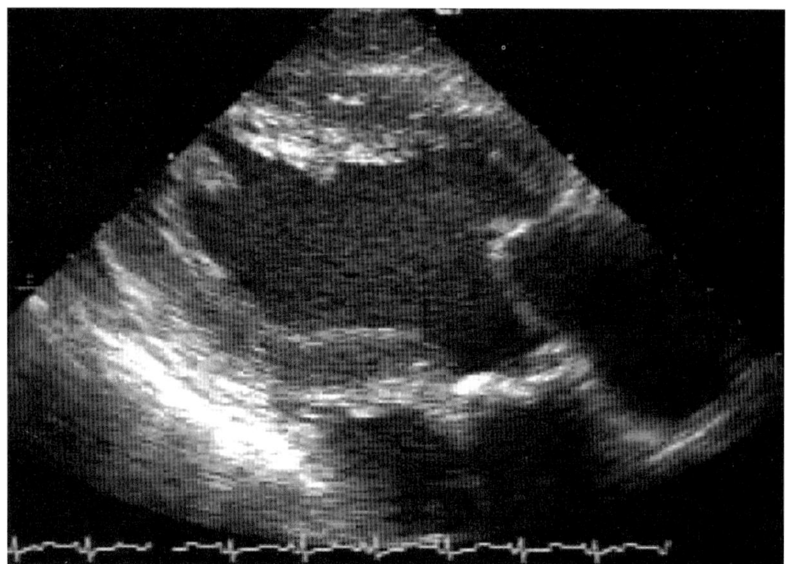

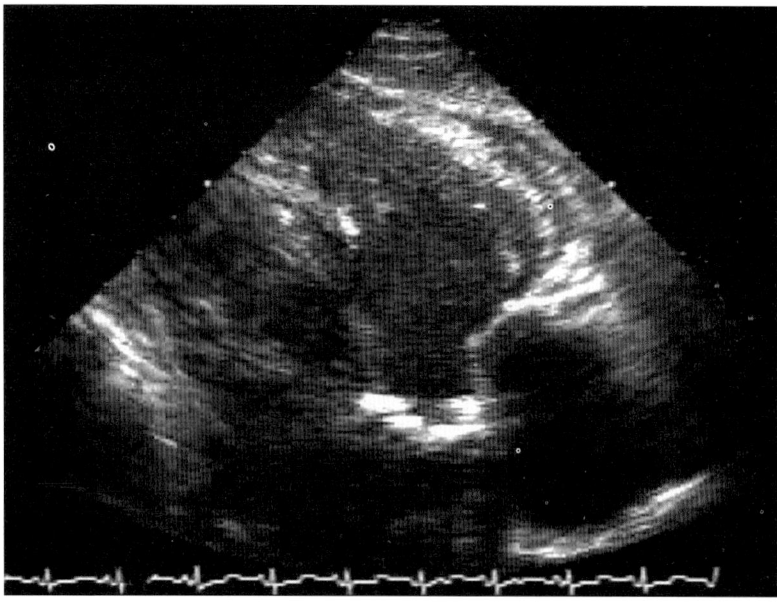

12. The images in Question 11 are especially useful to evaluate Doppler flow velocity through

A. the aortic valve.

B. the tricuspid valve.

C. the mitral valve.

D. the left ventricular outflow tract.

E. A and D.

13. In the accompanying transesophageal echocardiographic image, the structure indicated by the arrow is best described as

A. the posteromedial commissure.

B. the posterolateral commissure.

C. the anteromedial commissure.

D. the anterolateral commissure.

E. the left posterior commissure.

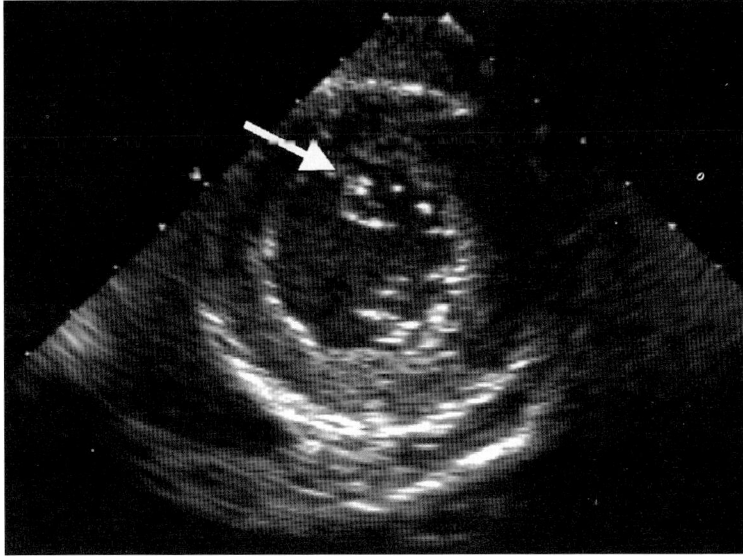

14. In the accompanying image, the arrow points to
   A. the left atrial appendage.
   B. the left lower pulmonary vein.
   C. the right lower pulmonary vein.
   D. the left upper pulmonary vein.
   E. the right upper pulmonary vein.

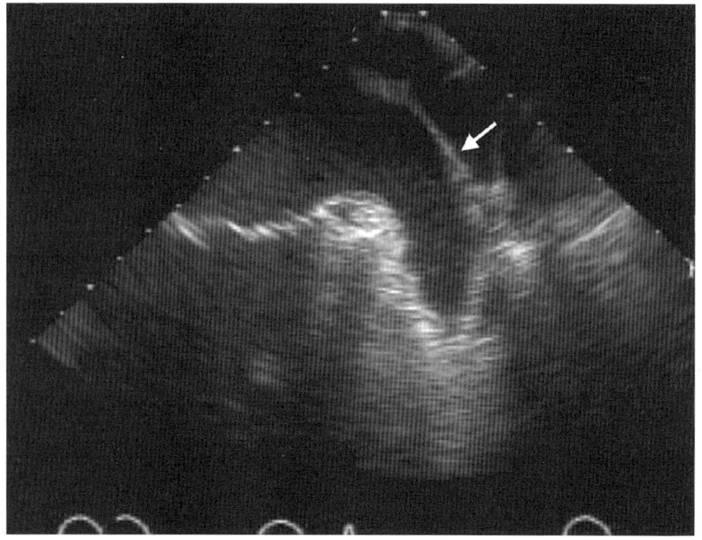

15. The sinotubular junction in the accompanying image is labeled with
   A. the letter A.
   B. the letter B.
   C. the letter C.
   D. the letter D.
   E. the letter E.

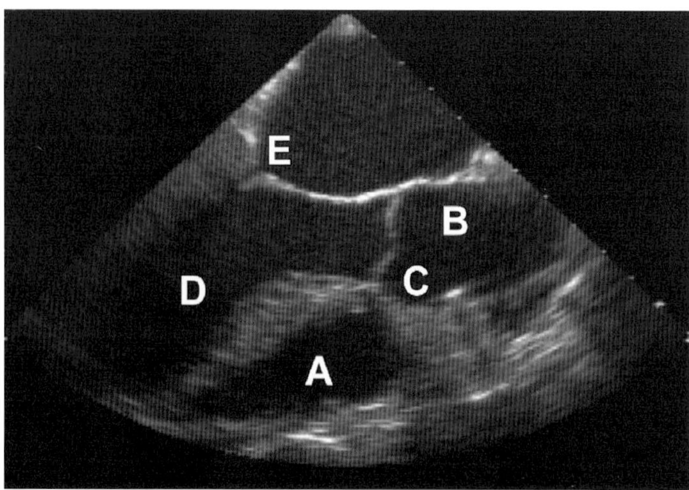

16. In the image accompanying Question 15, the cusp of the aortic valve that appears anteriorly or toward the bottom of the image display

A. is the noncoronary cusp.
B. is the left coronary cusp.
C. is the right coronary cusp.
D. may be the left or noncoronary cusp.
E. cannot be determined.

17. The cusp of the aortic valve that appears posteriorly in the image accompanying Question 15

A. is always the noncoronary cusp.
B. is always the left coronary cusp.
C. is always the right coronary cusp.
D. may be the left or noncoronary cusp.
E. may be the right or left coronary cusp.

18. In the accompanying image, the arrow points to

A. the dissected right coronary cusp.
B. the dissected left coronary cusp.
C. the dissected noncoronary cusp.
D. the left coronary artery.
E. the right coronary artery.

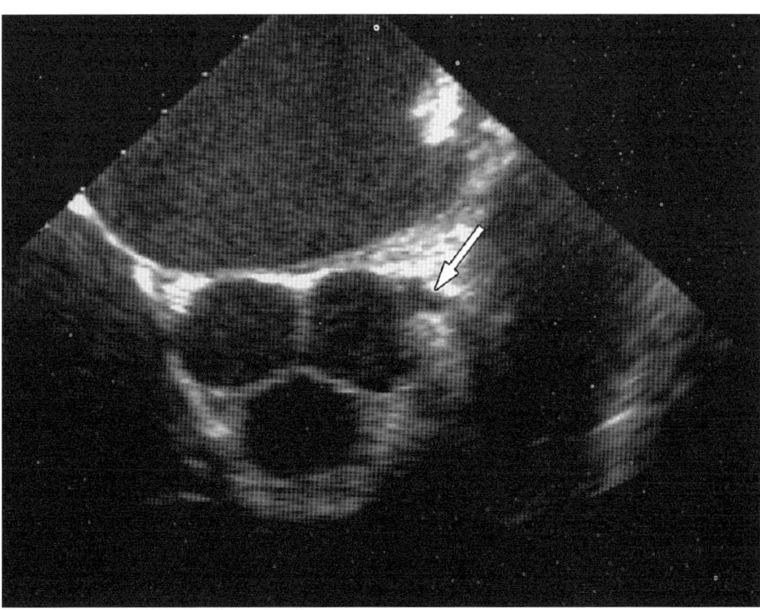

19. Most commonly, which one of the following views is used to assess left ventricular chamber size and wall thickness at end diastole?

A. Two-chamber view.
B. Four-chamber view.

C. Five-chamber view.
D. Transgastric mid short axis view.
E. Transgastric basal short axis view.

20. Which one of the following statements about pulmonary veins is true?
A. The left upper and lower pulmonary veins cannot be visualized simultaneously on a transesophageal echocardiographic image because the left upper pulmonary vein is higher than the left lower pulmonary vein.
B. The right upper and lower pulmonary veins cannot be visualized simultaneously on a transesophageal echocardiographic image because the right upper pulmonary vein is higher than the right lower pulmonary vein.
C. The left upper and lower pulmonary veins can be visualized simultaneously on a transesophageal echocardiographic image but the right upper and lower pulmonary veins cannot.
D. The right or left upper and lower pulmonary veins can be visualized simultaneously on a transesophageal echocardiographic image.
E. A and B.

21. In the accompanying image, the letter A labels
A. the descending thoracic aorta.
B. the left atrium.
C. the left lower pulmonary vein.
D. the right pulmonary artery.
E. the stomach.

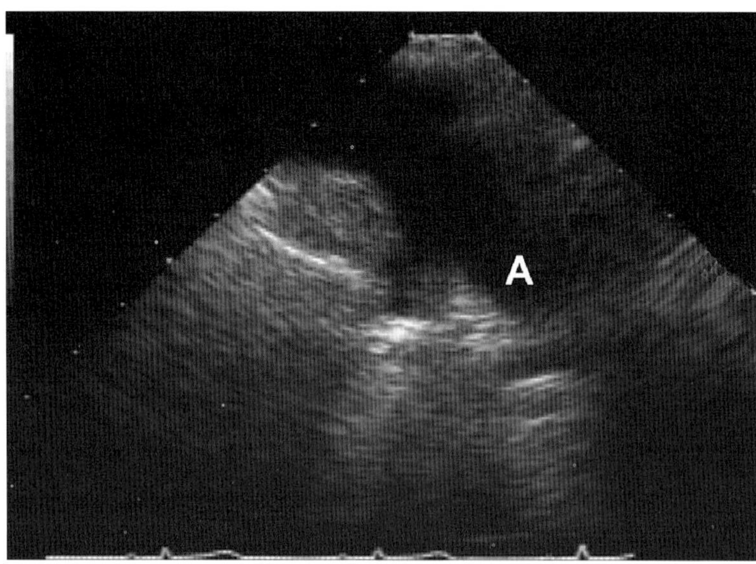

Figure from Seward et al. (34). Used with permission of Mayo Foundation for Medical Education and Research.

22. In the accompanying image, the letter A indicates
A. the inferior vena cava.
B. the superior vena cava.
C. the right upper pulmonary vein.
D. the left lower pulmonary vein.
E. the innominate vein.

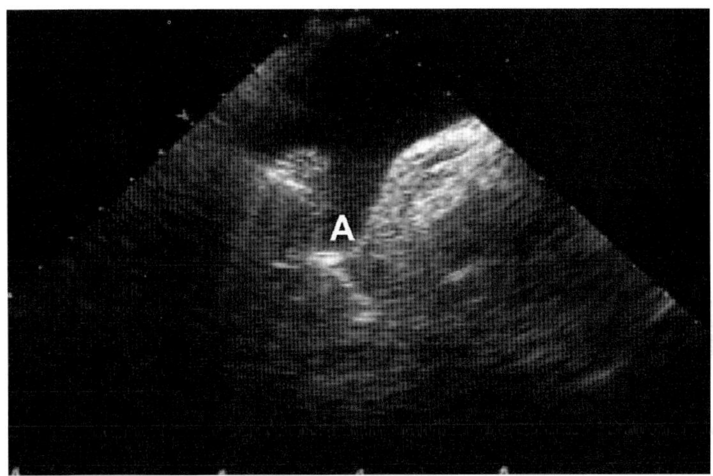

23. The image accompanying Question 22 is especially useful to evaluate
A. descending aortic dissection.
B. central line in superior vena cava.
C. aortic plaque.
D. anomalous pulmonary venous connection.
E. embolus in the distal left pulmonary artery.

24. According to recommendations from the American Society of Echocardiography, which one of the following statements about the phases of the cardiac cycle and the timing of events relative to electrocardiography is true?
A. In the two-chamber view, the end-diastolic image is the frame synchronized at the end of the PR interval on the electrocardiogram.
B. In the four-chamber view, the end-diastolic image is the frame synchronized with the peak of the R wave on the electrocardiogram.
C. In the five-chamber view, the end-systolic frame is synchronized with the beginning of the ST segment.
D. In the transgastric short axis view, the end-diastolic frame is synchronized at the Q wave or the beginning of the R wave.
E. None of the above.

25. The diameter of the aortic valve anulus is measured
A. from the trailing edge to the trailing edge of the aortic valve anulus during diastole.

B. from the leading edge to the trailing edge of the aortic valve anulus during diastole.

C. from the leading edge to the leading edge of the aortic valve anulus during diastole.

D. as the inner diameter of the aortic valve anulus during diastole.

E. at the points of attachment of the aortic valve cusps to the anulus during systole.

26. In the accompanying image, the arrow points to

A. the right atrium.

B. the right atrial appendage.

C. the right ventricle.

D. the right atrial aneurysm.

E. the right atrial pseudoaneurysm.

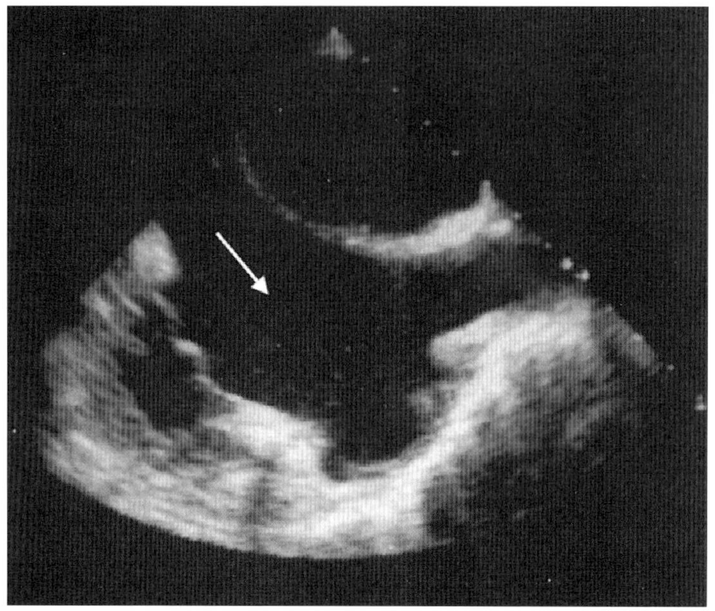

27. The accompanying transesophageal echocardiographic image is obtained with the probe in the mid esophagus. The arrow points to

A. the left main coronary artery.
B. the left anterior descending coronary artery.
C. the left circumflex coronary artery.
D. the right coronary artery.
E. the coronary sinus.

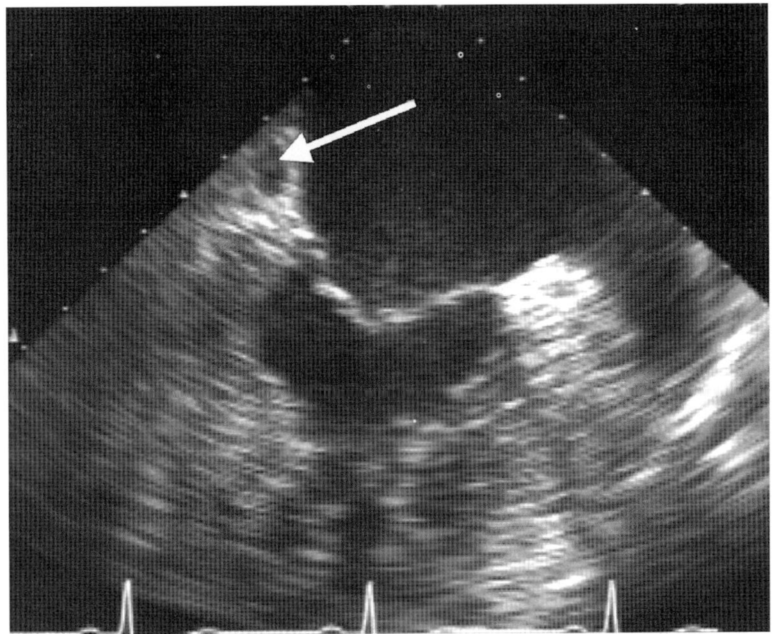

28. In the accompanying image, the arrow points to
A. the transverse sinus.
B. the oblique sinus.
C. the coronary sinus.
D. the atrial septal defect.
E. the secundum atrial septal defect.

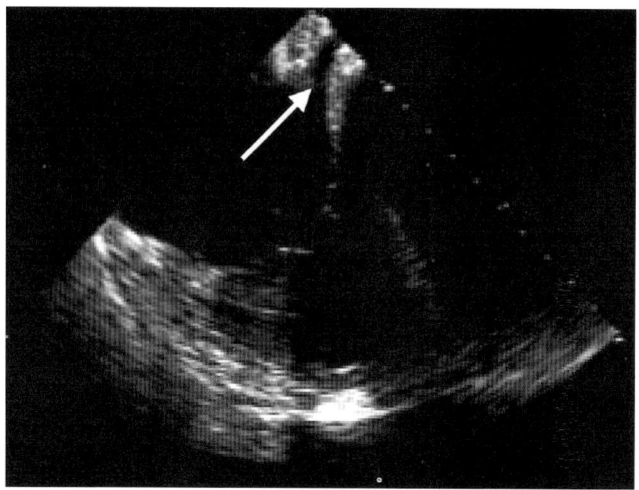

29. Color flow mapping of the image accompanying Question 28 shows flow
A. away from the transducer at 0.34 m/s.
B. away from the transducer at 3.4 m/s.
C. away from the transducer at 34 m/s.
D. toward the transducer at 34 m/s.
E. toward the transducer at 0.34 m/s.

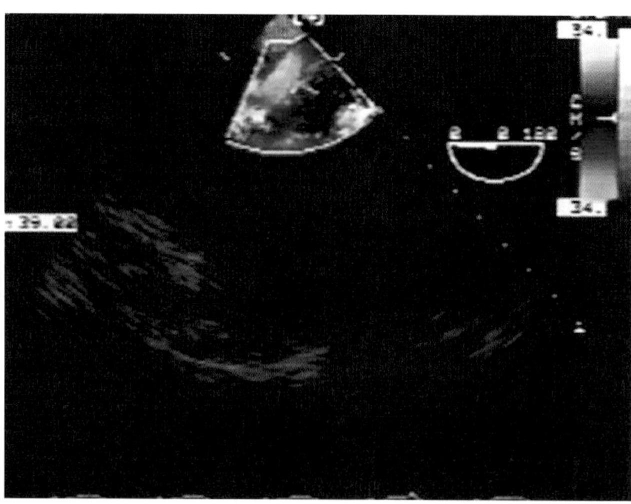

30. An 80-year-old patient undergoes mitral valve repair and coronary artery bypass graft surgery. The accompanying image is obtained during intraoperative transesophageal echocardiography. The letter X labels

A. the left ventricle.
B. the right atrium.
C. the left atrium.
D. the left atrial appendage.
E. the right atrial appendage.

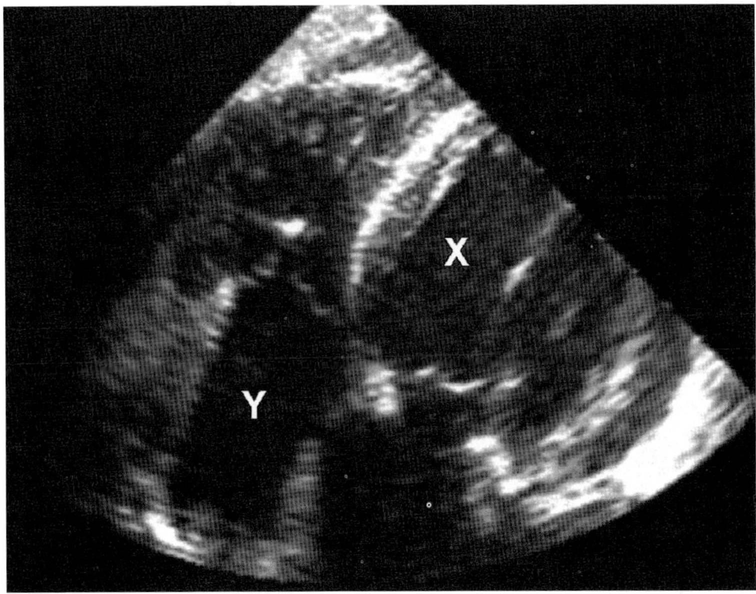

31. In the image accompanying Question 30, the cardiac chamber labeled by the letter Y is

A. the right atrium.
B. the right ventricle.
C. the left atrium.
D. the left ventricle.
E. the left ventricular outflow tract.

32. The image accompanying Question 30 is obtained with the transducer placed

A. at the level of aortic arch.
B. in the upper esophagus.
C. in the mid esophagus.
D. in the lower esophagus.
E. deep in the stomach.

33. Which one of the following structures in the accompanying figure is labeled with the letter X?

A. The descending thoracic aorta.
B. The ascending thoracic aorta.
C. The right pulmonary artery.
D. The left pulmonary artery.
E. The main pulmonary artery.

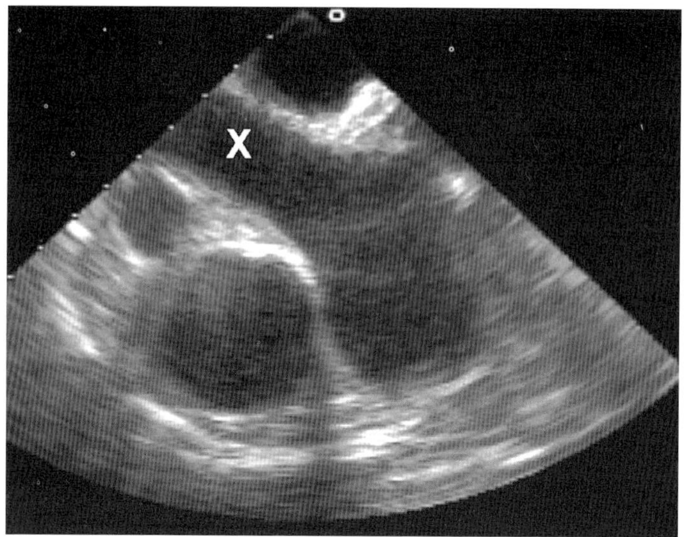

34. In the accompanying transesophageal echocardiographic image, the arrow indicates

A. the dissected proximal ascending aorta.
B. the ruptured right coronary cusp.
C. the ruptured left coronary cusp.
D. the right coronary artery.
E. the left coronary artery.

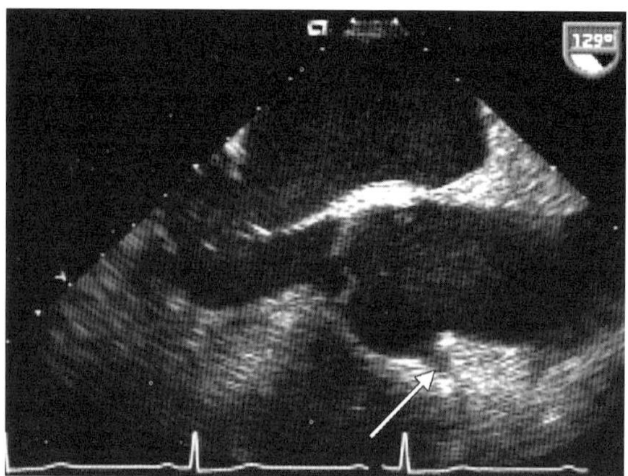

35. In the accompanying transesophageal echocardiographic image, the arrow points to
A. the right atrial pseudoaneurysm.
B. the right atrial appendage.
C. the right atrial aneurysm.
D. the right ventricular aneurysm.
E. the right atrial cyst.

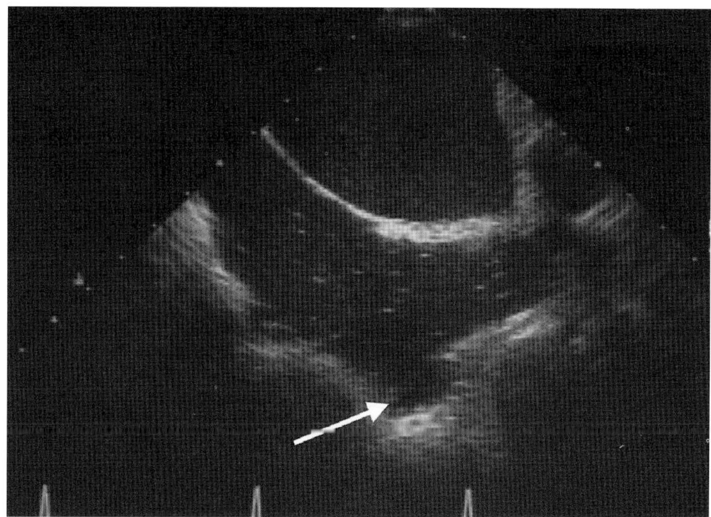

36. Normally, the right ventricle
A. does not exceed two-thirds of the left ventricle in a four-chamber view.
B. has a crescent shape in a transgastric short axis view.
C. has wall thickness less than 5 mm at the end of diastole.
D. has its apex not beyond that of the left ventricle in a four-chamber view.
E. has all of the above.

37. According to the Carpentier nomenclature,
A. the posterior mitral leaflet is divided into three scallops, and the anterior leaflet is divided into two scallops.
B. the anterior mitral leaflet is divided into three scallops, and the posterior leaflet is divided into two scallops.
C. the posterior mitral leaflet is divided into three scallops, and the anterior mitral leaflet is not divided.
D. the anterior mitral leaflet is divided into three scallops, and the posterior mitral leaflet is not divided.
E. the posterior mitral leaflet is divided into three scallops, and the anterior mitral leaflet is divided into three corresponding segments.

38. Which one of the following is usually visualized in a four-chamber view?
A. The posterior elements of the mitral leaflets.
B. The anterior element of the anterior mitral leaflet.

C. The anterior element of the posterior mitral leaflet.
D. A1 (lateral part).
E. P1 (lateral scallop).

39. In mid-esophageal five-chamber view, which one of the following is usually visualized?
A. A1 (lateral part) is to the left of the display, and P1 (lateral scallop) is to the right.
B. A1 (lateral part) is to the right of the display, and P1 (lateral scallop) is to the left.
C. A2 (middle part) is to the right of the display, and P2 (middle scallop) is to the left.
D. A3 (medial part) is to the left of the display, and P3 (medial scallop) is to the right.
E. A3 (medial part) is to the right of the display, and P3 (medial scallop) is to the left.

40. From the right to the left of the echocardiographic display screen, which of the following are visualized in a mid-esophageal commissural view?
A. A1 (lateral), A2 (middle), A3 (medial).
B. A1 (lateral), A2 (middle), P3 (medial).
C. A1 (lateral), P2 (middle), P3 (medial).
D. P1 (lateral), P2 (middle), P3 (medial).
E. P1 (lateral), A2 (middle), P3 (medial).

Answers & Discussion

1. Answer C

A four-chamber view is obtained with the transesophageal echocardiographic probe placed in the mid esophagus. Because the apex of the left ventricle is more inferior to the base, it may not be included in a four-chamber view if the tip of the probe is in the neutral position. This phenomenon is called foreshortening. It is important to realize that the left ventricular apex may not be visualized in a four-chamber view with the tip of the probe in the neutral position because of foreshortening. Anteflexion means flexing the tip of the probe anteriorly with the large control wheel. It usually makes the problem of foreshortening worse. To visualize and evaluate the left ventricular apex in a four-chamber view, the tip of the probe may require retroflexion (flexing the tip posteriorly) to direct the imaging plane through the apex. **Reference** 37.

2. Answer E

Most of the thoracic aorta can be routinely imaged with multiplane transesophageal echocardiography because it is adjacent to the esophagus as it passes vertically through the mediastinum. However, the distal ascending aorta and the proximal aortic arch usually cannot be visualized with transesophageal echocardiography because the air-filled left main bronchus and distal trachea are interposed between these regions and the esophagus. Air in the respiratory tract causes ultrasound waves to scatter, leading to diminished echocardiographic signals owing to attenuation. **References** 11 *(p 427)*; 23 *(p 197)*.

3. Answer D

The left ventricle (LV) is divided into three levels along its length. These are basal, mid, and apical levels. The tip of the papillary muscles represents the border between the mid and the basal levels, and the base of the papillary muscles represents the border between the mid and the apical levels. The mid level is the only portion containing the papillary muscles.

In patients with left ventricular hypertrophy, thickened walls and reduced chamber size may cause confusion, whether the image is obtained at the mid or the apical level. In such a situation, it is helpful to look for the papillary muscles to determine whether the image is a mid or an apical short axis view. If the papillary muscle is present, the image is a transgastric mid short axis view. In contrast, a transgastric apical short axis view does not contain papillary muscles. Therefore, the accompanying image is a transgastric mid short axis view because of the presence of the papillary muscles. **References** 10 *(pp 88–90)*; 11 *(pp 114, 116)*; 33; 37.

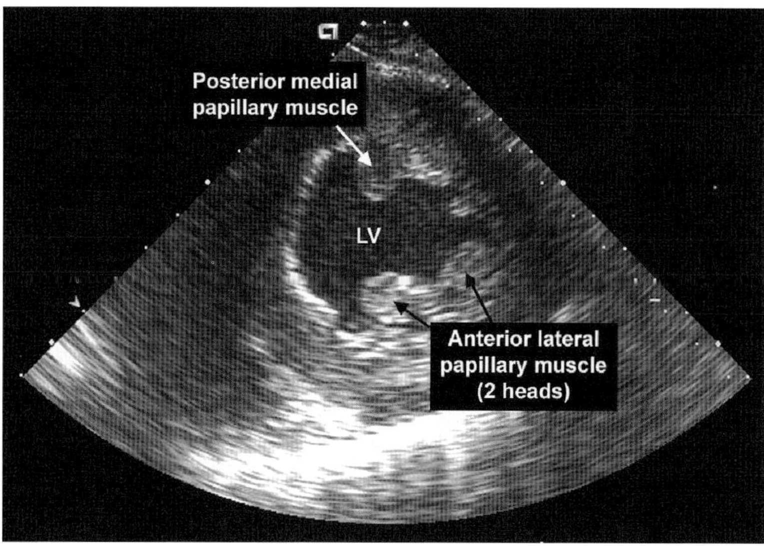

4. Answer E

In a mid-esophageal four-chamber view, the anterior mitral leaflet is on the left side of the image display and the posterior mitral leaflet is on the right. Usually, the anterior mitral leaflet is longer than the posterior leaflet in a mid-esophageal four-chamber view. **Reference** 37.

5. Answer E

6. Answer A

7. Answer E

The image shown in Question 5 is an upper esophageal aortic arch short axis view. This view is obtained with the transducer placed high in the upper esophagus, posterior to the aortic arch. It shows the longitudinal view of the main pulmonary artery, pulmonic valve, right ventricular outflow tract, mid aortic arch, and innominate vein.

This image is especially useful to evaluate Doppler velocity and pressure gradient across the pulmonic valve because this image allows the ultrasound beam to be aligned parallel to the blood flow through the pulmonic valve and main pulmonary artery.

Hence, the Doppler velocity and pressure gradient across the pulmonic valve are assessed more accurately. **References** 11 *(p 121)*; 37.

8. Answer B

The accompanying image is a mid-esophageal aortic valve short axis view obtained by placing the transducer in the mid esophagus with a multiplane angle at about 45°. This cross section is the only view that provides a simultaneous image of all three cusps of the aortic valve. The cusp adjacent to the atrial septum is the noncoronary cusp (NC). The right coronary cusp (RC) is located most anteriorly, and the left coronary cusp (LC) is on the right side of the display. LM indicates the left main coronary artery. **References** 11 *(pp 110–111, 117, 119)*; 37.

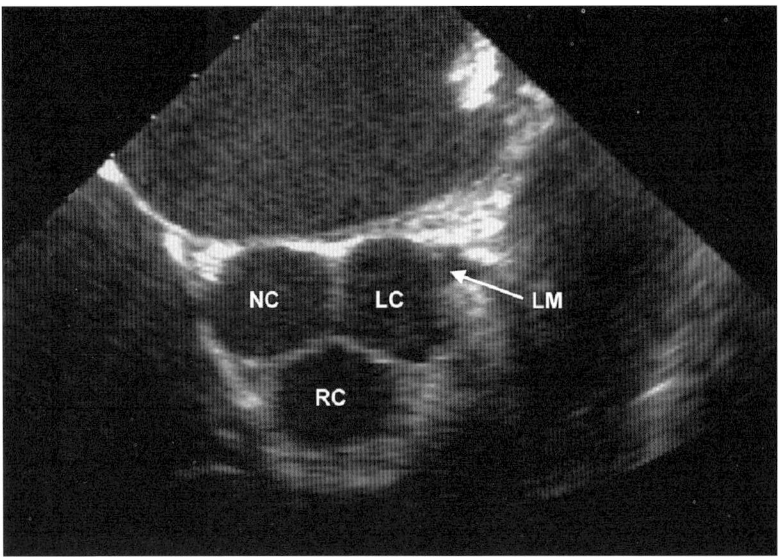

9. Answer D

The image in Question 9 is a mid-esophageal right ventricular inflow-outflow view. The image is developed by placing the transducer in the mid esophagus and rotating the multiplane angle to about 90°. The cross section shows the right ventricular outflow tract to the right side of the display and the inferior portion of the right ventricular free wall to the left. The arrow points to the tricuspid valve.

The tricuspid valve has three leaflets (anterior, posterior, and septal). The posterior leaflet of the tricuspid valve is on the left side of the display, and the anterior leaflet of the tricuspid valve is on the right. The septal leaflet of the tricuspid valve is not visualized in this image but can be seen in a four-chamber view. The mid-esophageal four-chamber view shows the septal leaflet to the right side of the display and the posterior leaflet to the left. (AV indicates aortic valve; LA, left atrium; PV, pulmonic valve; RA, right atrium; and RV, right ventricle.) **Reference** 37.

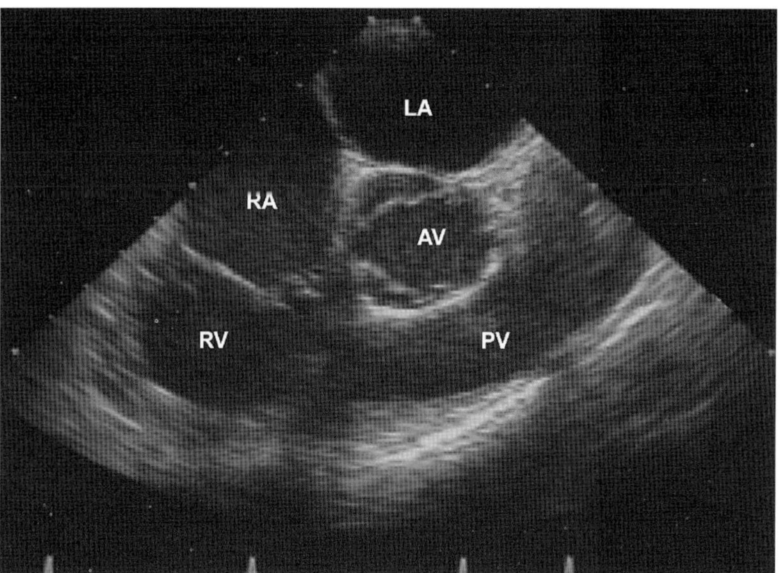

10. Answer A

The parasternal long axis measurement of the left atrium by transthoracic echocardiography at the level of the aortic valve is widely used to determine the left atrial dimension. In contrast to transthoracic echocardiography, transesophageal echocardiographic measurement of left atrial dimensions has not been standardized. Because the left atrium is imaged from a different perspective by transesophageal echocardiography than with transthoracic echocardiography, the planes of measurement are potentially different. Adequate and complete visualization of the left atrium may not be obtainable by transesophageal echocardiography because of the restricted position of the transducer within the esophagus and the variable apposition of the esophagus to the left atrium, resulting in limited, incomplete visualization of the left atrium in the scan sector. Block et al compared left atrial dimensions in four standard views by transthoracic echocardiography in 121 patients undergoing transesophageal echocardiography. The mid-esophageal basal short axis view at the level of the aortic valve with the transducer rotated 30° to 60° was the only transesophageal echocardiographic view in which complete left atrial dimensions could be reliably measured. The left atrial dimension measured by this view had the highest correlation to that measured by the corresponding transthoracic echocardiographic view. The reason for this relatively high correlation is the landmark provided by the aortic valve seen in the cross section, which ensures that the left atrial measurements are made at a similar level by both transthoracic and transesophageal echocardiographic techniques. **Reference** 4.

11. Answer E

12. Answer E

The accompanying transgastric images are obtained with the transducer placed in the stomach. The top image is the transgastric long axis view, which is developed from the transgastric mid-papillary short axis view by rotating the multiplane angle forward to about 90° until the aortic valve comes into view in the right side of the far field. The bottom image is the deep transgastric long axis view obtained by advancing the probe deeper into the stomach and anteflexing the probe. In the deep transgastric long axis view, the aortic valve is located in the far field at the bottom of the display with the left ventricular outflow directed away from the transducer.

The primary purpose of these two transgastric views of the aortic valve is to direct a Doppler beam parallel to the blood flow through the left ventricular outflow tract and the aortic valve, which is not possible from the mid-esophageal window. Doppler quantification of blood flow velocities through the left ventricular outflow tract and aortic valve are performed more accurately using transgastric views. Blood flow velocity in the left ventricular outflow tract is measured by positioning the pulsed wave Doppler sample volume in the center of the left ventricular outflow tract, just proximal to the aortic valve. Flow velocity through the aortic valve is measured by directing the continuous wave Doppler beam through the left ventricular outflow tract and across the aortic valve. Normal left ventricular outflow tract and aortic valve flow velocities are less than 1.5 m/s. (AV indicates aortic valve; LA, left atrium; and LV, left ventricle.) **Reference** 37.

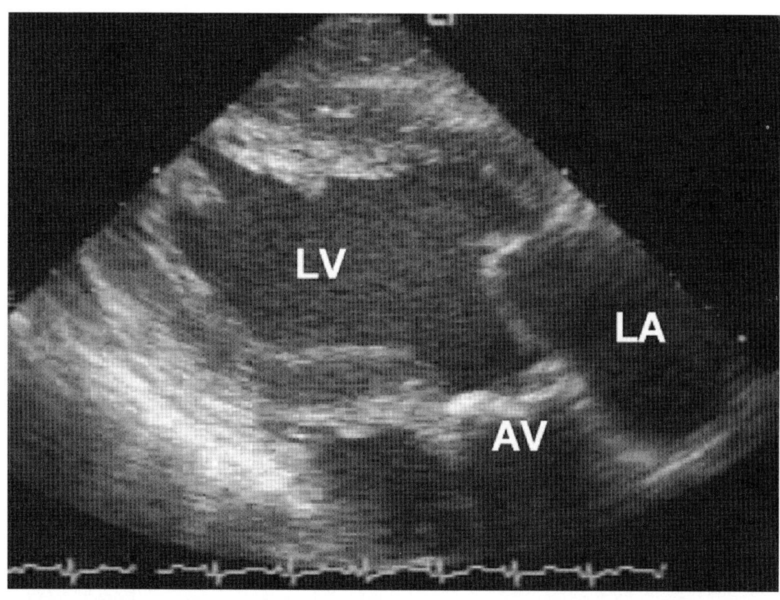

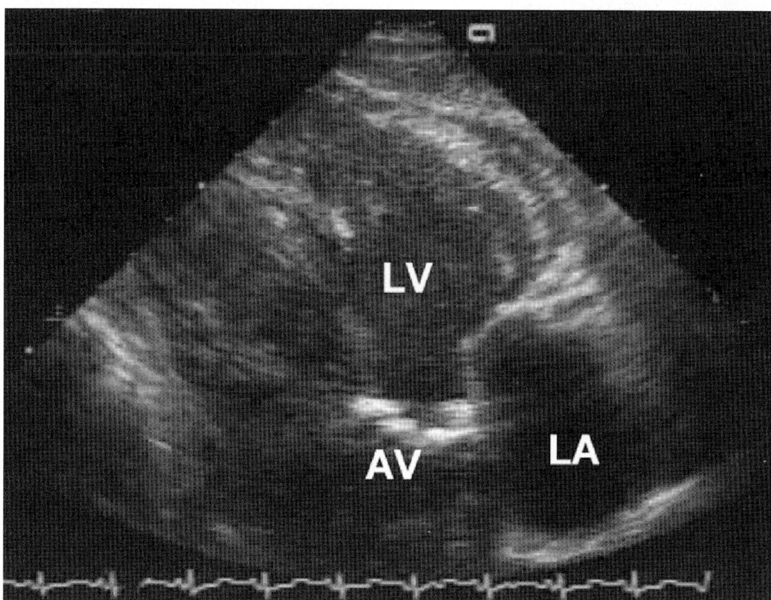

13. Answer A

In this transgastric basal short axis view, the posteromedial commissure is in the upper left of the display and the anterolateral commissure is to the lower right. In addition, the posterior leaflet of the mitral valve is to the right of the display and the anterior leaflet is to the left. Therefore, the arrow is pointing to the posteromedial commissure of the mitral valve. **Reference** 37.

14. Answer D

The image accompanying the question is obtained with the transducer in the mid esophagus. The arrow points to the left upper pulmonary vein, which enters the left atrium just lateral to the left atrial appendage. The image below resembles that shown in Question 14, with all structures labeled (Asc Ao, ascending aorta; LA, left atrium; LAA, left atrial appendage; LUPV, left upper pulmonary vein; PA, pulmonary artery; arrows, "Q-tip sign," the junction between LAA and LUPV). **Reference** 11 *(p 139)*.

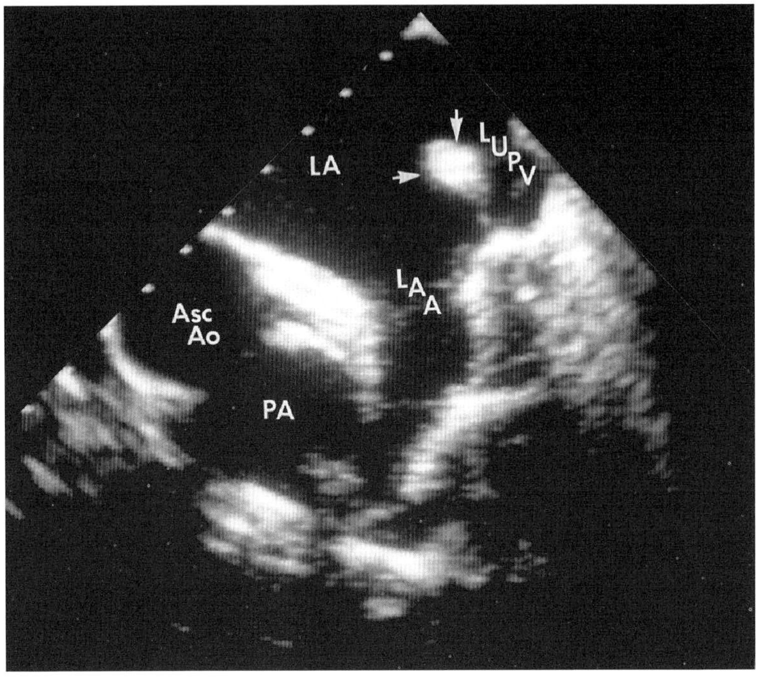

Figure from Seward et al. (35). Used with permission.

15. Answer B

16. Answer C

17. Answer D

The image in Question 15 is a mid-esophageal aortic valve long axis view, obtained with the array at about 120° to 160° until the left ventricular outflow tract, aortic valve, and proximal ascending aorta line up in the image. The sinotubular junction is labeled with the letter B and is the junction between the sinus of Valsalva and the proximal ascending aorta.

The cusp of the aortic valve that appears anteriorly or toward the bottom of the display is always the right coronary cusp, but the cusp that appears posteriorly in the cross section may be the left or the noncoronary cusp, depending on the exact location of the imaging plane as it passes through the valve. The mid-esophageal aortic long axis view is the best cross section for assessing the size of the aortic root by measuring the diameters of the aortic valve anulus, sinuses of Valsalva, sinotubular junction, and proximal ascending aorta. **Reference** 37.

18. Answer D

The accompanying image is an optimal short axis view of the aortic valve. It is obtained by placing the transducer in the mid esophagus and rotating the multiplane array to about 45°. The cusp on the right side of the display is the left coronary cusp. The arrow points to the left coronary artery with its ostium (LC, left coronary cusp; LM, left main coronary artery; NC, noncoronary cusp; RC, right coronary cusp). **References** 11 *(p 121)*; 34 *(p 545)*.

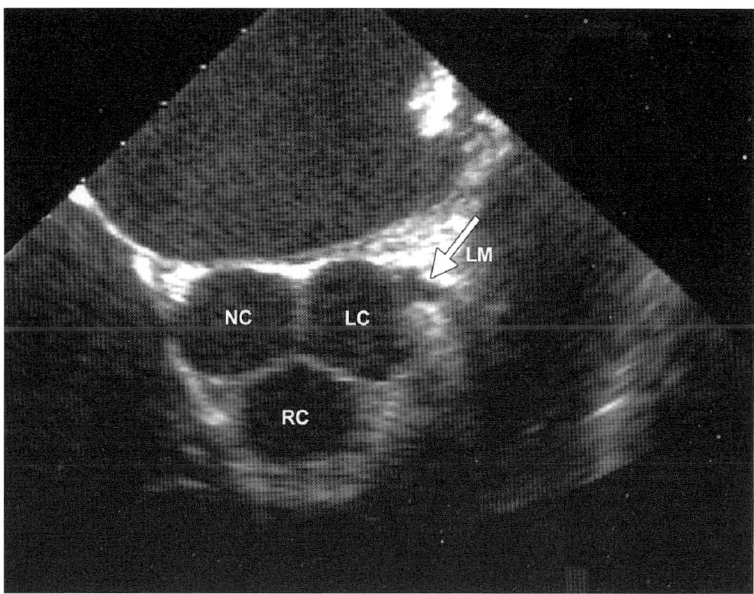

19. Answer D

Most commonly, the transgastric mid-esophageal short axis view is used for assessing left ventricular chamber size and wall thickness at the end of diastole, which is indicated by the Q wave or the onset of the R wave of the electrocardiogram. Normal left ventricular short axis diameter is less than 5.5 cm at the end of diastole and left ventricular wall thickness is less than 1.2 cm. (See also Question 24.) **References** 10 *(p 134)*; 37.

20. Answer D

21. Answer C

The right or left upper and lower pulmonary veins can be visualized simultaneously on the transesophageal echocardiography image.

To image the right pulmonary veins simultaneously, the multiplane array should be maintained at 70° to 80° and the shaft of the probe should be rotated rightward to view the Y configuration of the right upper and lower pulmonary veins as they enter the left atrium. To image the left pulmonary veins simultaneously, the array should be positioned at 100° to 110° and the shaft of the probe should be rotated toward the left to view the Y configuration of the left upper and lower pulmonary veins emptying into the left atrium. Therefore, the letter A labels the left lower pulmonary vein. **References** 11 *(pp 115–116, 120)*; 23 *(pp 31–32)*; 34.

22. Answer C

23. Answer D

This is an upper esophageal view with the array at 0°. The letter A indicates the right upper pulmonary vein located anterior to the right pulmonary artery and medial to the superior vena cava. Any anomalous connection of this vein to superior vena cava usually can be visualized in this view.

The typical anomalous pulmonary venous connection of the right upper pulmonary vein occurs in the medial superior vena cava, resulting in a "teardrop" appearance of the superior vena cava. **References** 1; 11 *(p 118)*; 34.

24. Answer D

According to the American Society of Echocardiography recommendation, the end-diastolic image is the frame synchronized with the Q wave or the onset of the R wave of the electrocardiogram. Usually, the transgastric mid short axis view is used for evaluation of left ventricular chamber size. The end-diastolic dimension of the left ventricle is best determined by measuring the chamber size in the transgastric short axis view at the Q wave or the onset of the R wave of the electrocardiogram. When the transgastric mid short axis view is used to evaluate the left ventricular end-systolic dimension, the frame synchronized with the smallest size of the left ventricle should be used to measure the end-systolic dimension. (See also Question 19.) **References** 10 *(p 134)*; 37.

25. Answer E

The diameter of the aortic valve anulus is measured at the points of attachment of the aortic valve cusps to the anulus during systole. Its normal range is 1.8 to 2.5 cm. **Reference** 37.

26. Answer A

The image accompanying the question is a longitudinal view with the transducer placed in the mid esophagus at 90°. The arrow in the image points to the right atrium. The completely labeled image is seen here (IVC, inferior vena cava; LA, left atrium; RA, right atrium; RAA, right atrial appendage; SVC, superior vena cava; TV, tricuspid valve). **References** 11 *(p 112)*; 34 *(p 535)*.

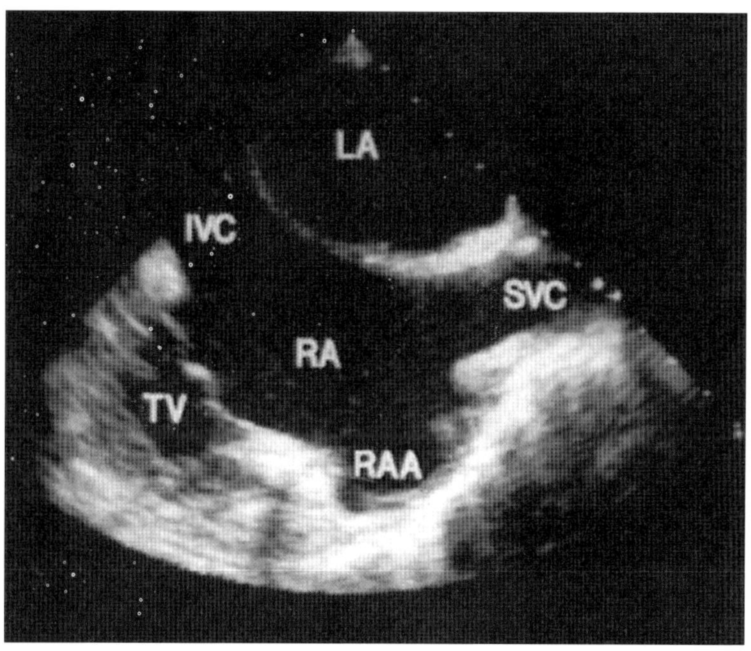

Figure from Seward et al. (34). Used with permission of Mayo Foundation for Medical Education and Research.

27. Answer E

In the mid-esophageal two-chamber view in Question 27, the left ventricular inferior wall is to the left of the display and the anterior wall is to the right. The structure indicated by the arrow is the coronary sinus. (See also Questions 28 and 29.) **Reference** 11 *(pp 39, 43)*.

28. Answer C

29. Answer A

The arrow in the image accompanying Question 28 points to the coronary sinus. This image is obtained by slightly advancing the probe from the mid-esophageal four-chamber view. The coronary sinus is located in the atrioventricular groove along the posterior surface of the heart and empties into the right atrium at the most inferior and posterior extent of the atrial septum adjacent to the septal leaflet of the tricuspid valve.

Conventionally, blue color in a color flow image is positioned in the lower part of the color map and represents negative Doppler frequency shifts caused by blood flow away from the transducer. In addition, the highest velocity away from the transducer (within the Nyquist frequency) is indicated by the color at the bottom of the color map. In the color flow image accompanying Question 29, the blue color has the velocity of 34 cm/s or 0.34 m/s as indicated by the color map. Therefore, the Doppler velocity of the blood flow in the coronary sinus is 0.34 m/s away from the transducer. **References** 11 *(pp 38, 42)*; 23 *(pp 20–22)*; 24 *(p 176)*; 26 *(p 77)*; 32 *(p 42)*.

30. Answer A

31. Answer A

32. Answer E

The image accompanying Question 30 is obtained with the transducer placed deep in the stomach and anteflexed. Because the transesophageal echocardiographic transducer images the heart from the apex to the base, this four-chamber view is reversed; that is, the cardiac chambers closer to the probe are the ventricles. Because the right heart is to the left of the display and the left heart to the right, the letter X indicates the left ventricle and the letter Y labels the right atrium. **Reference** 11 *(pp 45, 46)*.

33. Answer C

The image accompanying Question 33 is the mid-esophageal ascending aortic short axis view. It is a transverse plane view and shows the main pulmonary artery with its bifurcation. The right pulmonary artery is on the left side of the display and the left pulmonary artery on the right. Therefore, the letter X labels the right pulmonary artery. **References** 11 *(p 118)*; 34; 37.

34. Answer D

The image accompanying Question 34 is a mid-esophageal long axis view with the multiplane array at about 130°. Because the right coronary cusp with its ostium is located anteriorly or at the bottom of the image, the arrow points to the proximal part of the right coronary artery that originates from the corresponding ostium. **References** 11 *(p 180)*; 37.

35. Answer B

The image accompanying Question 35 is a bicaval view with the multiplane array at about 90°. The arrow points to the right atrial appendage. The superior vena cava is located on the right side of the display and the inferior vena cava to the left. Both superior and inferior venae cavae enter the right atrium. **References** 11 *(p 112)*; 34 *(p 535)*.

36. Answer E

During transesophageal echocardiography, the right ventricle is commonly evaluated by a mid-esophageal four-chamber view and a transgastric short axis view. In a four-chamber view, the right ventricular chamber size should not exceed two-thirds of the left ventricular chamber size, and its apex does not exceed the left ventricular apex in normal subjects. In a transgastric short axis view, a normal right ventricle has a crescent appearance, and the end-diastolic wall thickness of less than 5 mm is considered normal. In patients with severe right ventricular dysfunction, transesophageal echocardiography demonstrates severe hypokinesis or akinesis of the right ventricular free wall, enlargement of the right ventricle with the right ventricular apex reaching to or beyond the left ventricular apex, a change in shape of the right ventricle from crescent to round, and a flattening or bulging of the ventricular septum toward the left ventricle. **References** 10 *(pp 158–163)*; 42 *(pp 901–919)*.

37. Answer E

According to the Carpentier nomenclature of the mitral valve, the posterior leaflet is divided into three scallops: P1, P2, and P3, as shown in the accompanying figure. P1 is adjacent to the anterolateral commissure, near the left atrial appendage. P3 is adjacent to the posteromedial commissure. The anterior leaflet is also divided into three segments: A1, A2, and A3, located opposite the corresponding scallops of the posterior leaflet. P1 corresponds to the anterolateral scallop of the posterior mitral leaflet in the classic anatomic nomenclature, P2 to the middle scallop, and P3 to the posteromedial scallop. A1, A2, and A3 correspond to the anterolateral, middle, and posteromedial segments of the anterior mitral leaflet, respectively. (Ao indicates aortic; L, left coronary cusp; N, noncoronary cusp; R, right coronary cusp.) **Reference** 19.

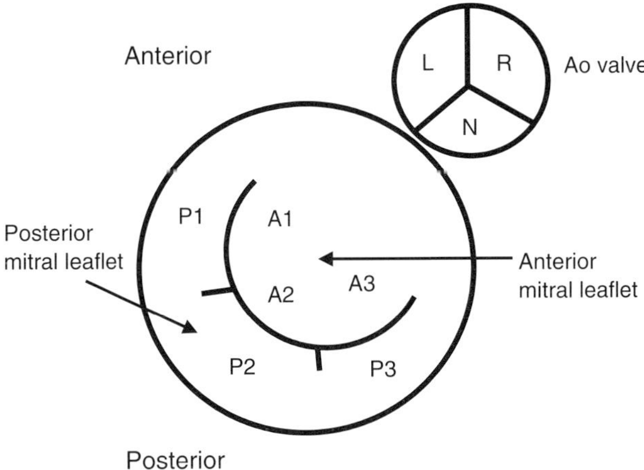

From Lambert et al. (19). Used with permission.

38. Answer A

During transesophageal echocardiography, the four-chamber view generally shows the posterior elements of the mitral leaflets. The anterior elements of the mitral leaflets usually cannot be visualized. Because A1 and P1 are located anteriorly, they are not visualized in a four-chamber view. **Reference** 19.

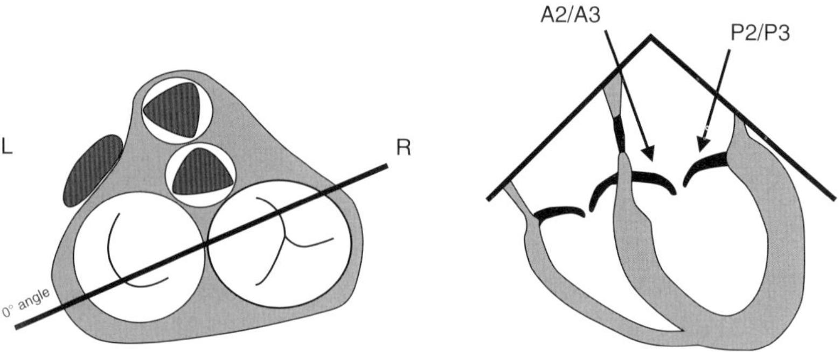

Figure from Lambert et al. (19). Used with permission.

39. Answer A

In the mid-esophageal five-chamber view, the anterior mitral leaflet (A1) is on the left side of the display and the posterior mitral leaflet (P1) on the right side of the display. Generally, the five-chamber view shows anterior elements of the mitral leaflets although the specific scallops visible depend on the image plane. The posterior elements of the mitral leaflets (A3 and P3) are usually not visualized in a five-chamber view. **Reference** 19.

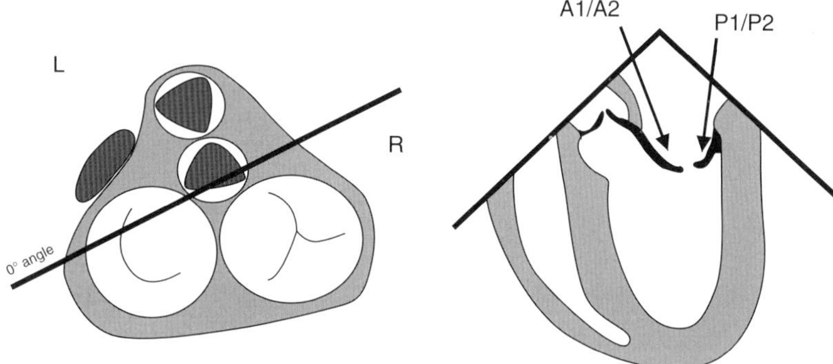

Figure from Lambert et al. (19). Used with permission.

40. Answer E

In the mid-esophageal commissural view, P1, A2, and P3 are visualized from the right to the left side of the display screen. Three scallops and two coaptation points are seen in this image: P1, P3, and a variable amount of A2, which disappears during diastole. **Reference** 19.

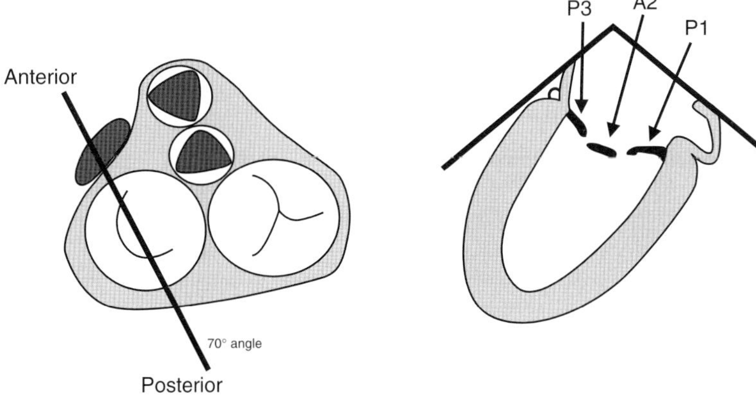

Figure from Lambert et al. (19). Used with permission.

Chapter 9

Myocardial Ischemia and Segmental Ventricular Function

Questions

Multiple choice (choose the *one* best answer):

1. To accurately describe the location and extent of regional wall motion abnormalities, which one of the following is recommended by the American Society of Echocardiography/Society of Cardiovascular Anesthesiologists guidelines for performing comprehensive intraoperative multiplane transesophageal echocardiography?
   A. A 12-segment model of the left ventricle.
   B. A 14-segment model of the left ventricle.
   C. A 16-segment model of the left ventricle.
   D. An 18-segment model of the left ventricle.
   E. A 20-segment model of the left ventricle.

2. According to the American Society of Echocardiography/Society of Cardiovascular Anesthesiologists guidelines for performing comprehensive intraoperative multiplane transesophageal echocardiography, which one of the following statements about the numeric scoring system of ventricular wall motion is true?
   A. Mild hypokinesis has a score of 1.
   B. Severe hypokinesis has a score of 2.
   C. Dyskinesis has a score of 3.
   D. Akinesis has a score of 4.
   E. Aneurysmal segment has a score of 5.

3. If the surgeon occludes the distal left anterior descending coronary artery, which one of the following best describes what may be observed on transesophageal echocardiography?
   A. Hypokinesis of the apical anterior segment.
   B. Hypokinesis of the apical inferior segment.
   C. Hypokinesis of the apical lateral segment.
   D. Hypokinesis of the apical septal segment.
   E. All of the above.

4. All of the following are complications of myocardial infarction detected by echocardiography ***except***
A. papillary muscle dysfunction.
B. ventricular septal defect.
C. mitral stenosis with diastolic doming of the mitral valve leaflets.
D. ventricular aneurysm.
E. left ventricular free wall rupture.

5. Which one of the following is the pathophysiologic mechanism of acute mitral regurgitation after myocardial infarction?
A. Mitral anulus dilation.
B. Papillary muscle dysfunction.
C. Papillary muscle rupture.
D. B and C.
E. All of the above.

6. During intraoperative transesophageal echocardiography, a 72-year-old patient has the hypokinetic segment shown in the accompanying image (arrow). According to the American Society of Echocardiography/Society of Cardiovascular Anesthesiologists guidelines for performing comprehensive intraoperative multiplane transesophageal echocardiography, this hypokinetic segment is
A. the anterolateral segment.
B. the lateral segment.
C. the anterior segment.
D. the posterior segment.
E. the inferior segment.

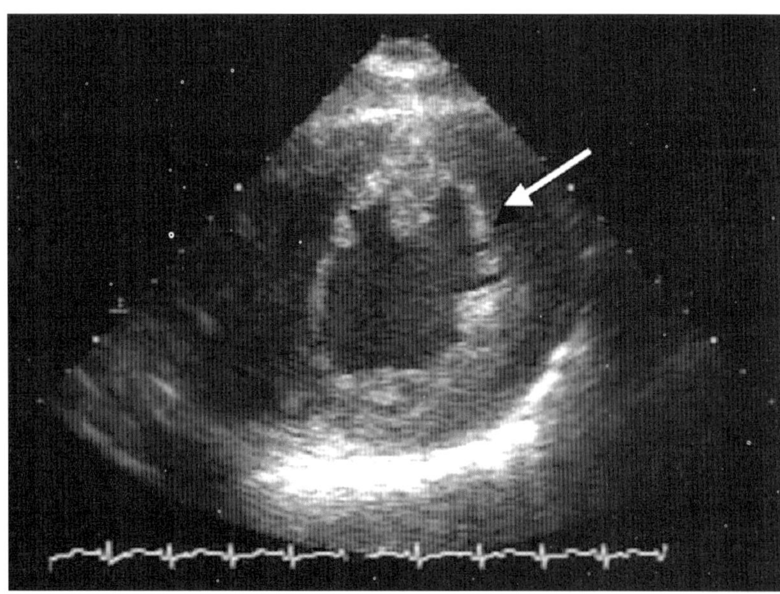

7. Most likely, the patient described in Question 6 has severe stenosis of
   A. the right coronary artery.
   B. the circumflex coronary artery.
   C. the left anterior descending coronary artery.
   D. the posterior descending artery.
   E. an undetermined structure.

8. If the surgeon occludes the first diagonal artery, which one of the following occurs?
   A. Regional wall motion abnormality of the basal anterior segment.
   B. Akinesis of the left ventricular apex.
   C. Dyskinesis of the lateral segment.
   D. Severe hypokinesis of the inferior segment.
   E. Hypokinesis of the right ventricle.

9. Generally, papillary muscle rupture occurs more frequently with
   A. anterior myocardial infarction.
   B. inferior myocardial infarction.
   C. anteroseptal myocardial infarction.
   D. lateral segment infarction.
   E. apical myocardial infarction.

10. Which one of the following about papillary muscle rupture is true?
   A. Anterolateral papillary muscle has a much higher incidence of rupture than does posteromedial papillary muscle because of its muscle thickness.
   B. Posteromedial papillary muscle has a much higher incidence of rupture than does anterolateral papillary muscle because of its muscle thickness.
   C. Anterolateral papillary muscle has a much higher incidence of rupture than does posteromedial papillary muscle because of its single blood supply.
   D. Posteromedial papillary muscle has a much higher incidence of rupture than does anterolateral papillary muscle because of its single blood supply.
   E. Both anterolateral and posteromedial papillary muscles have the same incidence of rupture.

11. A 68-year-old patient with chest pain becomes acutely short of breath. On physical examination, the patient has a loud systolic murmur with a thrill. His blood pressure is 88/46 mm Hg. Papillary muscle rupture is suspected. During transesophageal echocardiography in this patient, color flow imaging most likely will visualize
   A. mild mitral regurgitation with an eccentric jet toward the anterior leaflet due to the ruptured papillary muscle.
   B. moderate mitral regurgitation with an eccentric jet toward the posterior leaflet due to the ruptured papillary muscle.
   C. moderately severe mitral regurgitation with a regurgitant jet in an unpredictable direction.
   D. severe mitral regurgitation with a central jet.
   E. severe mitral regurgitation with an eccentric jet in the opposite direction of the flail leaflet segment.

12. The patient described in Question 11 should
  A. receive conservative medical therapy.
  B. receive medical management with elective surgical repair of the ruptured papillary muscle later.
  C. receive medical management with elective mitral valve replacement later.
  D. be brought to the operating room for mitral valve replacement or repair as soon as possible.
  E. be scheduled for elective surgical repair or replacement of the ruptured papillary muscle after he becomes hemodynamically stable.

13. In patients with ruptured papillary muscle due to myocardial infarction,
  A. the myocardial infarction is always large.
  B. the associated regional wall motion abnormality is always large.
  C. the completely ruptured papillary muscle may be visualized as a triangular mass attached to the corresponding mitral leaflet within the left atrium during systole.
  D. the ruptured papillary muscle may be visualized in four-chamber view but not in any transgastric view.
  E. all of the above are present.

14. Which one of the following statements about postinfarct ventricular free wall rupture is true?
  A. Most ventricular free wall ruptures occur within the first 3 hours after an acute myocardial infarction.
  B. Ventricular free wall rupture occurs more frequently after multiple myocardial infarctions in the same region.
  C. Left and right ventricles have a similar incidence of postinfarct free wall rupture.
  D. Typically, the site of ventricular rupture is located in the terminal distribution of the infarcted vessel.
  E. Both hypertension and left ventricular hypertrophy predispose the patient to ventricular rupture.

15. All of the following statements about echocardiographic features of ventricular free wall rupture are true ***except***
  A. pericardial effusion and thrombus in the pericardial space can be visualized.
  B. dynamic inversion of the right atrium is generally absent.
  C. rupture always occurs at the center of the myocardial infarction.
  D. a Doppler signal may not always be present.
  E. color flow mapping may show to-and-fro blood flow across the rupture site.

16. Postinfarct ventricular septal defect
  A. can be detected by a positive contrast test with agitated saline.
  B. occurs rarely with anterior wall infarction.
  C. is never multiple but always has a serpiginous course.
  D. most commonly occurs after multiple myocardial infarctions.
  E. typically is localized to the apical half of the septum in patients with anterior infarction.

17. Compared with a left ventricular pseudoaneurysm, a true ventricular aneurysm
A. has a narrowed neck with higher risk to rupture.
B. has a broad neck and is unlikely to rupture.
C. has a narrowed neck and is unlikely to rupture.
D. has a broad neck with higher risk to rupture.
E. is less common than pseudoaneurysm.

18. If the surgeon occludes the first septal perforator during off-pump coronary artery bypass graft surgery, intraoperative transesophageal echocardiography detects a regional wall motion abnormality of
A. the basal anteroseptal segment.
B. the mid anteroseptal segment.
C. the basal inferoseptal segment.
D. the mid inferoseptal segment.
E. the apical septal segment.

19. Normal left ventricular wall motion or regional wall motion means that
A. the left ventricle has good translational movement.
B. the heart moves around and the left ventricular wall thickens about 10% during systole.
C. the distance between the endocardial and epicardial borders increases more than 30% during systole.
D. the ventricular movement is visualized by transesophageal echocardiography, regardless of its myocardial thickening during the cardiac cycle.
E. the heart rotates rhythmically.

20. Which one of the following statements about regional wall motion analysis is true?
A. Hypokinesis is defined as a myocardial segment moving outward during systole.
B. An akinetic segment does not thicken but may move.
C. Dyskinesis is defined as a myocardial segment moving outward during diastole.
D. Normally, the percentage of thickening of the ventricular septum should be more than that of the free wall of the left ventricle.
E. Because akinesis means no movement, an akinetic segment is a fixed segment and never moves.

21. A 65-year-old patient with an acute myocardial infarction has severe hypotension. The accompanying images show the transesophageal echocardiographic appearance (LV, left ventricle; RV, right ventricle). The cardiologist's diagnosis is

A. pericardial tamponade.
B. ruptured right ventricular free wall with pericardial effusion.
C. ruptured left ventricular free wall with pericardial effusion.
D. ventricular septal defect.
E. left ventricular aneurysm.

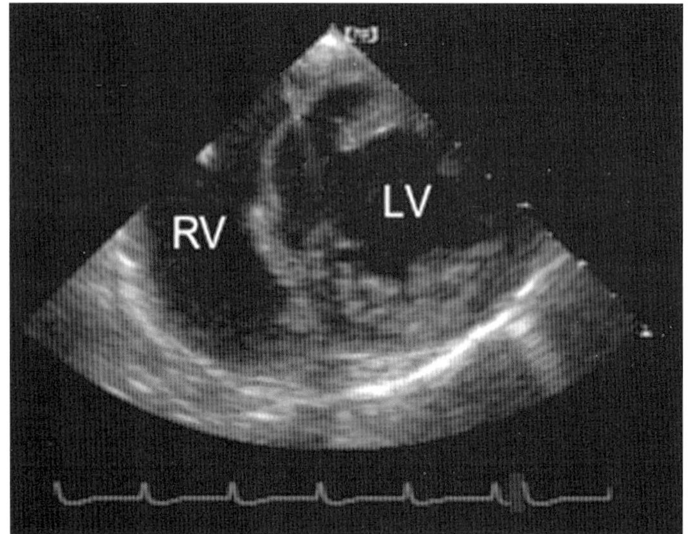

A

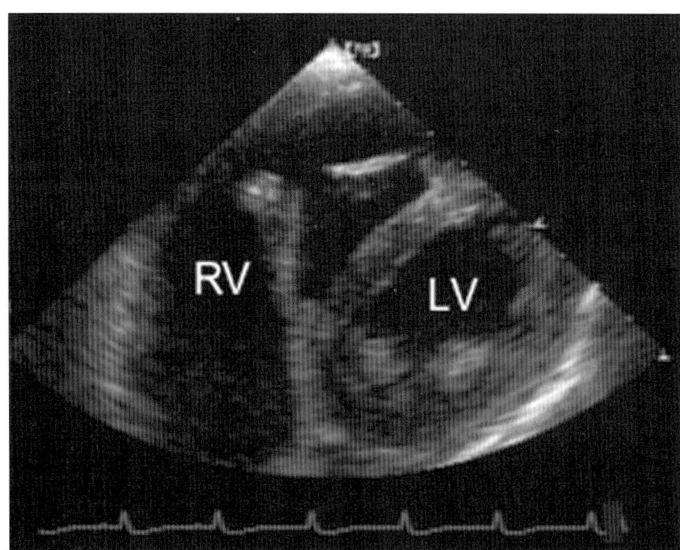

B

22. In the accompanying image, the letter X labels the akinetic segment and the letter Y labels the dyskinetic segment. According to the American Society of Echocardiography/Society of Cardiovascular Anesthesiologists guidelines for performing comprehensive intraoperative multiplane transesophageal echocardiography, which one of the following statements about these segments is true?

A. The akinetic segment is the inferior segment.
B. The dyskinetic segment is the inferolateral segment.
C. The anterior segment has a score of 3.
D. The inferolateral segment has a score of 4.
E. The lateral segment has a score of 5.

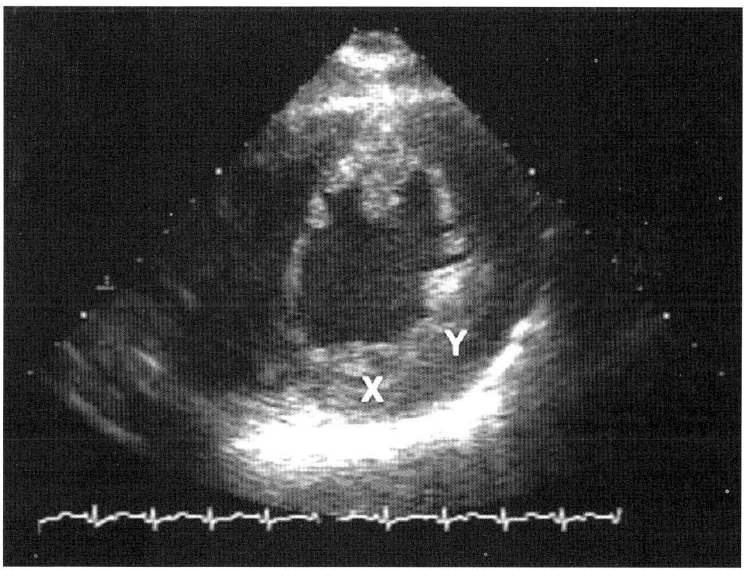

23. Akinesis of the segment labeled with the letter X in the image accompanying Question 22 is caused by severe stenosis of

A. the left anterior descending coronary artery.
B. the posterior descending artery.
C. the first diagonal.
D. the second diagonal.
E. the circumflex coronary artery.

24. Transesophageal echocardiography in a 62-year-old patient shows a hypokinetic segment, as indicated by the arrow in the accompanying image. According to the American Society of Echocardiography/Society of Cardiovascular Anesthesiologists guidelines for performing comprehensive intraoperative multiplane transesophageal echocardiography, this is
A. the posterior segment.
B. the inferior segment.
C. the anterior segment.
D. the lateral segment.
E. the septal segment.

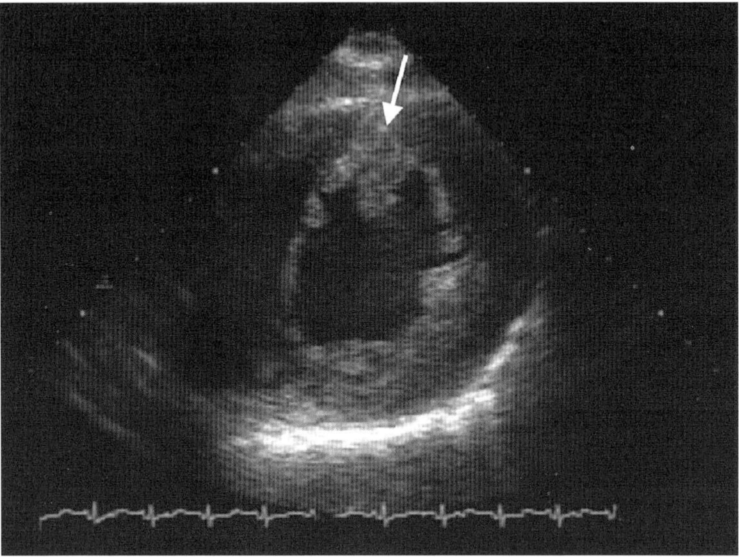

25. The segmental hypokinesis shown in the image accompanying Question 24 is caused by severe stenosis of
A. the left coronary artery.
B. the left main coronary artery.
C. the left anterior descending coronary artery.
D. the posterior descending artery.
E. the left circumflex coronary artery.

26. If air bubbles are present when the patient described in Question 24 is taken off cardiopulmonary bypass, which one of the following coronary arteries is most likely to have an air embolism?
A. The right coronary artery.
B. The left coronary artery.
C. The left anterior descending coronary artery.
D. The circumflex coronary artery.
E. The left main coronary artery.

27. If the patient in Question 24 has a coronary air embolism, intraoperative transesophageal echocardiography would most likely show hypokinesis of

A. the mid anterior segment.

B. the basal posterior segment.

C. the apical lateral segment.

D. the entire left ventricle.

E. the right ventricle.

28. Intraoperative transesophageal echocardiography reveals that the segment in the accompanying image shown with an arrow moved paradoxically during systole. From this image, the cardiologist can conclude that

A. the mid anteroseptal segment is aneurysmal.

B. the basal inferoseptal segment is aneurysmal.

C. the mid-anteroseptal segment is dyskinetic.

D. the basal septal segment is dyskinetic.

E. the mid-septal segment is dyskinetic.

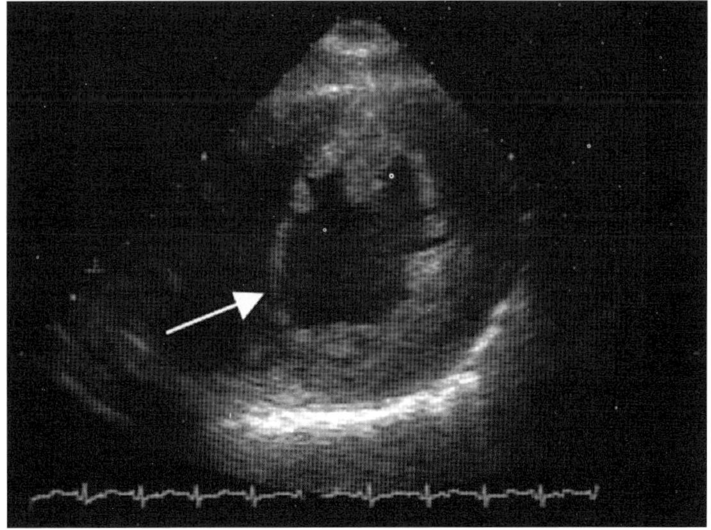

29. The regional wall motion abnormality in the image accompanying Question 28 is caused by severe stenosis of

A. the right coronary artery.

B. the circumflex coronary artery.

C. the left anterior descending coronary artery.

D. the posterior descending artery.

E. an undetermined structure.

30. The wall motion score index is

A. the sum of the total wall motion scores of all 16 segments divided by the patient's body weight.

B. the sum of the total wall motion scores of all 16 segments divided by the patient's body surface area.
C. the sum of the total wall motion scores of all 16 segments.
D. the sum of the wall motion scores divided by 16 segments.
E. the sum of the wall motion scores divided by the number of segments visualized.

31. A wall motion score index of
A. 16 represents normal left ventricular function.
B. 8 is common in the presence of normal left ventricular function.
C. 4 is associated with hyperkinetic ventricular segments.
D. 2 is compatible with a poorly contracting left ventricle and low ejection fraction (<30%).
E. 1 is a prognostic indicator for increased risks of serious complications after myocardial infarction.

32. If the second diagonal branch coronary artery is occluded, which one of the following can be observed on intraoperative transesophageal echocardiography?
A. Severe hypokinesis of the basal posterior segment.
B. Regional wall motion abnormality of the mid anterior segment.
C. Dyskinesis of the apical lateral segment.
D. Akinesis of the basal septal segment.
E. Normal left ventricular function but hypokinesis of the right ventricle.

33. During intraoperative transesophageal echocardiography in a 66-year-old patient, the accompanying two-chamber view is obtained with the transducer placed in the mid esophagus. The arrow indicates the hypokinetic left ventricular wall. Which one of the following statements about this image is true?

A. The anterior wall is hypokinetic.
B. The posterior wall is hypokinetic.
C. The inferior wall is hypokinetic.
D. The septal wall is hypokinetic.
E. The lateral wall is hypokinetic.

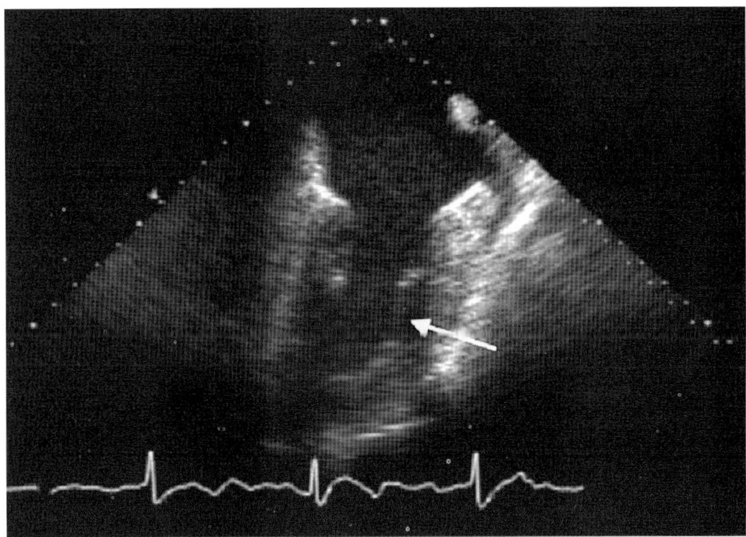

34. If this is the only hypokinetic ventricular wall, the cause of the hypokinesis in the image accompanying Question 33 is best described as severe stenosis of

A. the right coronary artery.
B. the posterior descending artery.
C. the left main coronary artery.
D. the left anterior descending coronary artery.
E. the left circumflex coronary artery.

35. A 78-year-old patient with frequent chest pain undergoes transesophageal echocardiography. Regional wall motion abnormality is observed in the area of the arrow, as shown in the accompanying two-dimensional image. From this image, the cardiologist can conclude that the patient has hypokinesis of

A. the septal wall.
B. the inferoseptal wall.
C. the posteroseptal wall.
D. the anteroseptal wall.
E. the entire ventricular septum.

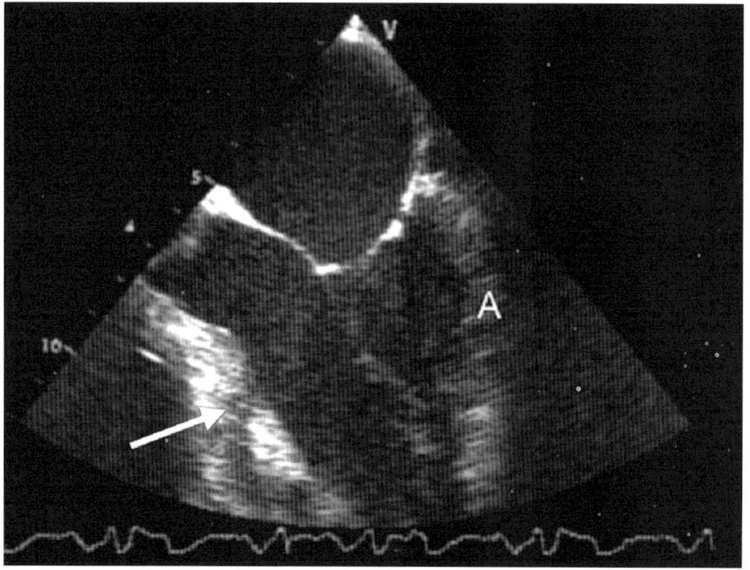

36. The left ventricular free wall on the right side of the image accompanying Question 35 (labeled with the letter A) is

A. the anterior wall.
B. the posterior wall.
C. the inferior wall.
D. the lateral wall.
E. the septal wall.

37. During intraoperative transesophageal echocardiography, the accompanying mid-esophageal four-chamber view revealed left ventricular hypokinesis, as indicated by the arrow. According to the American Society of Echocardiography/Society of Cardiovascular Anesthesiologists guidelines for performing comprehensive intraoperative multiplane transesophageal echocardiography, the hypokinesis most likely is due to severe stenosis of

A. the right coronary artery.

B. the posterior descending coronary artery.

C. the left anterior descending coronary artery.

D. the circumflex coronary artery.

E. an undetermined structure.

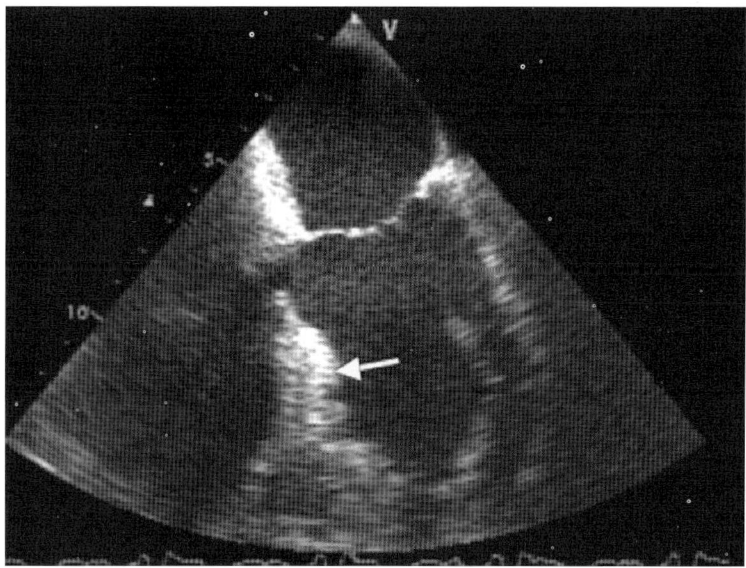

38. In patients with severe stenosis of the left circumflex coronary artery, which one of the following can be visualized in the accompanying transgastric two-chamber view?
A. Regional wall motion abnormality of the lateral wall.
B. Hypokinesis of the mid inferolateral segment.
C. Akinesis of the apical lateral segment.
D. Dyskinesis of the basal posterior segment.
E. None of the above.

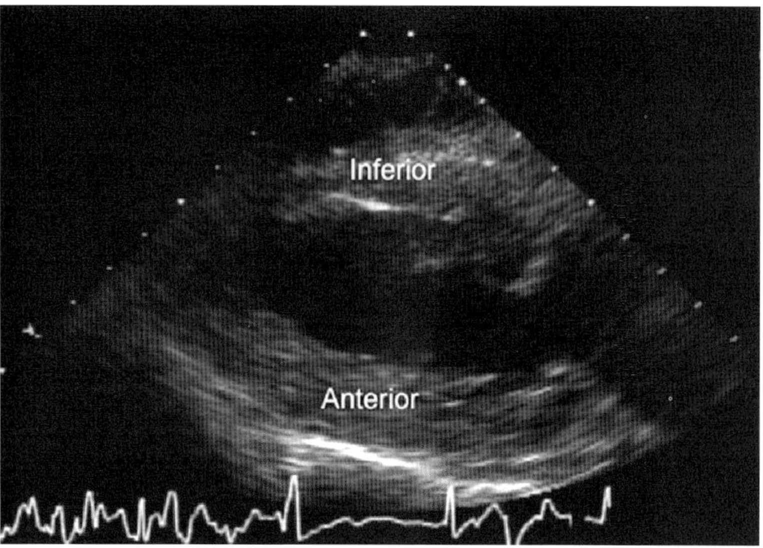

39. Differential diagnosis for regional wall motion abnormalities detected by preoperative transesophageal echocardiography includes
A. right ventricular volume overload.
B. left bundle branch block.
C. permanent pacemaker.
D. all of the above.
E. none of the above.

40. A 78-year-old patient undergoes coronary artery bypass graft surgery for his coronary artery disease. After the aortic cross-clamp is removed, a left ventricular wall motion abnormality is observed by intraoperative transesophageal echocardiography. The differential diagnosis includes
A. myocardial stunning.
B. poor myocardial protection.
C. air in the coronary artery bypass grafts.
D. the heart is not filled.
E. all of the above.

Answers & Discussion

1. Answer C

Left ventricular regional wall motion analysis is based on grading the contractility of individual segments. Segmental models of the left ventricle are necessary to accurately describe the location and extent of regional wall motion abnormalities detected by echocardiography. There are various left ventricular segmental models, depending on

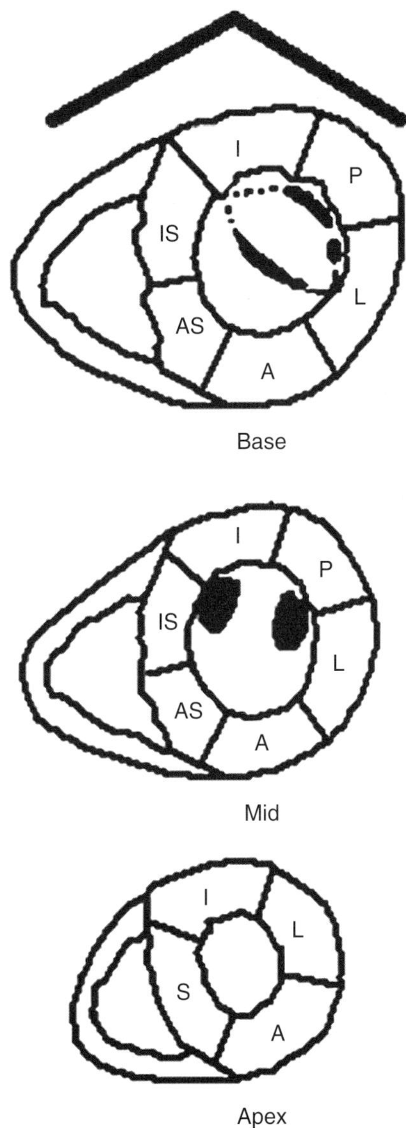

Figure from Shanewise et al. (37). Used with permission.

how the left ventricle is subdivided. The American Society of Echocardiography/Society of Cardiovascular Anesthesiologists guidelines for performing comprehensive intraoperative multiplane transesophageal echocardiography use a 16-segment model of the left ventricle, which is based on the recommendations proposed by the American Society of Echocardiography (ASE) Committee on Standards, Subcommittee on Quantitation of Two-Dimensional Echocardiograms. The ASE recommends this 16-segment model based on the following considerations:

1. Anatomic logic.
2. Easy identification of the segments using internal anatomic landmarks.
3. Relationship of the segments to known coronary arterial supply.
4. A uniform scoring system for grading the severity of segmental wall motion abnormalities.

This model, shown in the accompanying illustration, divides the left ventricle into three levels (basal, mid, and apical) and 16 segments. The basal and mid (papillary muscle) levels are each subdivided into six segments, and the apical level is subdivided into four segments (A, anterior; AS, anterior septum; I, inferior; IS, inferior septum; L, lateral; P, posterior; S, septal). **References** 10 *(pp 88–90)*; 11 *(pp 153–154)*; 23 *(pp 41–42)*; 33; 37.

2. Answer D

Analysis of left ventricular segmental function is based on visual assessment of the motion and thickening of a segment during systole. A numeric scoring system that depends on the contractility of the individual segments has been adopted to evaluate the severity of ventricular dysfunction. In this scoring system, higher scores indicate more severe wall motion abnormality. According to the American Society of Echocardiography/Society of Cardiovascular Anesthesiologists guidelines for performing comprehensive intraoperative multiplane transesophageal echocardiography, the recommended numeric scoring system for intraoperative transesophageal echocardiographic assessment of ventricular wall motion is 1 for normal; 2 for mild hypokinesis; 3 for severe hypokinesis; 4 for akinesis; and 5 for dyskinesis.

This numeric scoring system is different from that currently recommended by the American Society of Echocardiography, which has proposed the following scheme: 1 for a normally contracting segment (or hyperkinetic segment); 2 for hypokinesis; 3 for akinesis; 4 for dyskinesis; and 5 for an aneurysmal (that is, diastolically deformed) segment. In both scoring schemes, hyperkinesis is not distinguished from normal. **References** 10 *(pp 147–151, 452)*; 11 *(p 154)*; 25 *(p 200)*; 33; 37.

3. Answer E

According to the American Society of Echocardiography/Society of Cardiovascular Anesthesiologists guidelines for intraoperative transesophageal echocardiography, a 16-segment model of the left ventricle is used to describe the location and extent of regional wall motion abnormalities detected by transesophageal echocardiography. The typical regions of myocardium perfused by each of the major coronary arteries to the left ventricle are shown in the accompanying illustration (A, anterior; AS, anterior septum; CIRC, circumflex coronary artery; I, inferior; IS, inferior septum; L, lateral; LA, left atrium; LAD, left anterior descending coronary artery; LV, left ventricle; P, posterior; RA, right atrium; RC, right coronary artery; RV, right ventricle; S, septal).

Because the distal left anterior descending coronary artery provides the blood supply to all four apical segments of the left ventricle, its occlusion causes ischemia in the left ventricular apex, leading to hypokinesis of all apical segments. **Reference** 37.

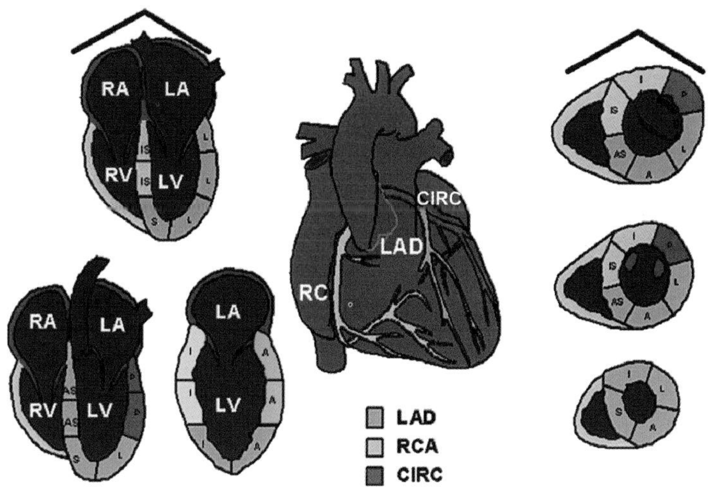

Figure from the Society of Cardiovascular Anesthesiologists. Used with permission.

4. Answer C

Complications after myocardial infarction include papillary muscle dysfunction or rupture with mitral regurgitation, ventricular septal defect, left ventricular free wall rupture, ventricular aneurysm, and pseudoaneurysm. Typically, mitral stenosis with doming of the mitral valve leaflets in diastole is seen in rheumatic valvular disease. **References** 10 *(pp 466–482)*; 11 *(pp 170–178)*; 23 *(pp 77–85)*; 25 *(pp 205–209)*.

5. Answer E

There are three separate pathophysiologic mechanisms of acute mitral regurgitation after myocardial infarction: 1) left ventricular cavity and mitral anulus dilation, 2) papillary muscle dysfunction, and 3) papillary muscle rupture. It is important to recognize the exact underlying cause of ischemic mitral regurgitation because papillary muscle rupture usually mandates urgent mitral valve replacement or repair. Mitral regurgitation due to papillary muscle dysfunction or anulus dilation may improve with afterload reduction, coronary revascularization, or both. **References** 10 *(pp 478–480)*; 11 *(pp 172–174)*; 23 *(pp 80, 82)*; 25 *(pp 205–206)*.

6. Answer D

7. Answer B

The image accompanying Question 6 is a transgastric mid short axis view. According to the 16-segment model recommended by the American Society of Echocardiography/Society of Cardiovascular Anesthesiologists guidelines, this hypokinetic segment is the posterior segment, which generally receives its blood supply from the circumflex coronary artery. Therefore, this patient most likely has severe stenosis of the circumflex coronary artery. **References** 10 *(pp 88–90)*; 11 *(pp 153–154)*; 23 *(pp 41–42)*; 32; 37.

8. Answer A

The first diagonal arises from the left anterior descending coronary artery and provides blood supply to the basal anterior segment. If the surgeon occludes the first diagonal, the basal anterior segment becomes ischemic, leading to regional wall motion abnormality. The left ventricular apex and the lateral segment receive their blood supply from the distal left anterior descending coronary artery and the circumflex coronary artery, respectively. Both the right ventricle and the inferior segment of the left ventricle receive their blood supply from the right coronary artery. **Reference** 2.

9. Answer B

10. Answer D

Papillary muscle rupture occurs more frequently with inferior myocardial infarction. Compared with the anterolateral papillary muscle that has a dual blood supply, the posteromedial papillary muscle has about a 10-fold higher incidence of rupture because of its single blood supply. **References** 10 *(pp 478–480)*; 11 *(pp 172–175)*; 23 *(pp 80, 82)*; 25 *(p 205–206)*.

11. Answer E

12. Answer D

Transesophageal echocardiography can be used to establish the diagnosis of papillary muscle rupture with mitral regurgitation. Because of the ruptured papillary muscle, the unsupported mitral leaflet segment becomes flail, leading to severe mitral regurgitation that is easily demonstrated by color flow imaging. Generally, the mitral regurgitation jet is eccentric, in the opposite direction of the flail leaflet segment. In patients with a posteromedial papillary muscle rupture, the posterior mitral leaflet is unsupported and becomes flail, resulting in an eccentric mitral regurgitation jet toward the anterior mitral leaflet. Conversely, in patients with anterolateral papillary muscle rupture, the anterior mitral leaflet is unsupported and becomes flail, resulting in an eccentric mitral regurgitation jet toward the posterior mitral leaflet.

In the setting of papillary muscle rupture, the mitral valve usually is replaced rather than repaired. Because patients with severe mitral regurgitation due to papillary muscle rupture generally present with hemodynamic decompensation, emergency mitral valve replacement, with or without coronary revascularization, is necessary for survival. Therefore, to optimize this patient's chance of survival, surgery should be performed as soon as possible. The long-term survival rate is excellent after successful surgery. **References** 10 *(pp 478–480)*; 11 *(pp 172–175)*; 23 *(pp 80, 82)*; 25 *(pp 205–206)*.

13. Answer C

In patients with postinfarct papillary muscle rupture, the four-chamber view readily demonstrates the ruptured portion of the papillary muscle, which may be either partial or complete. The accompanying image A shows a complete rupture, with the papillary muscle head (arrow) in the left atrium (LA) (LV indicates the left ventricle), and image B shows a partial rupture seen in the transgastric long axis view. The two portions of the papillary muscle (arrows) are barely held together by a thin strand of muscle (small arrows). During systole, the completely ruptured papillary muscle head may be visualized as a triangular mass attached to the corresponding flail mitral leaflet within the left atrium. Papillary muscle rupture can also be visualized from the transgastric views; in fact, the rupture is easier to localize from the transgastric longitudinal long axis view.

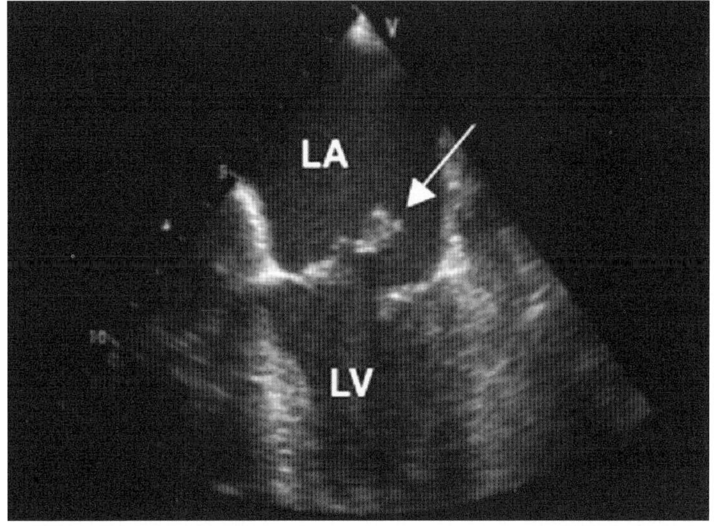

A

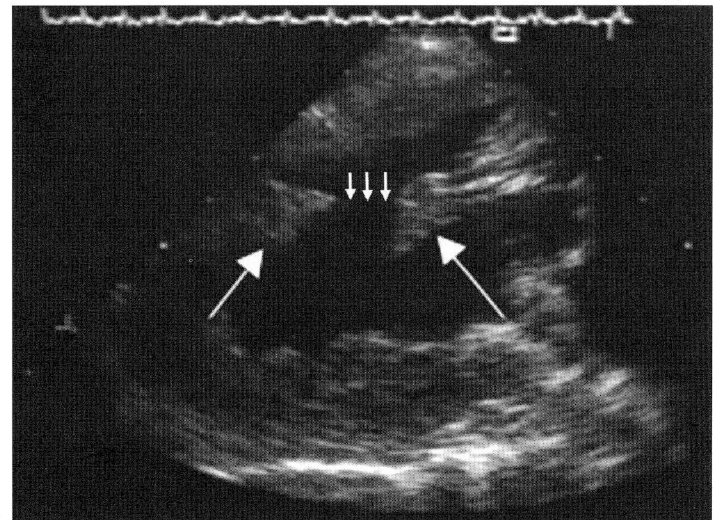

B

Although mitral regurgitation due to papillary muscle rupture is severe, patients usually have a small infarct in the distribution of the right or circumflex coronary artery, and hence, the associated regional wall motion abnormality is not large. **References** 10 *(pp 478–480)*; 11 *(pp 172–175)*; 23 *(pp 80, 82)*; 25 *(pp 205–206)*.

14. Answer D

Ventricular free wall rupture accounts for about 10% of in-hospital deaths attributable to myocardial infarction. It occurs more frequently in women and elderly patients. Because of the differences in the intracavitary pressures, rupture of the left ventricle is much more common than that of the right ventricle, and atrial rupture is extremely rare. Usually, ventricular rupture occurs after a first myocardial infarction. Prior myocardial infarction in the same distribution forms scar tissue that is more resistant to rupture. Prior myocardial infarction in a different distribution may result in a generally more dysfunctional left ventricle that is less able to generate the force to rupture the free wall, especially the infarcted scar tissue. In fact, most ventricular ruptures occur within the first 3 to 6 days after myocardial infarction, before scar formation. Hypertension may predispose the patient to ventricular rupture due to higher intracavitary pressure. But left ventricular hypertrophy itself may be protective because thicker myocardial walls mean more myocardial fibers must be disrupted. The location of the free wall rupture is typically in the terminal distribution of the infarcted vessel and often occurs in the apex. **References** 23 *(p 78)*; 25 *(pp 207–208)*.

15. Answer C

The echocardiographic features of ventricular free wall rupture include the following:

1. Pericardial effusion or hematoma with compression of cardiac chambers. Because there is free communication between the ventricular cavity and pericardium, free fluid or thrombus may be visualized in the pericardial space.
2. The dynamic inversion of the right atrium or the right ventricle that occurs in the typical tamponade on account of free fluid collection is generally absent because blood usually clots in the pericardial space after ventricular free wall rupture.
3. The free wall rupture typically occurs at the junction of myocardial infarction and normal zones. The site of rupture sometimes is identifiable but frequently cannot be identified.
4. Color flow mapping may show to-and-fro blood flow across the rupture site. However, a Doppler signal may not always be present.

The accompanying images show left ventricular free wall rupture. Part A, Apical effusion (arrow); B, zoom of apex showing fluid and thrombus (arrow); and C, surgical view showing infarct area (dark myocardium, small arrows) and rupture site (large arrow) with blood jet. **References** 23 *(p 78)*; 25 *(pp 207–208)*.

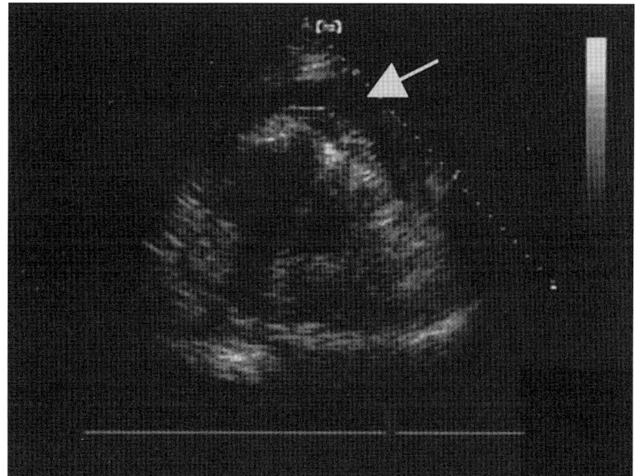

A

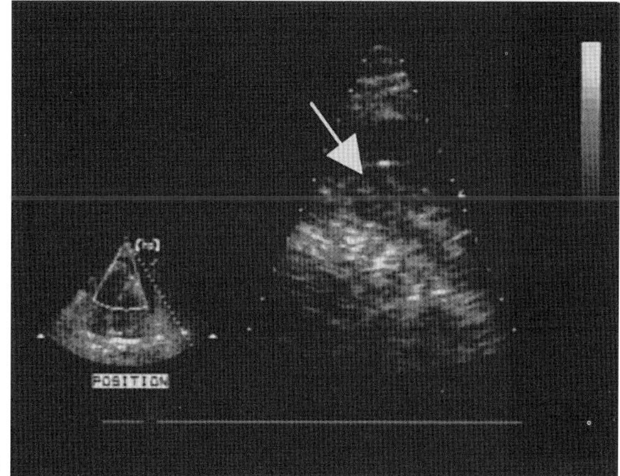

B

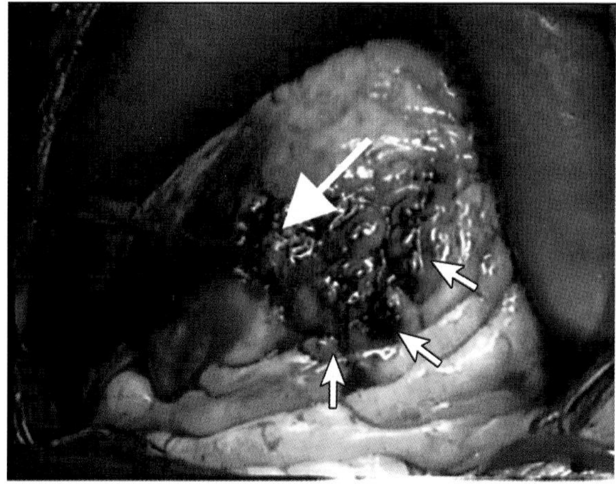

C

16. Answer E

Ventricular septal defect occurs in 1% to 3% of all acute myocardial infarctions. About 75% of ventricular septal defects occur after the first myocardial infarction. Two-thirds of postinfarct ventricular septal defects occur with anterior wall myocardial infarctions, although they also occur with inferior myocardial infarctions. When a ventricular septal defect is present, the right ventricle is frequently involved with infarction. Generally, the prognosis is poorer in patients with an inferoseptal defect because of more extensive right ventricular involvement with infarction. Typically, septal ruptures associated with anterior infarctions are relatively well circumscribed and localized to the apical half of the left ventricle. Inferoseptal ruptures most often occur within the basal half of the septum and can be complex, serpiginous, and poorly delineated by two-dimensional imaging. Sometimes, multiple ventricular septal ruptures occur after a myocardial infarction. Color flow imaging helps to demonstrate the intracardiac shunt caused by the postinfarct ventricular septal defect. Because the left ventricular pressure is higher than the right ventricular pressure, the shunt is typically left to right, and a contrast test with agitated saline shows a negative defect in the contrast bubbles in the right ventricle. **References** 10 *(pp 471, 473–475)*; 11 *(pp 171–172)*; 23 *(pp 78–80)*; 25 *(pp 206–207)*.

17. Answer B

A left ventricular pseudoaneurysm forms after a left ventricular free wall rupture is contained within the adherent pericardium. Typically, a pseudoaneurysm is characterized by a small neck communication between the left ventricle and the aneurysmal cavity. The ratio of the diameter of entry and the maximal diameter of the pseudoaneurysm is less than 0.5. Because myocardial elements are not present in the wall of a pseudoaneurysm, there is a high risk for the pseudoaneurysm to expand further and rupture, leading to immediate death.

True aneurysms are more common than pseudoaneurysms. In contrast to a pseudoaneurysm, a true ventricular aneurysm typically has a broad neck communication between the left ventricle and the aneurysmal cavity. Because of the myocardial elements in the wall of the true aneurysm, it is unlikely for a true aneurysm to rupture. **References** 10 *(pp 468–471)*; 11 *(p 177)*; 23 *(p 83)*; 25 *(pp 207–208)*.

18. Answer A

The first septal perforator arises from the proximal left anterior descending coronary artery and provides the blood supply to the basal anteroseptal segment. Therefore, intraoperative transesophageal echocardiography detects a wall motion abnormality of the basal anteroseptal segment if the surgeon occludes the first septal perforator during off-pump coronary artery bypass graft surgery. **Reference** 11 *(p 200)*.

19. Answer C

20. Answer B

Normally, the left ventricular free wall thickness increases more than 30% during systole; that is, in normal wall motion, the distance between the endocardial and epicardial borders increases more than 30% during systole. In normal subjects, the percentage of thickening of the ventricular septum is somewhat less than that of the free wall of the left ventricle. According to the American Society of Echocardiography/Society of Cardiovascular Anesthesiologists guidelines for performing comprehensive intraoperative multiplane transesophageal echocardiography, hypokinesis occurs when the systolic wall thickening is less than 30% but greater than 10%. When the systolic wall thickening is less than 10%, it is called severe hypokinesis. Akinesis means the myocardium does not thicken at all during systole. Dyskinesis is defined as outward movement of a myocardial segment during systole, usually in association with systolic wall thinning.

Ventricular wall thickening is not the same as ventricular or segmental movement. Left ventricular movement includes translation and rotation, which do not represent left ventricular function. Even though no wall thickening occurs, an akinetic segment may move because of being dragged by the other segments. The major advantages of using wall thickening to assess regional wall motion abnormalities are that wall thickening is unaffected by translation or rotation, independent of a center of reference, and unaffected by shape changes. The major disadvantages of using wall thickening to evaluate ventricular function are that the epicardium may be poorly defined and wall thickening does not correlate with other techniques. **References** 23 *(pp 73–75)*; 33; 37.

21. Answer D

The patient described in Question 21 has a postinfarction ventricular septal defect. The accompanying transesophageal echocardiographic images are transgastric short axis views, at the base and mid to apex levels. Part A shows the base of the left ventricle (LV) with rupture into the septum (arrow). Part B (toward the apex of the left ventricle) shows exit (arrow) into the right ventricle (RV). Part C is the surgical view of the ventricular septal defect (arrow). **References** 10 *(p 471)*; 11 *(pp 171–173)*; 23 *(pp 78, 80–81)*.

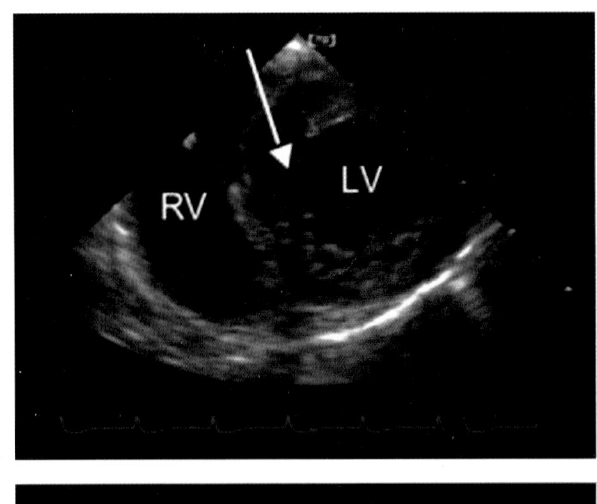
RV
LV
A

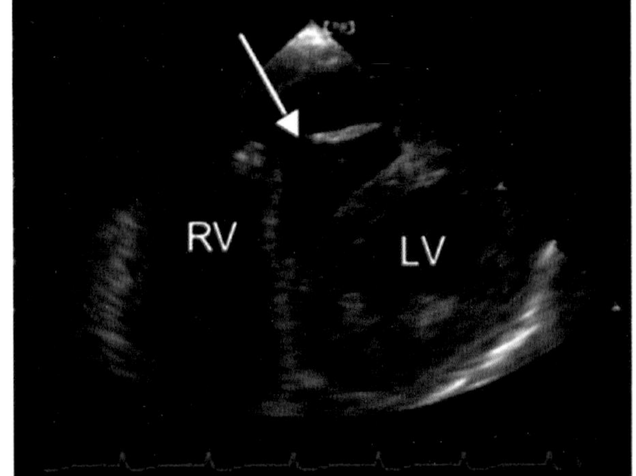
RV
LV
B

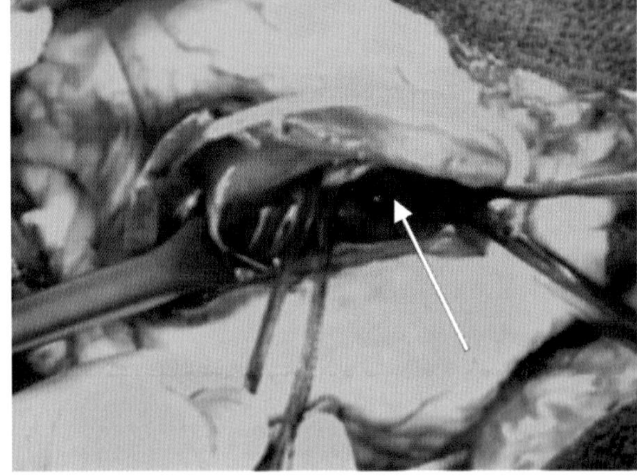
C

22. Answer E

23. Answer A

In the image accompanying Question 22, the akinetic segment labeled with the letter X is the anterior segment, and the dyskinetic segment labeled with the letter Y is the lateral segment. According to the American Society of Echocardiography/Society of Cardiovascular Anesthesiologists guidelines for intraoperative transesophageal echocardiography, akinesis has a score of 4 and dyskinesis has a score of 5. Therefore, the anterior segment is akinetic with a score of 4, and the lateral segment is dyskinetic with a score of 5. Because the anterior segment receives its blood supply from the left anterior descending coronary artery, akinesis of this segment is produced by severe stenosis or occlusion of the left anterior descending coronary artery. **Reference** 37.

24. Answer B

25. Answer D

According to the 16-segment model recommended by the American Society of Echocardiography/Society of Cardiovascular Anesthesiologists guidelines for performing comprehensive intraoperative multiplane transesophageal echocardiography, the patient described in Question 24 has a hypokinetic inferior segment. Generally, the inferior segment receives its blood supply from the posterior descending artery, which arises from the right coronary artery in 80% of the population. Therefore, this patient most likely has severe stenosis of the posterior descending coronary artery. **References** 25 *(p 198)*; 37.

26. Answer A

27. Answer E

Air bubbles tend to enter the right coronary artery because of the anatomic position of the right coronary ostium. Air embolism of the right coronary artery when the patient is taken off cardiopulmonary bypass causes ischemia of the myocardium in the distribution of the right coronary artery, resulting in hypokinesis. Because the right ventricle receives its blood supply from the right coronary artery, it would become hypokinetic if an air embolism in the right coronary artery occurred when coming off cardiopulmonary bypass. Therefore, intraoperative transesophageal echocardiography most likely shows hypokinesis of the right ventricle. **Reference** 2.

28. Answer C

29. Answer C

The image accompanying Question 28 is a transgastric mid short axis view because of the presence of papillary muscles. The dyskinetic segment in this image is the mid anteroseptal segment. Dyskinesis of this segment is caused by decreased blood supply due to stenosis of the second septal perforator, which arises from the left anterior descending coronary artery. **References** 10 *(pp 447–454)*; 11 *(p 168)*; 37.

30. Answer E

31. Answer D

The wall motion score index reflects overall left ventricular function. It is the sum of the wall motion scores divided by the number of visualized segments.

For this index to be reliable and meaningful, it is important that all or nearly all segments be visualized. A wall motion score index of 1.0 is normal; 1.1 to 1.4 indicates mild dysfunction; 1.5 to 2.4, moderate dysfunction; and 2.5 or higher, severe dysfunction. Decreased left ventricular function is associated with an increased wall motion score index.

The wall motion score index has been correlated with the extent of myocardial ischemia and infarction, as determined by perfusion imaging and autopsy. A wall motion score index of less than 1.5 describes a near-normal ventricle, a score higher than 1.7 usually indicates a perfusion defect of more than 20%, and a score higher than 2.0 is compatible with a poorly contracting left ventricle and low ejection fraction (<30%). Also, the wall motion score index is a prognostic indicator for post–myocardial infarction. Generally, a wall motion score index higher than 2.0 early after myocardial infarction is associated with increased risk of serious complications. **References** 11 *(p 154)*; 23 *(pp 42, 74–75)*.

32. Answer B

The second diagonal arises from the left anterior descending coronary artery, distal to the first diagonal. Because the second diagonal provides blood supply to the mid anterior segment, its occlusion causes a regional wall motion abnormality of the mid anterior segment, which can be visualized by transesophageal echocardiography. **Reference** 25 *(p 200)*.

33. Answer A

34. Answer D

The image accompanying Question 33 is a mid-esophageal two-chamber view. The hypokinetic wall indicated by the arrow is the anterior wall of the left ventricle, which receives its blood supply from the left anterior descending coronary artery. The left main coronary artery bifurcates and gives rise to the left circumflex and left anterior descending coronary arteries. Because the left circumflex coronary artery provides blood supply to the posterior and lateral walls, hypokinesis of the left ventricular anterior wall alone is caused by severe stenosis of the left anterior descending coronary artery, not the left main coronary artery. **References** 25 *(pp 197–201)*; 37.

35. Answer D

36. Answer B

According to the American Society of Echocardiography/Society of Cardiovascular Anesthesiologists guidelines for performing comprehensive intraoperative multiplane transesophageal echocardiography, the hypokinetic ventricular wall indicated by the arrow in the image accompanying Question 35 is the anteroseptal wall and the free ventricular wall on the left side of the display screen is the posterior wall.

Generally, the anteroseptal wall receives its blood supply from the left anterior descending coronary artery, and the posterior wall receives its blood supply from the circumflex coronary artery. Hence, hypokinesis of the anteroseptal wall in this 78-year-old patient is produced by severe stenosis of the left anterior descending coronary artery. **References** 25 *(pp 197–201)*; 37.

37. Answer C

According to the American Society of Echocardiography/Society of Cardiovascular Anesthesiologists guidelines for performing comprehensive intraoperative multiplane transesophageal echocardiography, the hypokinetic wall indicated by the arrow in the image accompanying Question 37 is the septal wall, which receives its blood supply from the left anterior descending coronary artery. Therefore, the hypokinesis of the septal wall in this patient is most likely caused by severe stenosis of the left anterior descending coronary artery. **Reference** 37.

38. Answer E

In a transgastric two-chamber view, the left ventricular wall, located at the top of the image adjacent to the probe, is the inferior wall, and the other wall, located anteriorly or at the bottom of the image accompanying Question 38, is the anterior wall. The inferior wall receives its blood supply from the right coronary artery (posterior descending artery), and the anterior wall receives its blood supply from the left anterior descending coronary artery. The left circumflex coronary artery has its distribution in the posterior and lateral segments, which are not visualized in the transgastric two-chamber view. Therefore, regional wall motion abnormalities due to circumflex stenosis cannot be visualized in the transgastric two-chamber view. **Reference** 37.

39. Answer D

Regional wall motion abnormalities may be produced by nonischemic causes as well as myocardial ischemia. Left bundle branch block exaggerates septal motion abnormalities. Placement of a permanent pacemaker produces apical and septal abnormalities. Right ventricular volume overload may also produce septal wall abnormalities. **References** 23 *(p 97)*; 42 *(p 658)*.

40. Answer E

All the choices listed in this question are possible causes of left ventricular hypokinesis after the aortic cross-clamp is removed. It is important to realize that an empty left ventricle prevents accurate analysis of wall motion, which leads to a false impression of ventricular hypokinesis. In such a situation, the heart should always be filled before making any diagnosis or conclusion. Stunned myocardium occurs when ischemic muscle is reperfused and is still viable but not functioning. The stunned myocardium shows reversible regional wall motion abnormalities after reperfusion of a transiently occluded coronary artery, and eventually myocardial function returns. Myocardial stunning frequently occurs after cardiopulmonary bypass, giving the appearance of global hypokinesis during intraoperative transesophageal echocardiography. Poor myocardial protection during cardiopulmonary bypass is certainly a possible cause of left ventricular hypokinesis after the cross-clamp is removed. Air embolism may occur during coronary artery bypass graft surgery, leading to regional wall motion abnormalities in its distribution. **References** 10 *(pp 464–465)*; 23 *(p 98)*.

Chapter 10

Assessing Heart Valves During the Perioperative Period

Questions

Multiple choice (choose the *one* best answer):

1. The normal mitral valve area is
A. 1.0 to 1.5 cm^2.
B. 1.5 to 2.0 cm^2.
C. 2.0 to 2.5 cm^2.
D. 4.0 to 6.0 cm^2.
E. 6.0 to 7.0 cm^2.

2. The normal aortic valve area is
A. 1 to 2 cm^2.
B. 2 to 3 cm^2.
C. 3 to 4 cm^2.
D. 4 to 5 cm^2.
E. 5 to 6 cm^2.

3. The normal tricuspid inflow has
A. a peak velocity greater than 2 m/s and a peak gradient greater than 7.5 mm Hg.
B. a peak velocity of 2 m/s or less and a peak gradient of 7.5 mm Hg or less.
C. a mean velocity greater than 2 m/s and a mean gradient greater than 7.5 mm Hg.
D. a mean velocity of 2 m/s or less and a mean gradient of 7.5 mm Hg or less.
E. a peak velocity less than 1 m/s and a mean gradient less than 2 mm Hg.

4. The most common cause of mitral stenosis is
A. rheumatic valvular disease.
B. degenerative valvular calcification.
C. vegetations.
D. drug toxicity.
E. congenital mitral stenosis.

5. The severity of aortic stenosis can be evaluated by all of the following ***except***
A. the aortic valve area.
B. the peak aortic flow velocity.
C. the left ventricular outflow tract peak velocity.
D. the ratio of the left ventricular outflow tract to the aortic valve time velocity integral.
E. the mean pressure gradient across the aortic valve.

6. The most common form of aortic stenosis is caused by
A. rheumatic valvular disease.
B. degenerative valvular calcification.
C. vegetations.
D. bicuspid aortic valve.
E. subaortic stenosis.

7. Which one of the following ages is more likely to have rheumatic mitral stenosis?
A. 5 years old.
B. 15 years old.
C. 40 years old.
D. 55 years old.
E. 85 years old.

8. In developed countries, the latency from the occurrence of acute rheumatic fever to the onset of symptoms of mitral stenosis is approximately
A. 20 to 40 days.
B. 20 to 40 weeks.
C. 20 to 40 months.
D. 20 to 40 years.
E. more than 40 to 50 years.

9. The typical echocardiographic features of rheumatic mitral stenosis include
A. a "hockey stick" appearance of the anterior mitral leaflet in the long axis view during diastole.
B. a "fish mouth" orifice in transgastric basal short axis view.
C. thickened and calcified mitral leaflets and subvalvular apparatus.
D. increased left atrial size.
E. all of the above.

10. Which one of the following parameters is consistent with severe mitral stenosis?
A. Peak pressure gradient of 10 mm Hg.
B. Mitral valve area of 1.2 cm^2.
C. Pressure half-time of 240 ms.
D. Mean pressure gradient of 7 mm Hg.
E. None of the above.

11. Which one of the following patients has severe aortic stenosis?
A. A 50-year-old woman has a ratio of the left ventricular outflow tract to the aortic valve time velocity integral less than 0.25.

B. A 60-year-old man has an aortic valve area greater than 1.5 cm^2.
C. An 80-year-old woman has a mean pressure gradient less than 25 mm Hg.
D. A 90-year-old man has a peak aortic valve velocity of 250 cm/s.
E. None of the above.

12. An 87-year-old patient has aortic stenosis and left ventricular dysfunction (decreased ejection fraction). During intraoperative transesophageal echocardiography, the severity of aortic stenosis is best evaluated by
A. the ratio of the left ventricular outflow tract time velocity integral to the aortic valve time velocity integral.
B. the peak pressure gradient across the aortic valve.
C. the mean pressure gradient across the aortic valve.
D. the peak aortic valve velocity.
E. the mean aortic valve velocity.

13. In patients with systolic anterior motion of the mitral valve after mitral repair, the coaptation site of the mitral valve is
A. the tip of the mitral leaflets.
B. the edge of the mitral leaflets on the atrial surface.
C. the edge of the mitral leaflets on the ventricular surface.
D. the body of the anterior mitral leaflet on the atrial surface.
E. the body of the posterior mitral leaflet on the ventricular surface.

14. In patients with mitral stenosis, M-mode echocardiography demonstrates
A. a normal E-F slope.
B. a shortened E-F slope.
C. a prolonged E-F slope.
D. a shortened D-E slope.
E. a prolonged D-E slope.

15. A 70-year-old patient with concomitant mitral stenosis and severe aortic regurgitation undergoes transesophageal echocardiography. The Doppler study reveals a mitral inflow pressure half-time of 200 ms. Most likely, the pressure half-time of mitral inflow in this patient is
A. not affected by the presence of the aortic regurgitation.
B. shortened because of the aortic regurgitation.
C. prolonged because of the aortic regurgitation.
D. sometimes prolonged and sometimes shortened because of the aortic regurgitation.
E. none of the above.

16. Which one of the following statements about the patient described in Question 15 is true?
A. The mitral valve area in this patient is best evaluated by the pressure half-time method.

B. The pressure half-time method overestimates the severity of mitral stenosis in this patient.
C. The pressure half-time method underestimates the severity of mitral stenosis in this patient.
D. The patient has moderate mitral stenosis because the calculated mitral valve area is 1.1 cm^2.
E. The patient has severe mitral stenosis because the mitral valve area is equal to the pressure half-time divided by the constant 220, or 0.9 cm^2.

17. All of the following patients have severe mitral regurgitation ***except***
A. A 50-year-old patient has a mitral regurgitant volume of 65 mL.
B. A 60-year-old patient has pulmonary vein systolic flow reversals during transesophageal echocardiography.
C. A 70-year-old patient has a regurgitant fraction of 60%.
D. An 80-year-old patient with chest pain has a papillary muscle rupture on two-dimensional echocardiography.
E. A 90-year-old patient has an effective regurgitant orifice of 20 mm^2.

18. The mitral valve area can be calculated by the continuity equation, dividing the left ventricular outflow tract stroke volume by the mitral valve time velocity integral. In patients with concomitant mitral stenosis and mitral regurgitation, this continuity equation
A. is the most accurate method to calculate the mitral valve area.
B. overestimates the severity of mitral stenosis.
C. slightly underestimates the severity of mitral stenosis because of the presence of mitral regurgitation.
D. severely underestimates the severity of mitral stenosis because of the presence of mitral regurgitation.
E. is not accurate because of the presence of mitral stenosis.

19. In a 72-year-old patient with low cardiac output, transesophageal echocardiography reveals a peak velocity of 3.3 m/s through the aortic valve and a mean gradient of 37 mm Hg. The Doppler information suggests
A. a normal aortic valve without stenosis.
B. mild aortic stenosis.
C. moderate aortic stenosis because the mean gradient was less than 50 mm Hg.
D. moderate aortic stenosis because the peak aortic valve velocity was less than 4.5 m/s.
E. none of the above.

20. The most appropriate next step for the patient described in Question 19 is
A. to measure mean aortic valve velocity.
B. to measure peak aortic pressure gradient.
C. to repeat measurement of peak aortic valve velocity in a week.
D. to repeat measurement of mean aortic pressure gradient in a month.
E. dobutamine echocardiography.

21. After aortic valve replacement with a St. Jude prosthesis (St. Jude Medical, Inc, St. Paul, Minnesota), intraoperative transesophageal echocardiography detects a peak velocity of 2.5 m/s and a mean gradient of 14.4 mm Hg across the aortic prosthetic valve. The Doppler information is consistent with

A. a normal St. Jude prosthetic valve at the aortic position.
B. abnormal stenosis of the aortic prosthetic valve.
C. obstruction of the aortic prosthesis.
D. severe regurgitation through the aortic prosthesis.
E. none of the above.

22. The most common cause of aortic regurgitation is

A. degenerative calcification of the aortic valve.
B. rheumatic heart disease.
C. prosthetic valve dysfunction.
D. endocarditis.
E. dilated aortic root.

23. During transesophageal echocardiography in a patient with severe aortic stenosis, a central jet of mitral regurgitation is detected. Most likely, the mechanism of the mitral regurgitation in this patient is

A. rheumatic valvular disease.
B. mitral valve prolapse.
C. papillary muscle rupture.
D. chordal rupture.
E. increased left ventricular systolic pressure.

24. When color flow imaging is used to evaluate mitral regurgitation, it tends to

A. overestimate an eccentric jet.
B. overestimate a central jet.
C. underestimate an eccentric jet.
D. underestimate a central jet.
E. B and C.

25. In patients with aortic stenosis and coexisting severe aortic regurgitation, which one of the following methods is more reliable in evaluating the severity of aortic stenosis?

A. Cardiac catheterization.
B. The ratio of the left ventricular outflow tract time velocity integral to the aortic valve time velocity integral.
C. Peak velocity across the aortic valve.
D. Mean pressure gradient across the aortic valve.
E. All of the above.

26. The severity of aortic regurgitation

A. is best correlated with the length of the aortic regurgitant jet.
B. is not correlated with the area of the regurgitant jet in the aortic valve short axis view.

C. is well correlated with the width of the regurgitant jet at its origin relative to the diameter of the left ventricular outflow tract.
D. is most commonly estimated by the length of the aortic regurgitant jet in the aortic valve long axis view.
E. A and D.

27. Which one of the following Doppler spectra indicates severe aortic regurgitation?
A. Holosystolic flow reversal in the ascending thoracic aorta.
B. Holodiastolic flow reversal in the descending thoracic aorta.
C. Early diastolic flow reversal in the proximal ascending aorta.
D. Systolic flow reversal in the pulmonary veins.
E. Systolic flow reversal in the hepatic vein.

28. In a patient with concomitant aortic regurgitation and mitral stenosis, Doppler echocardiography records
A. aortic regurgitation flow during early ejection.
B. mitral stenosis flow during isovolumic relaxation time.
C. aortic regurgitation flow during isovolumic contraction time.
D. mitral stenosis flow during isovolumic contraction time.
E. aortic regurgitation flow during late ejection.

29. Vena contracta is
A. the narrowest portion of the mitral regurgitation jet downstream from the orifice.
B. the maximal length of the mitral regurgitation jet.
C. the circumference of the mitral effective regurgitant orifice.
D. the radius of the mitral effective regurgitant orifice.
E. the radius of the proximal isovelocity surface area.

30. An average vena contracta of 0.5 cm or more from two views is
A. never associated with severe mitral regurgitation.
B. always associated with a regurgitant fraction of 20% or more.
C. always associated with a regurgitant volume of 30 mL or more.
D. always associated with an effective regurgitant orifice more than 40 mm^2.
E. none of the above.

31. A 56-year-old patient with mitral stenosis undergoes transesophageal echocardiography. The proximal isovelocity surface area radius measures 0.8 cm at an aliasing velocity of 56 cm/s. The peak mitral inflow velocity was 2.3 m/s and the angle between the mitral leaflets on the atrial side is 160°. On the basis of this information, this patient has
A. a normal mitral valve area.
B. mild mitral stenosis.
C. moderate mitral stenosis.
D. severe mitral stenosis.
E. undetermined mitral valve area because the proximal isovelocity surface area method is used to evaluate the severity of mitral regurgitation.

32. A 67-year-old patient with left ventricular dysfunction is scheduled for dobutamine echocardiography. If this patient has true severe aortic stenosis, the dobutamine echocardiogram

A. will decrease the peak velocity and mean gradient across the aortic valve.
B. will increase the mean gradient and decrease the peak velocity across the aortic valve.
C. will not change the mean gradient and peak velocity across the aortic valve.
D. will not change the ratio of the left ventricular outflow tract to the aortic valve time velocity integral.
E. will increase the aortic valve area.

33. The continuous wave Doppler velocity signal through the aortic valve shown in the accompanying image is obtained from a 70-year-old man. On the basis of this Doppler spectrum (MG, mean gradient), the peak pressure gradient across the aortic valve is approximately

A. 30 mm Hg.
B. 60 mm Hg.
C. 90 mm Hg.
D. 120 mm Hg.
E. 150 mm Hg.

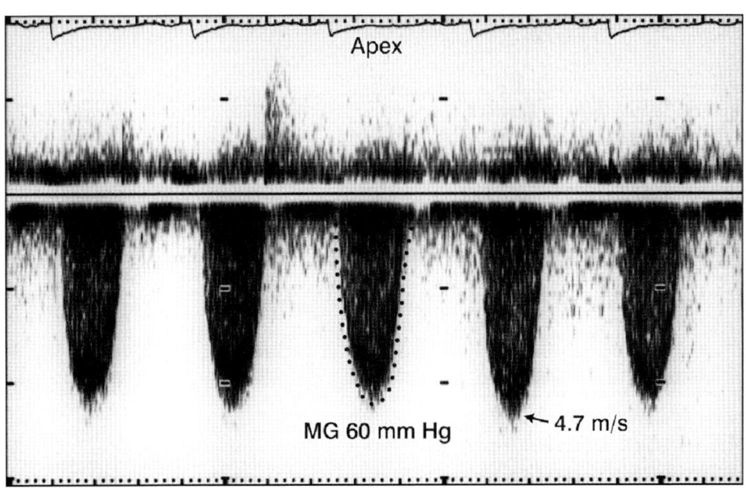

Figure from Oh et al. (23). Used with permission of Mayo Foundation for Medical Education and Research.

34. The patient whose Doppler is shown in Question 33 has

A. a normal aortic valve.
B. mild aortic stenosis.
C. moderate aortic stenosis.
D. severe aortic stenosis.
E. an undetermined condition.

35. The Duke criteria for infective endocarditis consist of major and minor criteria. All of the following are major criteria for infective endocarditis ***except***
A. positive blood culture.
B. temperature higher than 38.0°C.
C. new valvular regurgitation.
D. new partial dehiscence of the prosthetic valve.
E. oscillating intracardiac mass on the valve or supporting structures or in the path of regurgitant jets or on iatrogenic devices, in the absence of an alternative anatomic explanation.

36. All of the following are typical organisms for infective endocarditis ***except***
A. parainfluenza.
B. *Staphylococcus aureus.*
C. *Streptococcus viridans.*
D. the HACEK group (*Haemophilus* spp, *Actinobacillus actinomycetemcomitans, Cardiobacterium hominis, Eikenella* spp, and *Kingella kingae*).
E. *Streptococcus bovis.*

37. In patients with infective endocarditis, vegetations typically occur on
A. the ventricular surface of the mitral valve.
B. the ventricular surface of the tricuspid valve.
C. the ventricular surface of the aortic valve.
D. the pulmonary surface of the pulmonic valve.
E. the aortic surface of the aortic valve.

38. In patients with acute severe aortic regurgitation, the Doppler spectrum of the mitral inflow shows
A. increased early diastolic (E) velocity and decreased late diastolic (A) velocity with increased E/A ratio.
B. decreased E velocity and increased A velocity with decreased E/A ratio.
C. decreased E and A velocities with normal E/A ratio.
D. increased E and A velocities with normal E/A ratio.
E. no change of mitral E and A velocities.

39. Compared with mild aortic regurgitation, the Doppler signal of severe aortic regurgitation has
A. prolonged deceleration time and shortened pressure half-time.
B. shortened deceleration time and prolonged pressure half-time.
C. shortened deceleration time and pressure half-time.
D. prolonged deceleration time and pressure half-time.
E. the same deceleration time and pressure half-time.

40. In a 56-year-old patient with mitral regurgitation, the accompanying Doppler spectrum is obtained with the sample volume placed in the pulmonary vein. This Doppler spectrum indicates that the patient has

A. a normal flow pattern for the pulmonary vein.

B. mild pulmonic regurgitation.

C. severe pulmonic regurgitation.

D. severe mitral regurgitation.

E. mild mitral regurgitation.

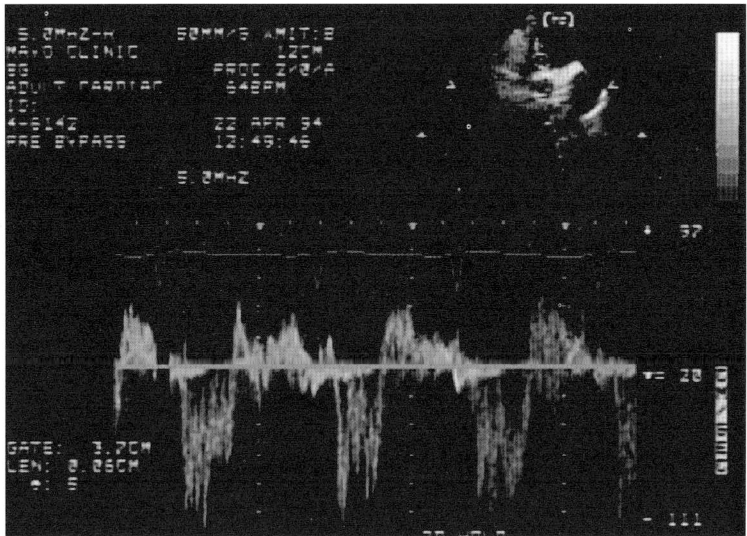

41. The accompanying two-dimensional transesophageal echocardiographic images were obtained during systole (A, without color flow; B, with color flow). The predominant lesion of this disease is

A. trivial mitral stenosis.
B. mild mitral regurgitation.
C. moderate aortic stenosis.
D. moderately severe aortic regurgitation.
E. severe tricuspid regurgitation.

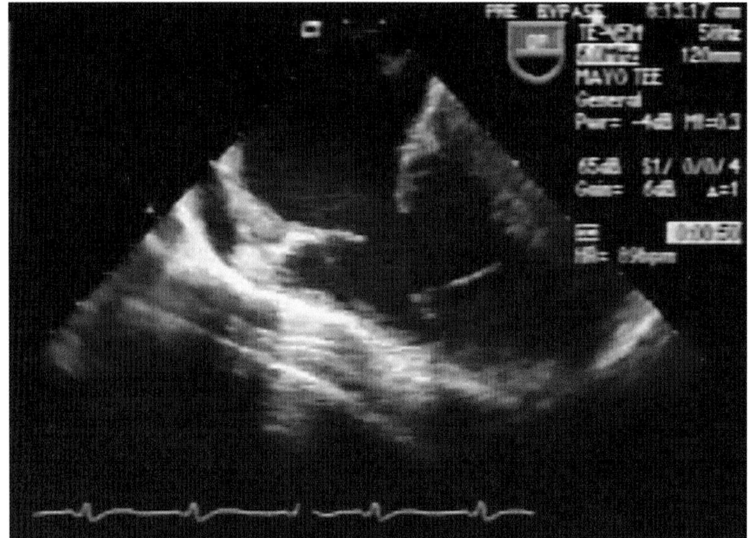

A

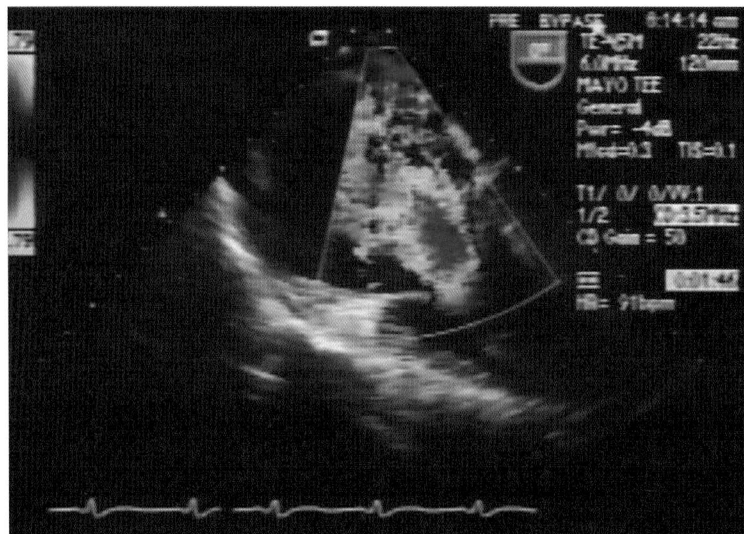

B

42. Most likely, the etiology of the valvular lesion shown in the image accompanying Question 41 is

A. Ebstein's anomaly.

B. carcinoid disease.

C. papillary muscle dysfunction.

D. ischemic disease.

E. dilated tricuspid anulus.

43. Frequently, patients with the valvular lesion shown in the image accompanying Question 41 also have an affected

A. mitral valve.

B. aortic valve.

C. pulmonic valve.

D. all of the above.

E. none of the above.

44. Which one of the following statements about tricuspid stenosis is true?

A. The pressure half-time method is used to calculate the mitral valve area but not the tricuspid valve area in tricuspid stenosis.

B. The constant of 220 ms is used to calculate the tricuspid valve area by the pressure half-time method.

C. The tricuspid inflow pressure half-time of 200 ms indicates severe tricuspid stenosis.

D. A mean gradient of 7 mm Hg across the tricuspid valve indicates normal tricuspid valve without stenosis.

E. A mean gradient of 7 mm Hg across the tricuspid valve indicates mild tricuspid stenosis.

45. A ratio of aortic regurgitant jet width to left ventricular outflow tract diameter

A. of 10% or more indicates moderate aortic regurgitation.

B. of 20% or more indicates moderately severe aortic regurgitation.

C. of 30% or more indicates severe aortic regurgitation.

D. indicates all of the above.

E. indicates none of the above.

46. Which one of the following suggests severe mitral regurgitation?

A. A left ventricular dimension of 5.5 cm at end diastole.

B. A left atrial size of 4.0 cm.

C. Decreased early mitral inflow diastolic velocity.

D. A central mitral regurgitation jet with color flow area 20% of the left atrial size.

E. An eccentric mitral regurgitation jet reaching the posterior wall of the left atrium.

47. Which one of the following statements about normal prosthetic valves is true?

A. The pressure gradient across a normal prosthetic valve is higher than that expected for a respective native valve.

B. The pressure gradient across a normal prosthetic valve is lower than that expected for a respective native valve.

C. A normal prosthetic valve should not be stenotic in comparison with the respective native valve.

D. Flow velocity across a normal prosthetic valve is the same as that expected for a respective native valve.

E. None of the above.

48. After the patient is taken off cardiopulmonary bypass, the accompanying two-dimensional images are obtained by intraoperative transesophageal echocardiography during systole (A), diastole (B), and color flow imaging (C). LA indicates the left atrium. The mitral prosthetic valve is

A. a normal bileaflet prosthesis.

B. a normal tilting-disk prosthesis.

C. a normal ball-cage prosthesis.

D. a dysfunctional bileaflet prosthesis.

E. a dysfunctional tilting-disk prosthesis.

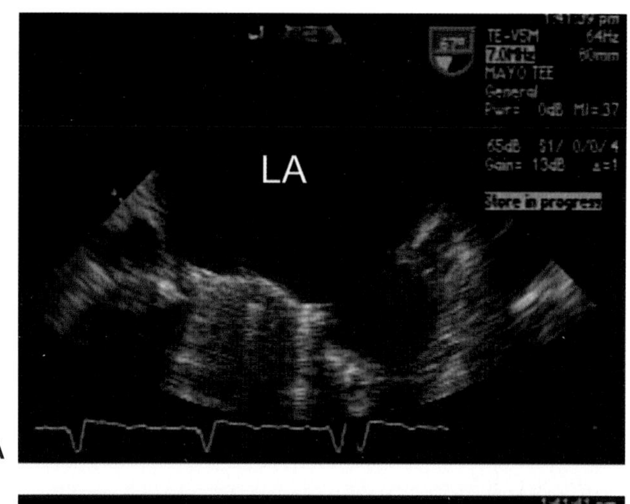
A
LA
TE-V5M 64Hz
MAYO TEE
General
Pwr= 0dB MI=.37
65dB S1/ 0/0/ 4
Gain= 13dB
Store in progress

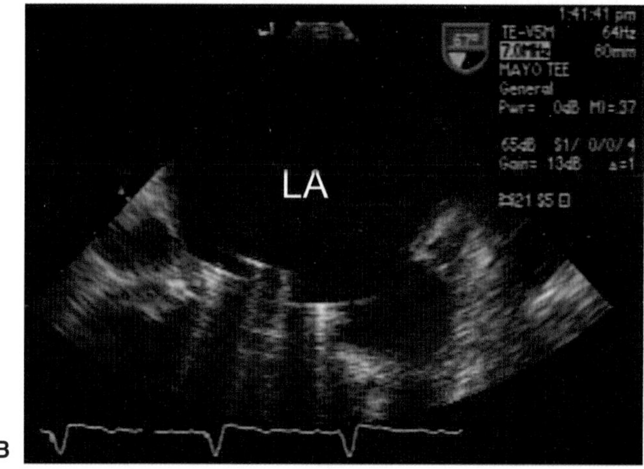
B
LA
1:41:41 pm
TE-V5M 64Hz
80mm
MAYO TEE
General
Pwr= 0dB MI=.37
65dB S1/ 0/0/ 4
Gain= 13dB

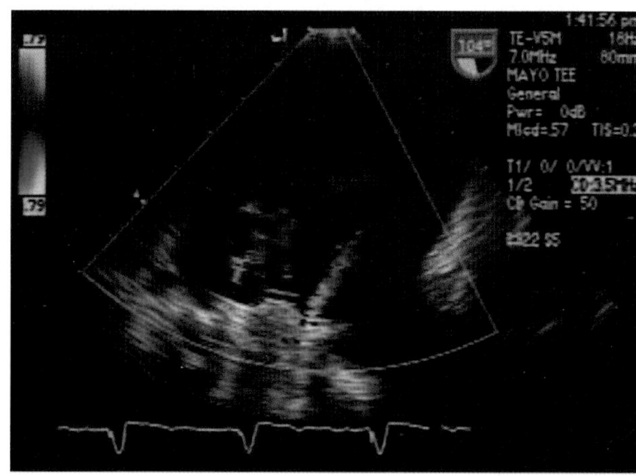
C
1:41:56 pm
TE-V5M 18Hz
7.0MHz 80mm
MAYO TEE
General
Pwr= 0dB
MIcd=.57 TIS=0.3
1/2
Cf Gain = 50

49. All of the following are consistent with severe tricuspid regurgitation ***except***
A. a tricuspid annular diameter of 3.8 cm.
B. a tricuspid inflow velocity greater than 1 m/s.
C. a color flow regurgitant jet area greater than 30% of the right atrial area.
D. a dense tricuspid regurgitant signal.
E. systolic flow reversal in the hepatic vein.

50. A 58-year-old patient with an aortic valve lesion undergoes preoperative transesophageal echocardiography. The accompanying Doppler spectrum shows holodiastolic flow (arrows) in the descending thoracic aorta (Desc Ao). This Doppler spectrum is consistent with
A. plaques in the descending aorta.
B. coarctation of the aorta.
C. severe aortic regurgitation.
D. severe aortic stenosis.
E. systemic hypertension.

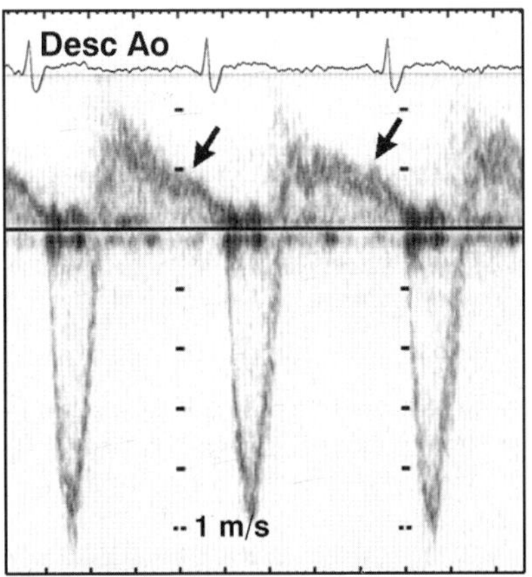

Figure from Oh et al. (23). Used with permission of Mayo Foundation for Medical Education and Research.

51. During transesophageal echocardiography in a 76-year-old patient, the Doppler study reveals the mitral inflow time velocity integral of 66 cm and the left ventricular outflow tract time velocity integral of 23 cm. The diameter of the patient's left ventricular outflow tract is 2.1 cm. The mitral valve area calculated by the continuity equation is approximately
A. 0.6 cm^2.
B. 1.2 cm^2.
C. 1.8 cm^2.
D. 2.4 cm^2.
E. 3.0 cm^2.

52. According to the above calculated mitral valve area, the diagnosis for the patient described in Question 51 is

A. normal mitral valve without any stenosis.

B. mild mitral stenosis.

C. moderate mitral stenosis.

D. severe mitral stenosis.

E. undetermined.

53. If the patient described in Question 51 also has severe aortic regurgitation, the calculated mitral valve severity is

A. underestimated because of the aortic regurgitation.

B. not affected by the presence of severe aortic regurgitation.

C. an accurate estimate of the severity of mitral stenosis.

D. an overestimate of the severity of mitral stenosis.

54. Normally, a mechanical prosthetic valve

A. does not have any regurgitation.

B. has mild perivalvular regurgitation.

C. has mild transvalvular and perivalvular regurgitation.

D. has "built-in" regurgitant jets.

55. Which one of the following patients most likely has mild aortic regurgitation?

A. A 90-year-old patient has aortic regurgitation pressure half-time of 420 ms.

B. An 80-year-old patient with chronic aortic regurgitation has a left ventricular diastolic dimension of 7.6 cm.

C. A 70-year-old patient has a dense continuous wave Doppler aortic regurgitation jet.

D. In a 60-year-old patient, the ratio of the regurgitant jet area to the left ventricular outflow tract area is 65%.

E. This cannot be determined.

56. The accompanying image is a continuous wave Doppler recording of mitral inflow and the tricuspid regurgitant jet. (DT indicates deceleration time; PAPs, systolic pulmonary artery pressures.) On the basis of this Doppler information, the mitral valve area

A. is less than 1 cm^2.

B. is approximately 1.5 cm^2.

C. is about 2.5 cm^2.

D. is obviously normal.

E. cannot be estimated.

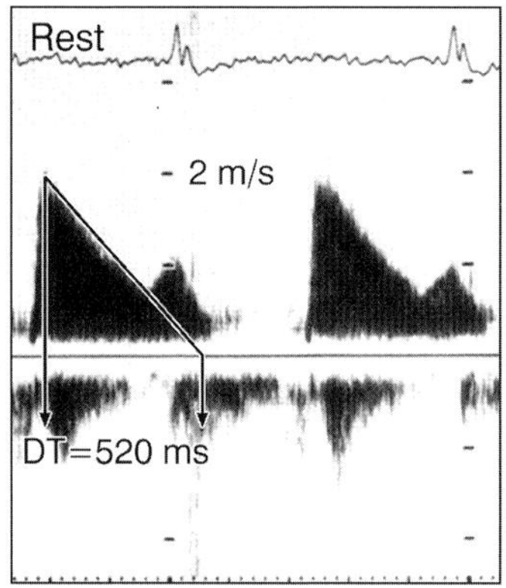

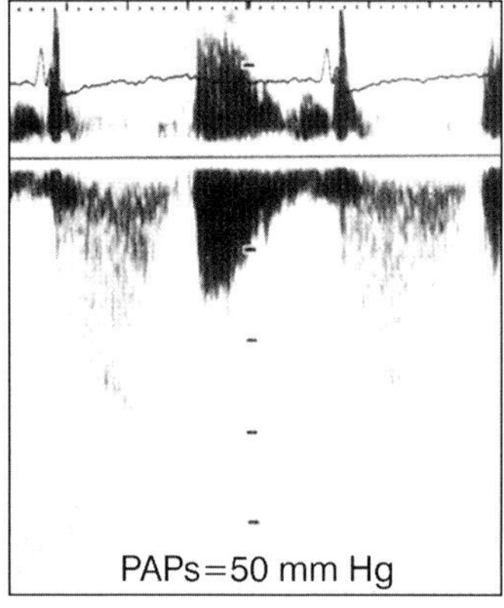

Figure from Oh et al. (23). Used with permission of Mayo Foundation for Medical Education and Research.

57. The Doppler spectrum accompanying Question 56 is consistent with
A. a normal mitral valve without any mitral stenosis.
B. mild mitral stenosis.
C. moderate mitral stenosis.
D. severe mitral stenosis.
E. an undetermined finding.

58. A 72-year-old patient with a history of mitral regurgitation undergoes transesophageal echocardiography. Compared with transesophageal echocardiography performed 2 years ago, the Doppler study now shows a lower velocity of mitral regurgitant flow, and the color flow imaging at an aliasing velocity of 70 cm/s shows much more severe mitral regurgitation. The clinician's conclusion is that
A. the patient's mitral regurgitation is improving over time because the mitral regurgitant velocity is lower than that 2 years ago.
B. the patient's mitral regurgitation became more severe over time.
C. the color flow imaging overestimates the severity of mitral regurgitation because the aliasing velocity is too high.
D. the color flow imaging overestimates the severity of mitral regurgitation because the aliasing velocity is too low.
E. the current Doppler study cannot be explained because the color flow imaging showed worsening mitral regurgitation.

59. The accompanying image of Doppler velocity is obtained with the ultrasound beam through the aortic prosthetic valve. (DT is deceleration time, and PHT, pressure half-time, both in milliseconds.) The Doppler spectrum is consistent with
A. mild aortic regurgitation.
B. mild aortic stenosis.
C. severe aortic regurgitation.
D. severe aortic stenosis.
E. an undetermined condition.

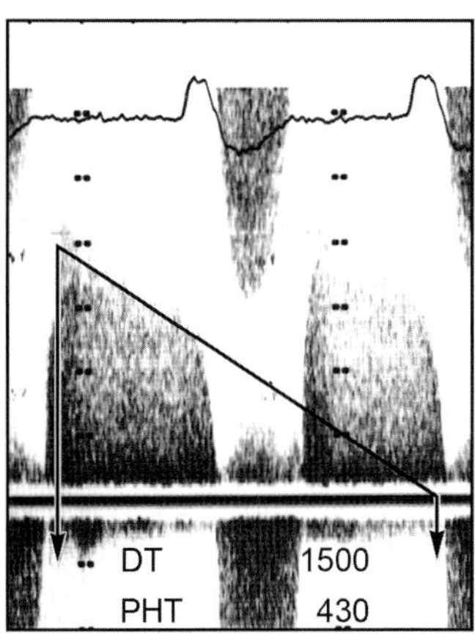

Figure from Oh et al. (23). Used with permission of Mayo Foundation for Medical Education and Research.

60. The accompanying Doppler spectra are obtained in a patient with aortic regurgitation. The patient has normal diastolic function before the development of aortic regurgitation. (A indicates late filling; AV, aortic valve; DT, deceleration time; E, early filling; MV, mitral valve; PHT, pressure half-time.) On the basis of the Doppler information, which one of the following statements about this patient is true?

A. The patient has chronic mild aortic regurgitation.
B. The patient has acute moderate aortic regurgitation.
C. The patient has chronic moderately severe aortic regurgitation.
D. The patient has acute severe aortic regurgitation.
E. The Doppler spectrum of mitral inflow does not provide any information about aortic regurgitation.

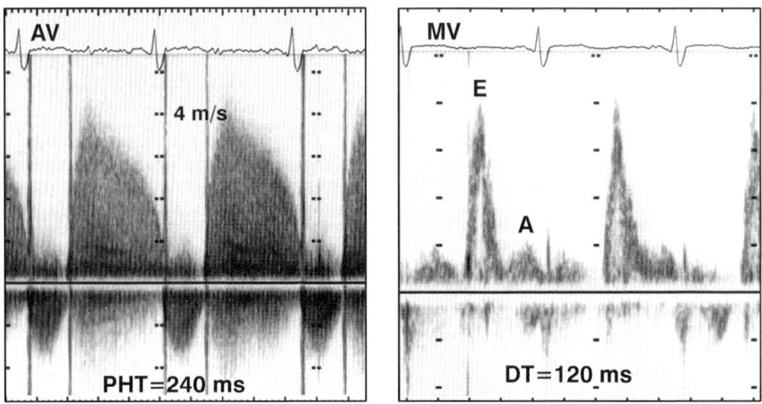

Figure from Oh et al. (23). Used with permission of Mayo Foundation for Medical Education and Research.

61. All the following statements about complications of mechanical prosthesis are true ***except***

A. thrombosis may occur in patients with a prosthetic valve, but hemolysis never happens.
B. mitral regurgitation through a prosthetic valve may cause hemolysis.
C. endocarditis may occur in patients with a prosthetic valve.
D. ring abscess may occur in patients with a prosthetic valve.
E. dehiscence is one of the complications of a prosthetic valve.

62. A 75-year-old patient with a left ventricular ejection fraction of 30% has an aortic valve velocity of 4.3 m/s and a left ventricular outflow tract velocity of 43 cm/s. The mean pressure gradient across the aortic valve is less than 50 mm Hg. Most likely, this patient has

A. a normal aortic valve without stenosis because the left ventricular ejection fraction is 30%.
B. mild aortic stenosis because the mean pressure gradient is less than 50 mm Hg.
C. moderate aortic stenosis because the aortic valve velocity is 4.3 m/s.

D. moderately severe aortic stenosis because the left ventricular outflow tract velocity is 43 cm/s.
E. severe aortic stenosis even though the mean pressure gradient is less than 50 mm Hg.

63. The accompanying transesophageal echocardiographic image is obtained in a febrile patient. (LA indicates left atrium; LV, left ventricle; MV, mitral valve.) The arrow points to
A. an infected congenital ventricular septal defect.
B. an acquired ventricular septal defect with infection.
C. an infected atrial septal defect.
D. a pseudoaneurysm of the mitral leaflet.
E. an abscess of the aortic and mitral valve intervalvular fibrosa.

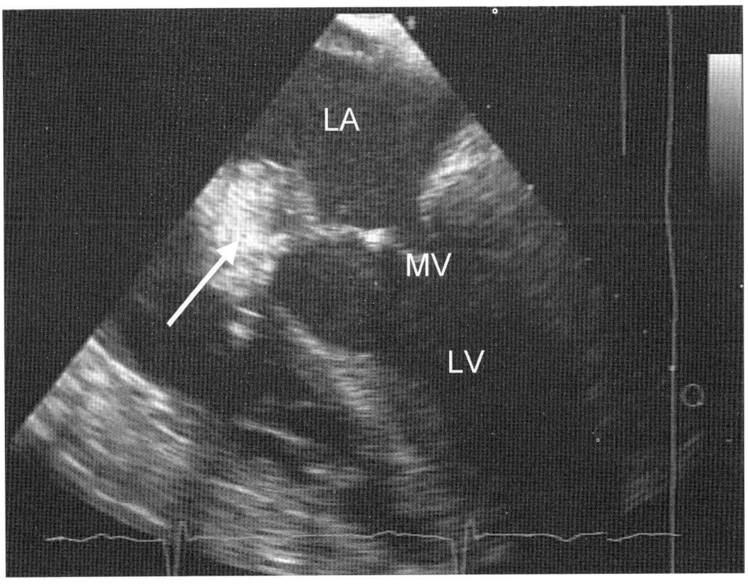

64. During transesophageal echocardiography in a patient with a history of mitral valve replacement, severe perivalvular regurgitation around the prosthesis is detected by color flow Doppler. The color map has aliasing at a velocity of 65 cm/s. The perivalvular regurgitation detected in this patient is
A. physiologic but underestimated.
B. pathologic but overestimated.
C. an ultrasound artifact because the aliasing velocity is too low.
D. a phenomenon called "ghosting."
E. none of the above.

65. A 58-year-old patient undergoes mitral valve replacement. Immediately after coming off cardiopulmonary bypass but before administration of protamine, a trace of perivalvular regurgitation with very low flow velocity is detected by intraoperative transesophageal echocardiography, despite the normal two-dimensional appearance of the prosthesis. Which one of the following statements about perivalvular regurgitation is true?

A. Perivalvular regurgitation is the volume displaced by an occluder during closure.
B. Perivalvular regurgitation is the "built-in" regurgitation to wash the hinge point.
C. Any degree of perivalvular regurgitation is always physiologic.
D. Any degree of perivalvular regurgitation is always pathologic.
E. Trace perivalvular regurgitation with very low flow velocity may not be pathologic, especially before the administration of protamine.

66. The next step of management for the patient described in Question 65 is to

A. replace the mitral prosthesis.
B. go back on cardiopulmonary bypass.
C. give protamine.
D. give heparin.
E. A, B, and D.

67. Which one of the following statements about the methods used to evaluate a mechanical prosthesis is true?

A. Planimetry is the most common method to evaluate the area of a mechanical prosthesis.
B. The pressure half-time method is the most accurate method to evaluate the area of a mechanical prosthesis.
C. The pressure half-time method may overestimate the area of a mitral prosthesis.
D. The continuity equation measures the size and the physical boundaries of a mitral prosthetic valve.
E. The continuity equation does not measure the effective orifice area of a mitral prosthesis.

68. Which one of the following is a normal regurgitant flow pattern for mechanical prostheses?

A. Two curved side jets for the Starr-Edwards prosthetic valve.
B. One central jet for the Bjork-Shiley prosthetic valve.
C. Two side and one central jet for the Medtronic-Hall prosthetic valve.
D. Two unequal side jets for the St. Jude prosthetic valve.
E. None of the above.

69. Valvular regurgitations commonly seen in the clinically normal population include all of the following ***except***

A. trivial pulmonary regurgitation in a 20-year-old man.
B. mild tricuspid regurgitation in a 30-year-old woman.
C. mild aortic regurgitation in a 40-year-old man.
D. mild mitral regurgitation in a 50-year-old woman.
E. mild pulmonary regurgitation in a 60-year-old man.

70. During transesophageal echocardiography in a 66-year-old patient, color flow imaging reveals mitral regurgitation. At an aliasing velocity of 36 cm/s, the proximal isovelocity surface area radius is 1 cm. The continuous wave Doppler detects the mitral regurgitation peak velocity of 450 cm/s and time velocity integral of 200 cm. The effective regurgitation orifice is approximately

A. 0.2 cm^2.

B. 0.3 cm^2.

C. 0.4 cm^2.

D. 0.5 cm^2.

E. undetermined.

71. The regurgitation volume in the patient described in Question 70 is approximately

A. 25 mL.

B. 50 mL.

C. 75 mL.

D. 100 mL.

E. undetermined.

72. The mitral regurgitation in the patient described in Question 70 is

A. trivial.

B. mild.

C. moderate.

D. moderately severe.

E. severe.

73. The accompanying two-dimensional echocardiographic image is obtained after a patient undergoing mitral valve surgery is taken off cardiopulmonary bypass. The patient had

A. mitral valve repair with anuloplasty.
B. mitral valve replacement with a bioprosthesis.
C. mitral valve replacement with a bileaflet mechanical prosthesis.
D. mitral valve replacement with a tilting-disk prosthesis.
E. mitral valve replacement with a stentless valve.

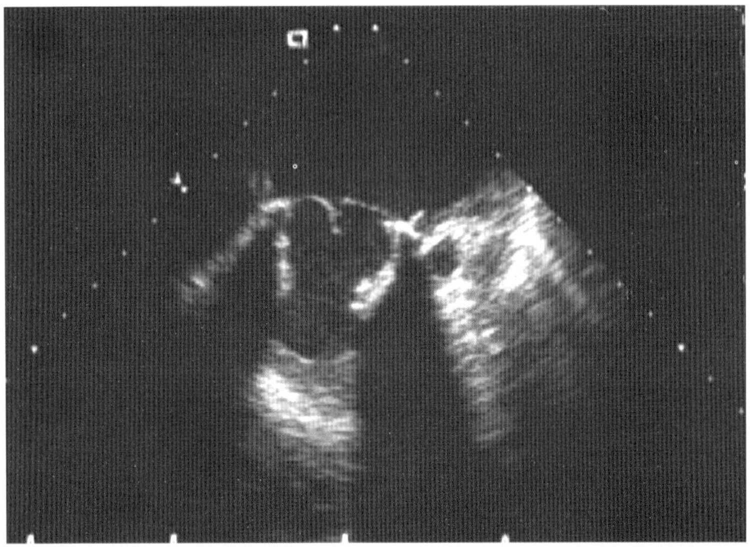

74. Which one of the following statements about a freestyle or stentless valve is true?

A. The stentless valve has a smaller effective orifice area than that of the same size stented valve.
B. If the size of the stentless valve and the stented valve are the same, their effective orifice areas are the same.
C. The effective orifice area of a stentless valve usually decreases slowly over time.
D. The mean pressure gradient across a stentless valve never changes over time.
E. The stentless valve provides low gradients and laminar flow similar to a native valve.

75. During transesophageal echocardiography in a febrile patient with a St. Jude mitral prosthesis, the two-dimensional image shows rocking movement of the prosthetic sewing ring (MR, mitral regurgitation). Color flow imaging in the accompanying figure shows

A. a normal regurgitant flow pattern for St. Jude prosthesis.
B. severe transvalvular regurgitation.
C. transvalvular mitral regurgitation with an eccentric jet.
D. transvalvular mitral regurgitation with a central jet.
E. perivalvular regurgitation.

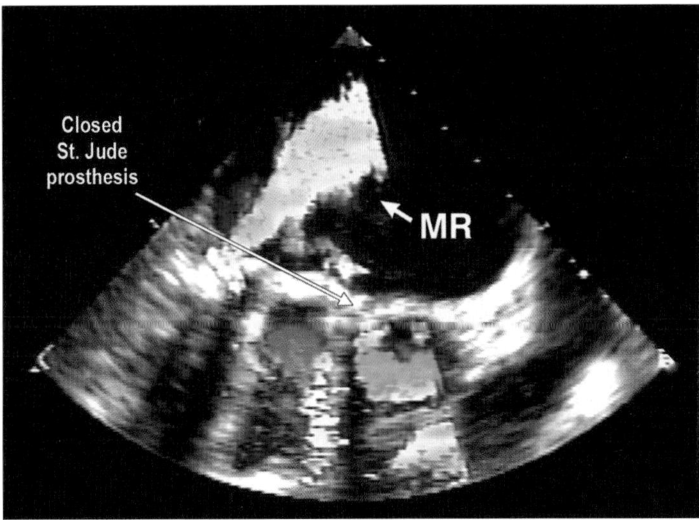

Figure from Oh et al. (23). Used with permission of Mayo Foundation for Medical Education and Research.

76. The regurgitation jet shown in the image accompanying Question 75 is caused by

A. normal closing volume.
B. incomplete valve leaflet closure.
C. annular dilation.
D. dehiscence of the sewing ring.
E. leaflet defect of the prosthetic valve.

77. Most likely, the patient shown in the image accompanying Question 75 has

A. a normal mitral prosthesis.
B. thrombosis on the mitral prosthesis.
C. endocarditis.
D. rheumatic valvular disease.
E. degeneration of the prosthetic valve.

78. A 68-year-old patient undergoes mitral valve repair. Before being taken off cardiopulmonary bypass, calcium chloride is administered, and dopamine, 4 μg/kg per minute, is started. Shortly after being taken off cardiopulmonary bypass, the patient has systolic blood pressure of 78 mm Hg. Intraoperative transesophageal echocardiography shows the accompanying image. Which one of the following best describes the cause of hypotension?

A. Residual mitral regurgitation.
B. Decreased myocardial contractility.
C. Iatrogenic mitral stenosis.
D. Systolic anterior motion of the anterior mitral leaflet.
E. Severe systemic vasodilatation.

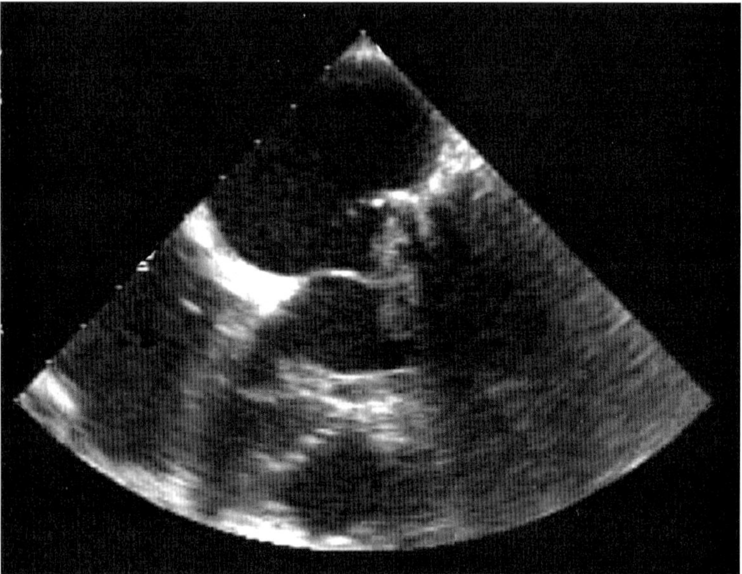

79. Based on the intraoperative transesophageal echocardiographic findings in the patient described in Question 78, the cardiologist should

A. tell the surgeon to return the patient to bypass to repair the mitral valve again.
B. tell the surgeon to return the patient to bypass to replace the mitral valve.
C. administer another gram of calcium chloride.
D. increase dopamine to 6 μg/kg per minute.
E. give fluids and stop the dopamine infusion.

80. The accompanying right heart view shows globular masses on the tricuspid valve (RA, right atrium; RV, right ventricle). This type of lesion may be associated with

A. immunocompromise.
B. right heart instrumentation.
C. injection drug use.
D. all of the above.
E. none of the above.

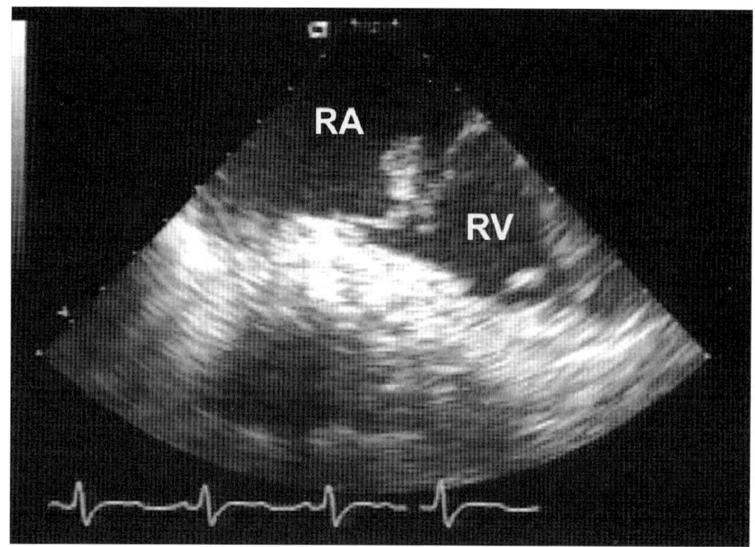

81. A 80-year-old patient undergoes open heart surgery for his aortic stenosis. The accompanying image is obtained before cardiopulmonary bypass. The cause of this patient's aortic stenosis is

A. a bicuspid aortic valve.

B. rheumatic valvular heart disease.

C. calcification of the aortic valve.

D. congenital abnormality of the aortic valve.

E. undetermined.

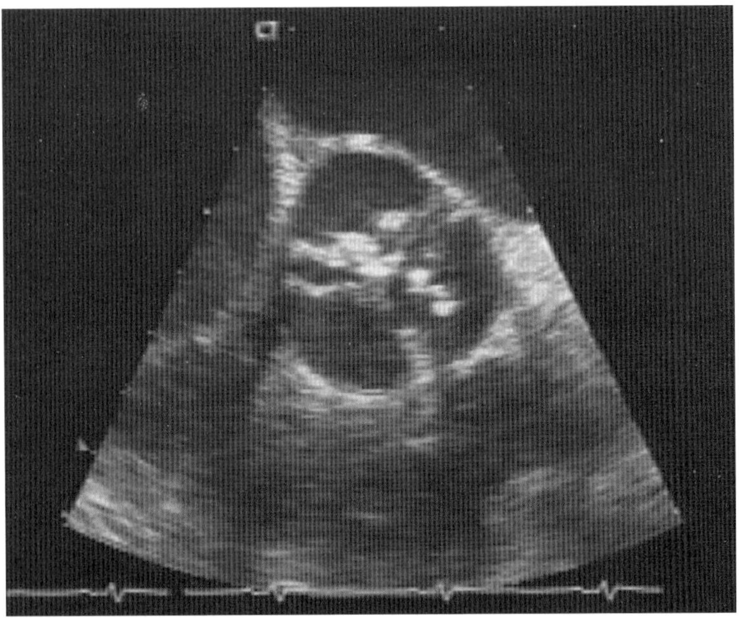

82. After the patient is taken off cardiopulmonary bypass, the accompanying transesophageal echocardiographic image shows that the patient underwent

A. aortic valve replacement with a ball-cage prosthesis.

B. aortic valve replacement with a tilting-disk prosthesis.

C. aortic valve replacement with a bileaflet prosthesis.

D. aortic valve replacement with a bioprosthesis.

E. a Ross procedure.

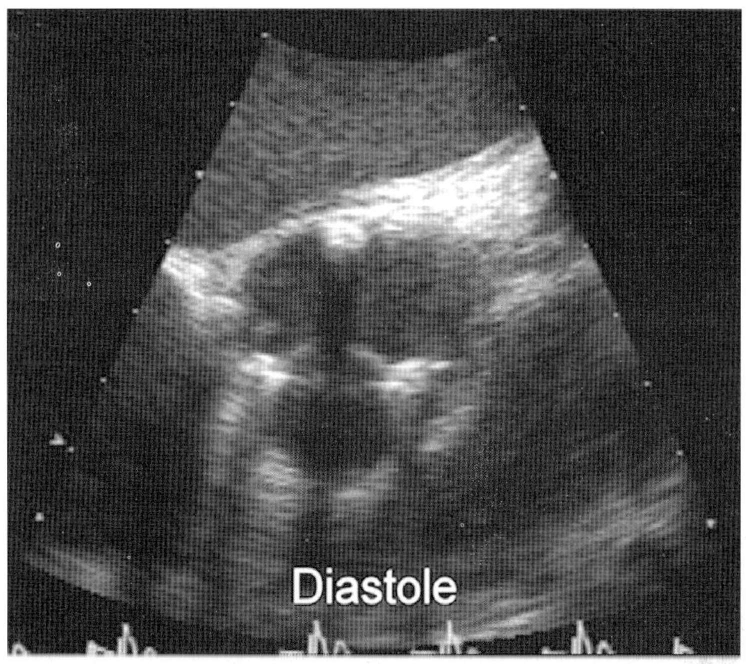
Diastole

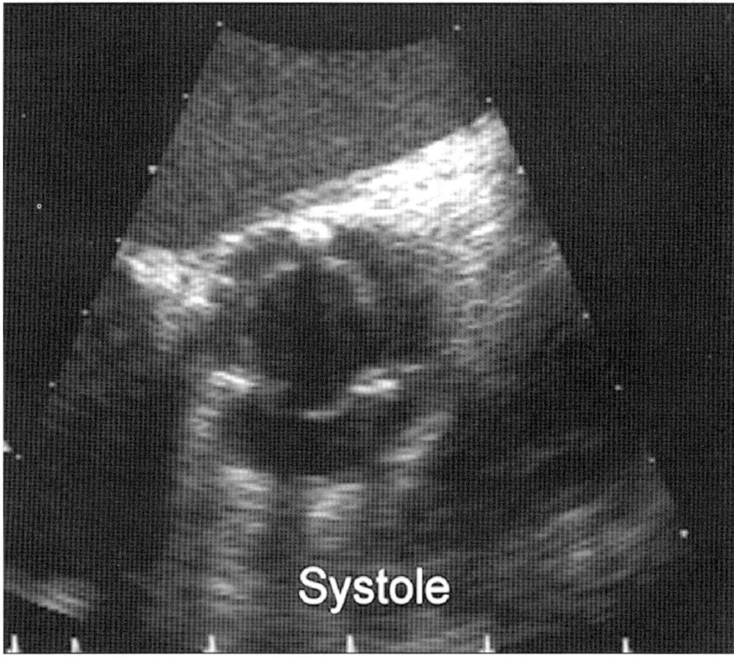
Systole

83. The dimensionless obstructive index used to evaluate the aortic prosthetic valve
   A. is the ratio of the left ventricular outflow tract to the aortic prosthesis velocity.
   B. is the ratio of the aortic prosthesis area to the left ventricular outflow tract area.
   C. indicates prosthetic obstruction if the index is 0.3 or higher.
   D. indicates a normal prosthetic valve without obstruction or stenosis if the index is 0.2 or lower.
   E. cannot be used to differentiate increased flow velocity across an aortic prosthesis because of prosthetic obstruction from increased velocity attributable to regurgitation.

84. After the patient is taken off cardiopulmonary bypass, the accompanying color flow image is obtained in a patient who underwent mitral valve replacement with a St. Jude prosthetic valve. (LA indicates left atrium.) The cardiologist should tell the cardiac surgeon
   A. to return the patient to bypass because there are three regurgitant jets.
   B. to replace the prosthetic valve because there is severe mitral regurgitation.
   C. there is no need to return the patient to bypass even though this is an abnormal St. Jude mitral valve with three mild regurgitant jets.
   D. the St. Jude mitral valve is normal because there is no regurgitant jet at all.
   E. this is a normal St. Jude mitral valve with normal regurgitant flow pattern.

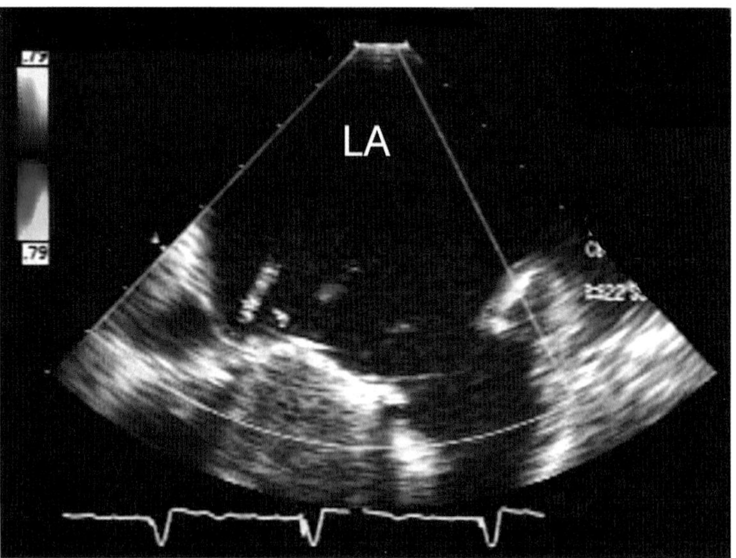

85. The accompanying two-dimensional images are obtained in a patient with a mitral prosthesis. (LA indicates left atrium.) This patient has

A. a normal tilting-disk prosthesis.
B. a dysfunctional tilting-disk prosthesis.
C. a normal bileaflet prosthesis.
D. a bileaflet prosthesis with one leaflet not closing.
E. a bileaflet prosthesis with both leaflets not opening.

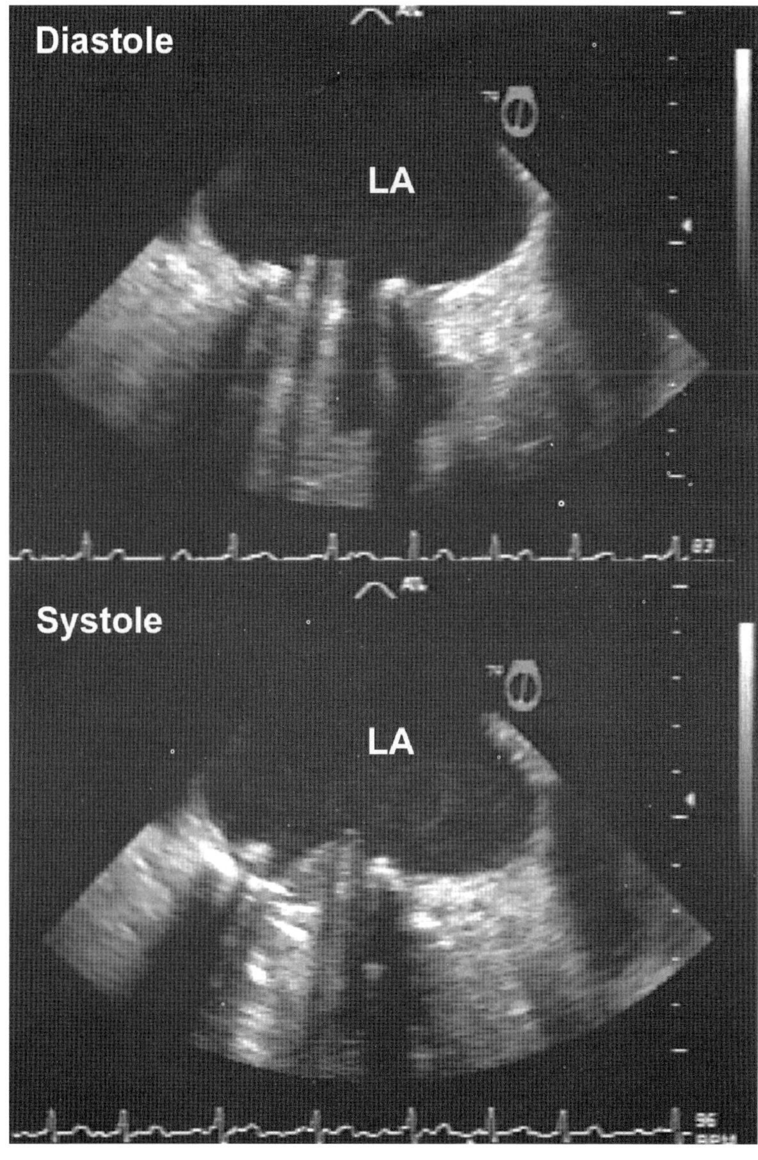

86. The accompanying transesophageal echocardiographic image is obtained in a febrile patient with normal left ventricular function. The intracardiac structures indicated by the arrows are highly mobile within the left ventricular outflow tract. Most likely, this patient has

A. aortic valve prolapse.

B. flail aortic cusp.

C. thrombus of the aortic valve.

D. subaortic stenosis.

E. infective endocarditis.

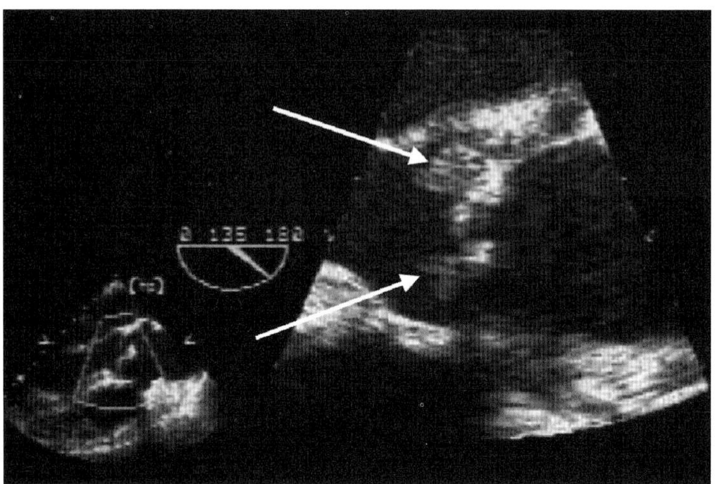

87. A 75-year-old woman with a small aorta undergoes aortic valve replacement with a 19-mm St. Jude prosthetic valve. After she is taken off cardiopulmonary bypass, a mean gradient of 20 mm Hg across the prosthetic valve is detected from a deep transgastric view. Two-dimensional imaging shows normal movement of the bileaflet prosthesis. The cardiologist should tell the surgeon

A. to return the patient to bypass and find out the cause of the stenosis.

B. to return the patient to bypass and replace the prosthetic valve.

C. the mean gradient indicates severe stenosis of the mechanical prosthesis.

D. the mean gradient of 20 mm Hg is normal in this patient.

E. the Doppler echocardiography overestimates the pressure gradient in deep transgastric view.

88. Color flow imaging in a 75-year-old patient reveals an eccentric mitral regurgitant jet with a distorted proximal isovelocity surface area. The mitral inflow time velocity integral was measured as 18 cm and the left ventricular outflow tract time velocity integral was 22 cm. The mitral anulus diameter was 3.8 cm and the left ventricular outflow tract diameter was 2.1 cm. Thus, the mitral regurgitation volume is approximately

A. 28 mL.

B. 48 mL.

C. 88 mL.

D. 128 mL.

E. undetermined because the proximal isovelocity surface area was distorted.

89. The mitral regurgitant fraction in the patient described in Question 88 is greater than

A. 30%.

B. 40%.

C. 50%.

D. 60%.

E. undetermined.

90. The patient described in Question 88 has

A. mild mitral regurgitation.

B. moderate mitral regurgitation.

C. moderately severe mitral regurgitation.

D. severe mitral regurgitation.

E. an undetermined condition.

91. A 56-year-old patient has the accompanying transesophageal echocardiographic images before bypass. (LA indicates left atrium; LV, left ventricle.) On the basis of these two-dimensional images, which one of the following best describes the mechanism of the mitral regurgitation in this patient?

A. Anterior mitral leaflet prolapse.

B. Flail anterior mitral leaflet.

C. Anterior mitral leaflet dysfunction due to ruptured papillary muscle.

D. Perforated posterior mitral leaflet.

E. Flail posterior mitral leaflet due to ruptured chordae tendineae.

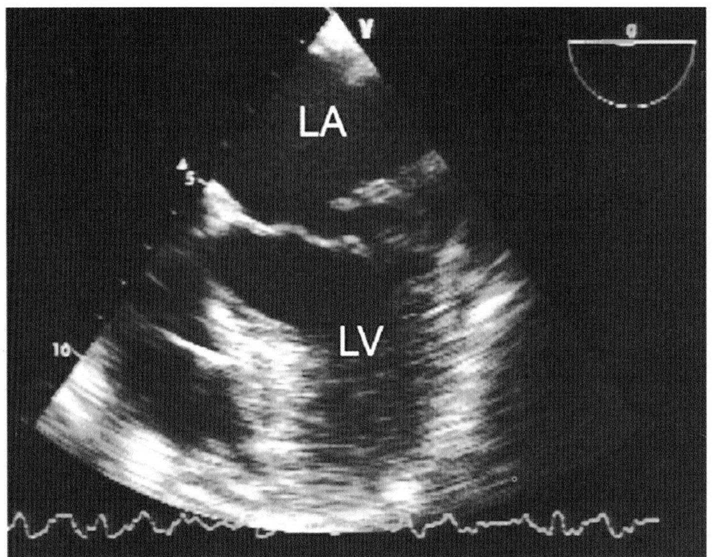

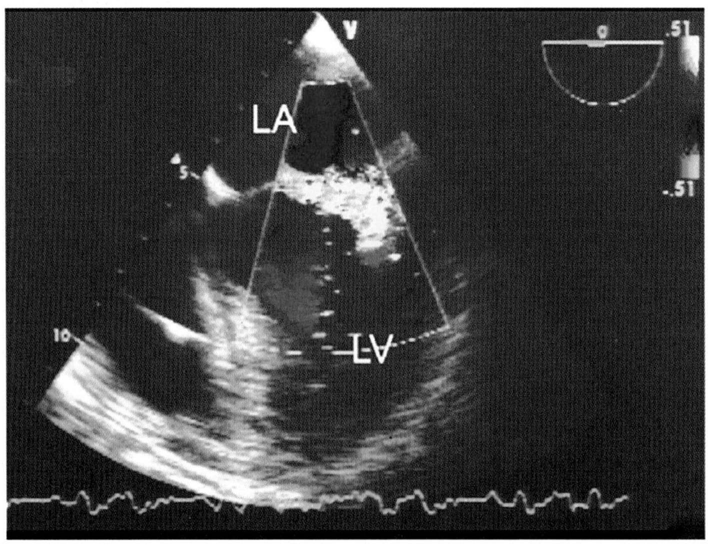

92. Most likely, the mitral regurgitation in the patient shown in Question 91 is

A. mild because the regurgitant jet area is relatively small.

B. moderate because the ratio of the regurgitant jet area to the left atrial area is less than 30%.

C. moderately severe because the ratio of the regurgitant jet area to the left atrial area is less than 50%.

D. severe even though the ratio of the regurgitant jet area to the left atrial area is no greater than 40%.

E. undetermined.

93. The accompanying transesophageal echocardiographic image (LA, left atrium; LV, left ventricle) further tells the cardiologist that the flail scallop is

A. A1 (the lateral scallop of the anterior mitral leaflet).

B. P1 (the lateral scallop of the posterior mitral leaflet).

C. A2 (the middle scallop of the anterior mitral leaflet).

D. P2 (the middle scallop of the posterior mitral leaflet).

E. A3 (the medial scallop of the anterior mitral leaflet).

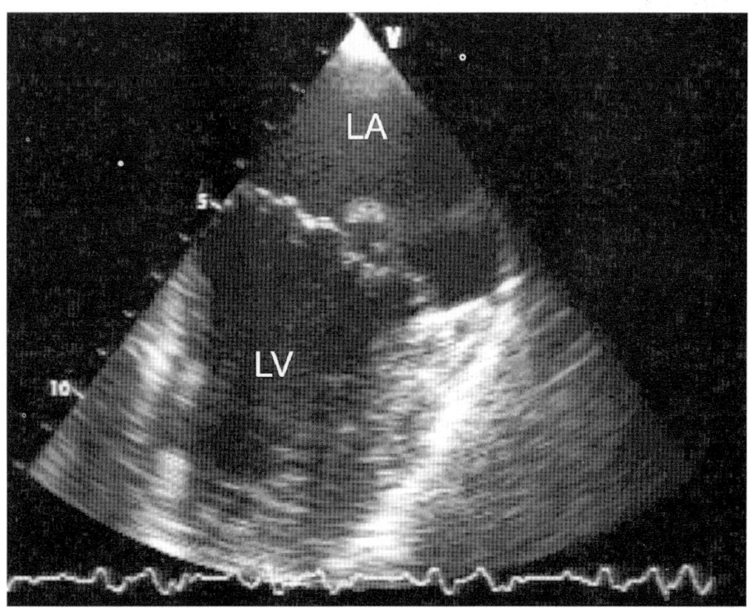

94. Another patient undergoes transesophageal echocardiography before bypass. The accompanying intraoperative transesophageal echocardiographic image (LA, left atrium; LV, left ventricle) shows

A. P2 (the middle scallop of the posterior mitral leaflet).
B. P1 (the lateral scallop of the posterior mitral leaflet).
C. P3 (the medial scallop of the posterior mitral leaflet).
D. A2 (the middle scallop of the anterior mitral leaflet).
E. A1 (the lateral scallop of the anterior mitral leaflet).

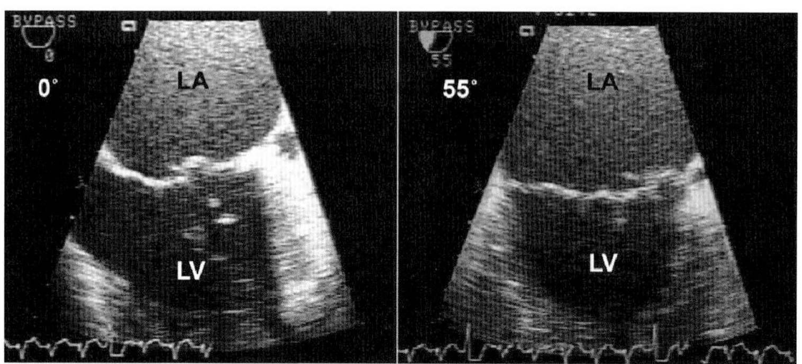

95. During transesophageal echocardiography in a 62-year-old patient with severe chronic anemia, the Doppler study reveals that the mean pressure gradient across the aortic valve is 52 mm Hg, both the left ventricular outflow tract velocity and the time velocity integral are increased, and the ratio of the left ventricular outflow tract to the aortic valve time velocity integral is 0.3. On two-dimensional imaging, the aortic valve does not appear to be severely stenotic. Which one of the following best describes the cardiologist's conclusion?

A. The patient has severe aortic stenosis because the mean gradient is greater than 50 mm Hg.
B. The two-dimensional imaging is not correct because the mean pressure gradient across the aortic valve indicates severe aortic stenosis.
C. The Doppler study is not correct because two-dimensional imaging does not reveal severe aortic stenosis.
D. Both two-dimensional imaging and Doppler information are incorrect.
E. The patient does not have severe aortic stenosis but has an increased cardiac output.

96. A 66-year-old patient with a Medtronic-Hall mitral prosthesis is scheduled for elective noncardiac surgery. The accompanying image is obtained during preoperative transesophageal echocardiography. (LA indicates left atrium; RA, right atrium.) It shows

A. a normal flow pattern for the prosthetic valve.

B. mild mitral regurgitation due to dysfunction of the prosthesis.

C. moderate mitral regurgitation due to dysfunction of the prosthesis.

D. moderately severe mitral regurgitation due to dysfunction of the prosthesis.

E. severe mitral regurgitation due to dysfunction of the prosthesis.

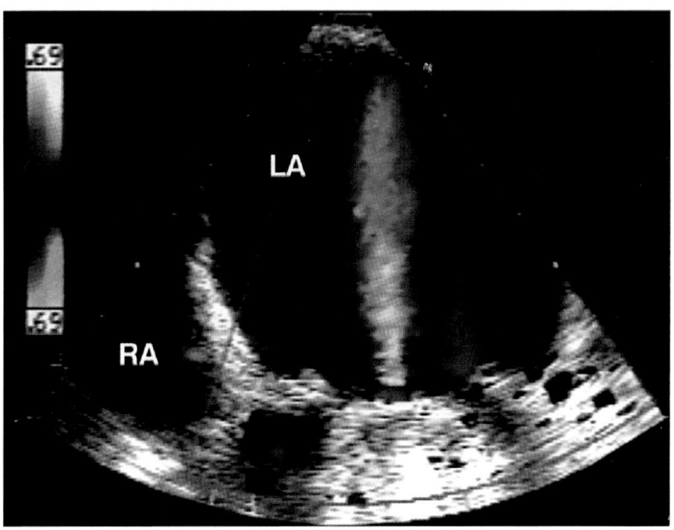

Figure from Oh et al. (23). Used with permission of Mayo Foundation for Medical Education and Research.

97. On the basis of the preoperative transesophageal echocardiographic findings accompanying Question 96, the cardiologist should

A. cancel the elective surgery because of the severe mitral regurgitation.

B. delay the surgery and evaluate the patient for severe mitral regurgitation.

C. reschedule the elective surgery because the patient should have aortic valve replacement first.

D. send the patient to a cardiac surgeon for aortic valve replacement after the elective surgery.

E. proceed with the scheduled elective surgery.

98. A 65-year-old man with mitral regurgitation undergoes transesophageal echocardiography. At an aliasing velocity of 32 cm/s, the proximal isovelocity surface area radius is greater than 1 cm. The patient's blood pressure is 116/58 mm Hg. The patient's mitral regurgitation is most likely

A. mild.

B. moderate.

C. moderately severe.
D. severe.
E. undetermined.

99. The accompanying Doppler image is obtained in a patient with aortic regurgitation. The measured deceleration time (DT) of the aortic regurgitant jet is 800 ms. The pressure half-time of the aortic regurgitant flow is
A. 120 ms.
B. 158 ms.
C. 230 ms.
D. 370 ms.
E. 450 ms.

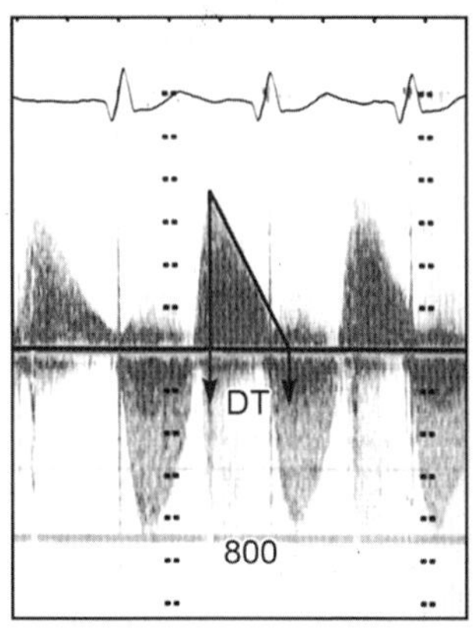

Figure from Oh et al. (23). Used with permission of Mayo Foundation for Medical Education and Research.

100. The Doppler information about the aortic regurgitation in Question 99 is consistent with
A. trivial aortic regurgitation.
B. mild aortic regurgitation.
C. moderate aortic regurgitation.
D. moderately severe aortic regurgitation.
E. severe aortic regurgitation.

101. After mitral valve repair, systolic anterior motion is detected intraoperatively in a patient with severe hypotension. The best pharmacologic management is
A. dopamine.
B. dobutamine.
C. epinephrine.
D. ephedrine.
E. phenylephrine.

102. The accompanying transesophageal echocardiographic image is obtained with the probe placed in the upper esophagus. Color flow imaging of this transesophageal echocardiographic view (LA indicates left atrium; RA, right atrium; RV, right ventricle) supports a diagnosis of

A. patent ductus arteriosus.
B. mild aortic regurgitation.
C. mild pulmonary regurgitation.
D. intrapulmonary shunt.
E. an undetermined condition.

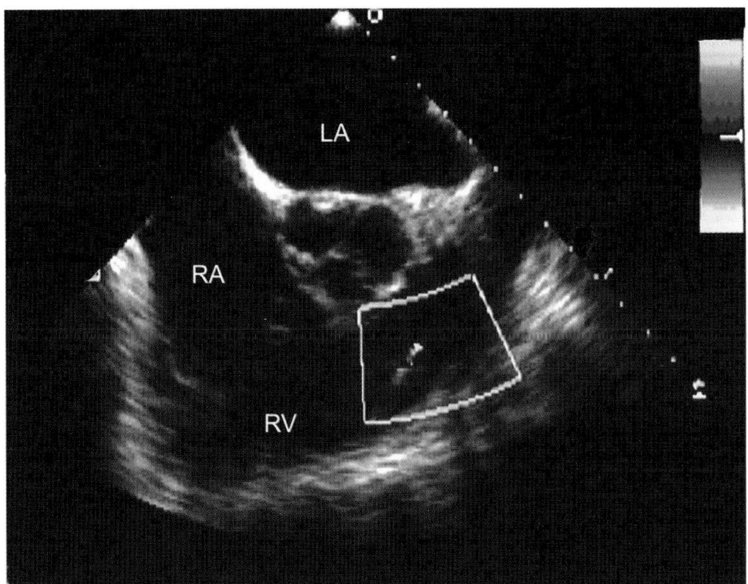

103. The accompanying M-mode echocardiogram (LV indicates left ventricle) typically is seen in patients with

A. aortic regurgitation.
B. aortic stenosis.
C. mitral regurgitation.
D. mitral stenosis.
E. mitral valve prolapse.

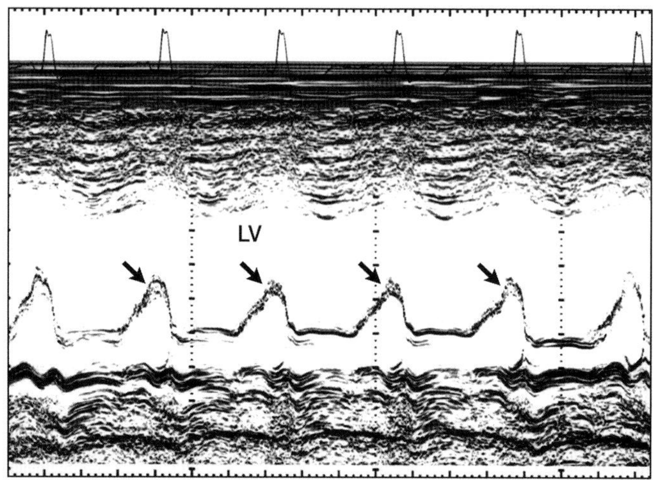

Figure from Oh et al. (23). Used with permission of Mayo Foundation for Medical Education and Research.

Answers & Discussion

1. Answer D

The normal mitral valve area measures 4.0 to 6.0 cm^2. Anatomically, the mitral valve is a complex structure composed of the mitral anterior and posterior leaflets, fibromuscular mitral anulus, chordae tendineae, papillary muscles, and left ventricular myocardium subjacent to the papillary muscles. Functional integrity of the mitral valve requires that each of these components performs appropriately and acts in concert with its other members. **References** 23 *(p 115)*; 24 *(pp 3–6)*; 42 *(pp 391–392)*.

2. Answer C

The normal aortic valve area is 3 to 4 cm^2. The normal aortic valve has three thin cusps and an unrestrictive systolic opening. During systole, the aortic valve opens with a leaflet separation about 2 cm. When the aortic valve is closed during diastole, each leaflet overlaps its neighbors by 2 to 3 mm, thus allowing a tight seal against backflow of blood despite substantial diastolic pressure in the aorta. **References** 23 *(p 104)*; 42 *(p 499)*.

3. Answer E

Normally, the tricuspid inflow has a peak velocity less than 0.5 to 1 m/s and a mean gradient less than 2 mm Hg. Because there is respiratory variation in tricuspid valve inflow velocity, it is best to determine Doppler flow velocity through the tricuspid valve in expiration. **References** 23 *(p 119)*; 42 *(pp 824–829)*.

4. Answer A

Rheumatic valvular disease remains the most common cause of mitral stenosis despite the declining incidence of rheumatic fever in Western nations. Isolated mitral stenosis occurs in 40% of all patients presenting with rheumatic heart disease, and a history of rheumatic fever can be elicited from about 60% of patients presenting with pure mitral stenosis. The uncommon causes of mitral stenosis include degenerative calcification, vegetation, drug toxicity, and congenital valvular stenosis. **References** 5; 11 *(p 188)*; 23 *(p 113)*; 42 *(p 403)*.

5. Answer C

The hemodynamic severity of aortic stenosis determined by two-dimensional and Doppler echocardiography is based on aortic valve area, peak aortic flow velocity, mean pressure gradient, and the ratio of the left ventricular outflow tract to the aortic valve time velocity integral. Left ventricular outflow tract peak velocity alone provides no information about the severity of aortic stenosis. **References** 11 *(pp 218, 222)*; 23 *(pp 104–113)*; 42 *(pp 514–527)*.

6. Answer B

The most common cause of aortic stenosis in adults is degenerative valvular calcification that immobilizes the aortic valve cusps. On two-dimensional echocardiography, the aortic cusps are thickened and calcified, resulting in a decreased systolic opening. The right coronary cusp appears by far the most commonly affected. Commissural fusion is most frequently noted between the right and noncoronary leaflets. During transesophageal echocardiography, it may be difficult to measure the area of the calcified aortic valve by planimetry, but the number of aortic cusps can usually be determined. **References** 5; 23 *(pp 104–113)*; 26 *(pp 232–233)*; 42 *(pp 512–513)*.

7. Answer D

8. Answer D

Mitral stenosis is usually the predominant feature of rheumatic mitral disease. The age distribution of mitral stenosis is bimodal, affecting the younger (20–30 years old) and the older (50–60 years old) age groups. Disease in the younger age group is characterized by a severe initial episode or recurrent episodes of rheumatic endocarditis that produce accelerated valve injury with rapid scarring and contracture of leaflets, leading to mitral stenosis. Mitral stenosis in the older age group is caused by a milder initial episode of rheumatic endocarditis with a gradual progression of leaflet injury. After the initial injury, leaflet calcification, thickening, and deformation are accelerated by the chronic effects of abnormal transvalvular blood flow. In developed countries, there is a long latent period of 20 to 40 years from the occurrence of rheumatic fever to the onset of symptoms of mitral stenosis. **References** 5; 24 *(pp 3–4)*.

9. Answer E

The typical two-dimensional echocardiographic features of rheumatic mitral stenosis are the "hockey stick" appearance of the anterior mitral leaflet in the long axis view during diastole and the "fish mouth" appearance of the mitral orifice due to fusion of the commissures seen in the short axis view. The "hockey stick" appearance is shown in the long axis view of the accompanying image (AV, aortic valve; LA, left atrium; LV, left ventricle; MV, mitral valve). During transesophageal echocardiography, the transgastric basal short axis view may visualize thickened and calcified mitral leaflets and subvalvular apparatus, increased left atrial size, with the potential for thrombus formation, and immobility of the posterior mitral leaflet. Increased left atrial size is secondary to increased left atrial pressure due to mitral stenosis. Sometimes, spontaneous contrast is observed, which is a sign of decreased flow and increased risk of thrombus formation. Immobility of the posterior mitral leaflet is observed in patients with rheumatic mitral stenosis, but it can also be seen in hypereosinophilia or ergot use. **References** 11 *(pp 188–192)*; 23 *(p 113)*; 26 *(pp 249–250)*.

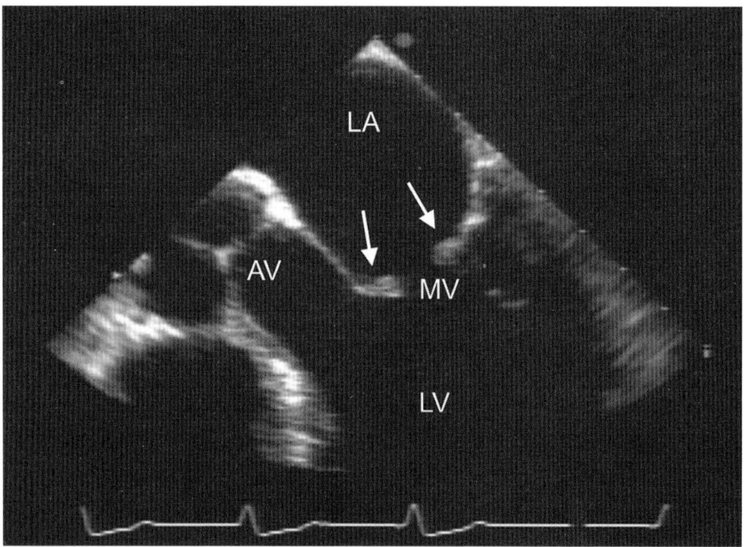

10. Answer C

Mitral stenosis is usually considered severe when the following two-dimensional and Doppler information is found: 1) mitral valve area of 1.0 cm^2 or less; 2) resting mean pressure gradient of 10 mm Hg or higher; and 3) pressure half-time of 220 ms or more. The pressure half-time of 240 ms correlates to a mitral valve area less than 1.0 cm^2 because the pressure half-time method empirically uses the constant 220 divided by pressure half-time to calculate the mitral valve area. **References** 11 *(pp 192–195)*; 23 *(pp 113–119)*.

11. Answer A

Generally, severe aortic stenosis is defined by the following criteria: an aortic valve area of 0.75 cm^2 or less; peak aortic valve velocity of 4.5 m/s or more; mean pressure gradient of 50 mm Hg or more; a ratio of left ventricular outflow tract to aortic valve time velocity integral of 0.25 or less. Therefore, the 50-year-old woman with the ratio less than 0.25 has severe aortic stenosis. **References** 5; 23 *(p 106)*; 42 *(pp 514–527)*.

12. Answer A

Generally, the flow velocity and pressure gradient across the aortic valve vary with changes in stroke volume. In patients with normal left ventricular function, a peak velocity of 4.5 m/s or more or a mean gradient of 50 mm Hg or more indicates severe aortic stenosis. However, when left ventricular systolic function and cardiac output are reduced, the peak aortic velocity and mean pressure gradient decrease correspondingly. In such patients, the peak aortic velocity may be less than 4.5 m/s and the mean pressure gradient may be less than 50 mm Hg, even though the aortic stenosis is severe. The ratio of the left ventricular outflow tract time velocity integral to the aortic valve time velocity integral is independent of any change in stroke volume because the left ventricular outflow tract and aortic valve velocities change proportionally. Therefore, among the choices listed as possible responses to this question, the ratio of the left ventricular outflow tract to the aortic valve time velocity integral or time velocity integral ratio is more reliable in estimating the severity of aortic stenosis in patients with decreased left ventricular function. **References** 23 *(pp 106–111)*; 42 *(pp 524–525)*.

13. Answer D

In the presence of systolic anterior motion of the mitral valve after mitral repair, the coaptation site (solid arrow in the accompanying image) of the anterior mitral leaflet (A in the figure; P is the posterior leaflet) is the body of the leaflet on the atrial side. The tip of the anterior mitral leaflet is pushed against the interventricular septum (dashed arrow is the septal contact), resulting in left ventricular outflow tract dynamic obstruction with an increased pressure gradient. (See also Questions 78, 79, and 101.) **References** 11 *(pp 514–515)*; 23 *(pp 238–240)*; 24 *(p 42)*.

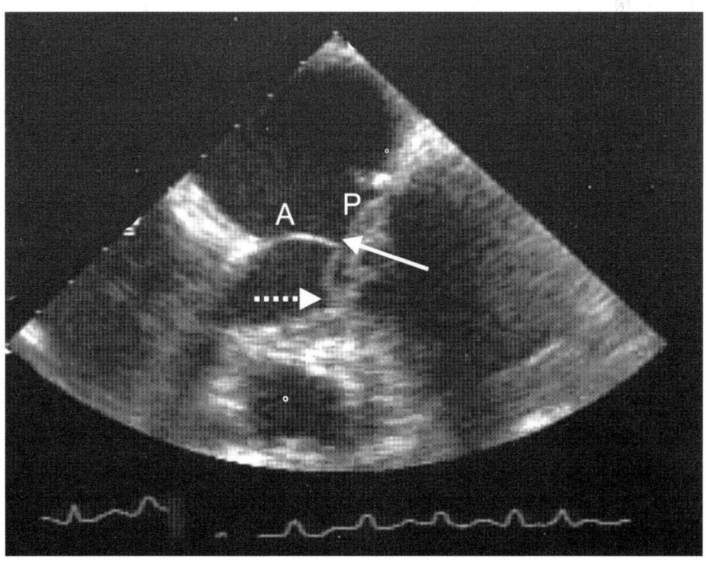

14. Answer C

On M-mode echocardiography, a normal mitral valve is usually labeled as illustrated in the accompanying image. The inflection begins with D, which indicates the end of systole, immediately before the opening of the valve. As the anterior mitral leaflet opens, it peaks at E. The point F indicates the end of the initial diastolic closing. In atrial systole, blood is propelled through the mitral orifice, and the mitral leaflets reopen. The peak of this phase of mitral valve motion is indicated as A. The valve begins to close with atrial relaxation. Complete closure occurs after the onset of ventricular systole at C. During systole, the leaflet gradually moves upward until the onset of mitral valve opening again occurs at D. The E-F slope is obtained by drawing a line through the E and F points. In patients with mitral stenosis, M-mode echocardiography demonstrates thickened mitral leaflets and a prolonged E-F slope. **References** 17 *(pp 5, 8)*; 23 *(p 114)*.

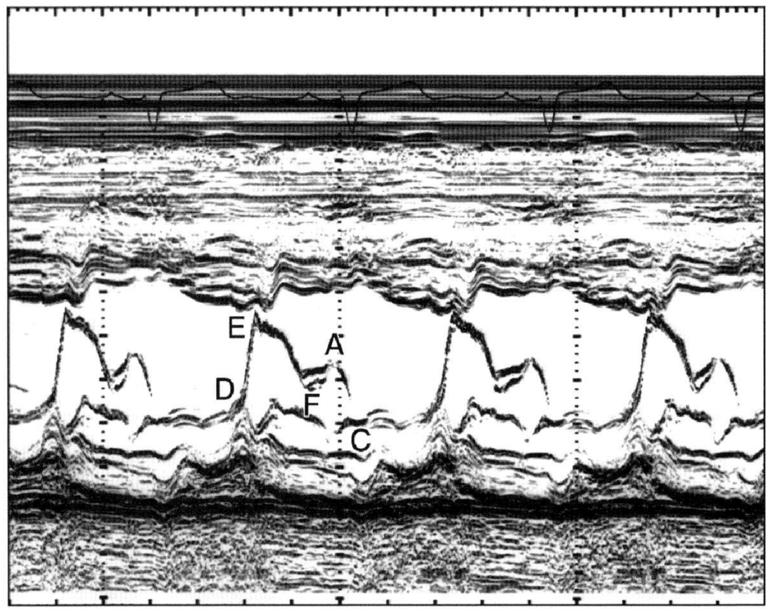

Figure from Oh et al. (23). Used with permission of Mayo Foundation for Medical Education and Research.

15. Answer B

16. Answer C

In patients with concomitant mitral stenosis and severe aortic regurgitation, a rapid increase in left ventricular diastolic pressure due to aortic regurgitation may shorten the pressure half-time. Because the mitral valve area is calculated as the constant 220 divided by the pressure half-time, decreased pressure half-time due to severe aortic regurgitation affects the mitral valve area, as calculated by the pressure half-time method, leading to a falsely increased mitral valve area and hence underestimation of the severity of mitral stenosis. **Reference** 23 *(pp 113–119)*.

17. Answer E

Generally, severe mitral regurgitation is indicated by the following criteria: 1) mitral regurgitation color flow jet reaching the posterior wall of the left atrium with a high aliasing velocity on the color map; 2) two-dimensional echocardiographic evidence of disruption of the mitral valve apparatus, such as papillary muscle rupture, or flail mitral leaflet; 3) pulmonary vein systolic flow reversals; 4) mitral regurgitation volume of 60 mL or more; 5) mitral regurgitation fraction of 55% or more; and 6) an effective regurgitant orifice of 0.4 cm^2 or more. The 90-year-old patient with an effective regurgitant orifice of 20 mm^2, or 0.2 cm^2, does not have severe mitral regurgitation because the criterion for severe mitral regurgitation is an effective regurgitant orifice of 0.4 cm^2 (40 mm^2) or more. **Reference** 23 *(pp 122–129)*.

18. Answer B

According to the continuity equation, "what comes in must go out"; thus, the mitral inflow volume should equal the left ventricular outflow tract stroke volume. The mitral flow volume is the product of the mitral valve area and the mitral time velocity integral. The continuity equation (inflow equaling outflow) can also be expressed as left ventricular outflow tract stroke volume equaling the product of the mitral valve area and the mitral time velocity integral or mitral valve area is the result of dividing the left ventricular outflow tract stroke volume by the mitral time velocity integral. The continuity equation assumes that the mitral inflow volume equals the left ventricular outflow tract stroke volume. However, this assumption is violated in the presence of mitral regurgitation because the mitral inflow volume is not the same as the left ventricular outflow tract stroke volume. In the presence of mitral regurgitation, left ventricular outflow tract stroke volume equals mitral inflow volume minus mitral regurgitant volume. Applying this concept to the continuity equation used to calculate the mitral valve area, the left ventricular outflow tract stroke volume is less than the actual mitral inflow volume because part of the mitral inflow volume regurgitates back into the left atrium. Therefore, the mitral valve area calculated by the continuity equation is falsely decreased in patients with severe mitral regurgitation; that is, the continuity equation overestimates the severity of mitral stenosis.

In patients with severe mitral regurgitation, the correct continuity equation to calculate the mitral valve area is the sum of the left ventricular outflow tract stroke volume and mitral regurgitant volume divided by the mitral time velocity integral. **Reference** 23 *(pp 62–63, 115)*.

19. Answer E

20. Answer E

In the presence of left ventricular dysfunction with decreased cardiac output, it may be difficult to distinguish functional or pseudo severe aortic stenosis from anatomic or true severe aortic stenosis. Low cardiac output decreases the effective orifice area because the dysfunctional left ventricle cannot generate enough pressure to open the aortic valve fully. Thus, functional or pseudo severe aortic stenosis may occur in patients with left ventricular dysfunction and low cardiac output. In patients with true severe aortic stenosis and reduced cardiac output, abnormal left ventricular function may decrease the peak velocity and the mean gradient across the aortic valve, resulting in a peak aortic velocity less than 4.5 m/s and a mean pressure gradient less than 50 mm Hg.

In both situations, gradual infusion of low-dose dobutamine while performing Doppler echocardiography to increase the stroke volume may be helpful in differentiating morphologically severe aortic stenosis from pseudo severe aortic stenosis. In patients with functional or pseudo severe aortic stenosis, dobutamine increases stroke volume, and hence, the aortic valve can be opened to a greater degree, leading to an increase in the aortic valve area. In patients with anatomic or true aortic stenosis, the aortic valve area cannot be increased by dobutamine infusion because of the aortic valve pathology. **Reference** 23 *(p 111)*.

21. Answer A

Normal prosthetic flow velocity and pressure gradients vary depending on the type and size of the prosthesis, the location, and the cardiac output. According to the normal Doppler values for various aortic prosthesis determined by the Mayo Clinic echocardiography laboratory, normal St. Jude aortic prostheses have an average peak velocity of 2.5 ± 0.6 m/s and a mean gradient of 14.4 ± 7.7 mm Hg. Therefore, the Doppler information in this question is consistent with a normal St. Jude prosthetic valve. **Reference** 23 *(pp 133, 136)*.

22. Answer A

The etiology of aortic regurgitation varies widely, and the most common cause is degenerative calcification of the aortic valve. Other causes of aortic regurgitation include a congenitally abnormal valve, a dilated aortic root, Marfan syndrome, endocarditis, aortic dissection, prosthetic valve dysfunction, and valvulopathy caused by combined use of fenfluramine and phentermine ("fen-phen"). **References** 11 *(p 223, 225)*; 23 *(p 119)*.

23. Answer E

Generally, a central regurgitation jet indicates that the mechanism of the valvular regurgitation is functional. In patients with severe aortic stenosis, the cause of functional mitral regurgitation is usually increased left ventricular systolic pressure. In such patients, there is no apparent morphologic abnormality of the mitral leaflets. After aortic valve replacement, the left ventricular systolic pressure is reduced and the mitral regurgitation frequently decreases or disappears. Therefore, when patients with severe aortic stenosis and some degree of mitral regurgitation undergo aortic valve replacement, intraoperative transesophageal echocardiography is useful to evaluate the severity of mitral regurgitation before and after aortic valve replacement and to assess the need for mitral valve repair or replacement. Mitral valve prolapse, papillary muscle rupture, and ruptured chordae usually cause an eccentric regurgitant jet due to the structural abnormalities of the mitral valve. Patients with rheumatic valvular disease typically have mitral stenosis with characteristic abnormalities of the mitral leaflets. **References** 11 *(pp 200–208)*; 23 *(pp 122–123)*.

24. Answer E

Color flow imaging is used to estimate the amount of the regurgitant jet. In patients with mitral regurgitation, the regurgitant jet area is compared with the size of the left atrium. This qualitative method tends to underestimate the severity of regurgitation when the jet is eccentric and overestimate the severity of regurgitation when the jet is central. Therefore, the regurgitant jet size on color flow imaging should be interpreted in the context of jet geometry and valvular structural abnormalities. **References** 10 *(pp 40–42)*; 23 *(p 123)*.

25. Answer B

In patients with aortic stenosis and coexisting severe aortic regurgitation, the ratio of the left ventricular outflow tract time velocity integral to the aortic valve time velocity integral reliably evaluates the severity of aortic stenosis. In the presence of severe aortic regurgitation, flow across the aortic valve increases with aortic regurgitation, as does the aortic pressure gradient. The increased flow is reflected in the left ventricular outflow tract and aortic valve velocities proportionally. Thus, the time velocity integral ratio remains the same for a given aortic valve area.

In the cardiac catheterization laboratory, the Gorlin formula is used to calculate the aortic valve area (AVA): AVA = cardiac output/C × SEP × the square root of pressure gradient, where C is the constant in the Gorlin formula, and SEP is the systolic ejection period. The Gorlin formula is sensitive to the presence of aortic regurgitation. With aortic regurgitation, the true aortic flow cannot be calculated by the usual Fick or indicator dilution output techniques. Therefore, cardiac catheterization is unreliable in this situation and tends to result in a lower calculated aortic valve area because of an underestimation of cardiac output. **References** 23 *(pp 104–113)*; 25 *(pp 408–411)*; 42 *(pp 419–420)*.

26. Answer C

Comparison of color flow imaging with aortic angiography showed that two parameters correlated well with the angiographic severity of aortic regurgitation: 1) the regurgitant jet area in an aortic valve short axis view relative to the short axis area of the left ventricular outflow tract, and 2) the width of the regurgitant jet at its origin relative to the diameter of the left ventricular outflow tract. However, the maximal extent or length of the regurgitant jet is poorly correlated with the angiographic severity of aortic regurgitation. **Reference** 23 *(pp 120–122)*.

27. Answer B

In the setting of severe aortic regurgitation, holodiastolic flow reversal can be demonstrated in the descending thoracic aorta and even in the abdominal aorta. In patients with mild aortic regurgitation, mild early diastolic flow reversal in the descending aorta may be seen. Systolic flow reversal in the pulmonary vein is observed in patients with severe mitral regurgitation, but not in patients with severe aortic regurgitation. Systolic flow reversal in the hepatic vein is a sign of severe tricuspid regurgitation. **References** 23 *(pp 120–122)*; 26 *(pp 282, 284)*.

28. Answer C

During Doppler study, the aortic regurgitant flow recorded by Doppler echocardiography begins immediately after aortic valve closure and ends at aortic valve opening. Physiologically, the time from the aortic valve closure to the aortic valve opening includes the diastolic period and the isovolumic contraction time. There are four phases during diastole: isovolumic relaxation time, the rapid filling phase, diastasis, and the late filling phase. The isovolumic contraction time is the time period between closure of the mitral valve and opening of the aortic valve. Aortic regurgitation can occur when the left ventricular pressure is still lower than the aortic pressure during the isovolumic relaxation time. Therefore, the aortic regurgitation flow is recorded during isovolumic relaxation time, the rapid filling phase, diastasis, the late filling phase, and isovolumic contraction time. The Doppler flow of mitral stenosis starts after the mitral valve opening and ends at mitral valve closure, that is, it is recorded during rapid filling, diastasis, and late filling phases but not during isovolumic relaxation and contraction times. **References** 11 *(pp 223–229)*; 17 *(p 67)*; 23 *(pp 119–122)*.

29. Answer A

30. Answer D

The effective regurgitant orifice is one of the markers for the severity of valvular regurgitation. Although direct visualization of the mitral effective regurgitant orifice is difficult, it can be closely approximated by measurement of the width of the vena contracta, which is the narrowest portion of the regurgitation jet downstream from the orifice. It has been reported that there are good correlations of the vena contracta width with the effective regurgitant orifice and the regurgitant volume. A vena contracta width greater than 0.5 cm is always associated with an effective regurgitant orifice greater than 40 mm^2 and a regurgitant volume greater than 60 mL, both of which indicate severe mitral regurgitation. A vena contracta less than 0.3 cm indicates mild regurgitation, and that of 0.3 to 0.5 cm requires additional methods, such as quantitative Doppler, to further clarify the severity of mitral regurgitation. **References** 23 *(p 124)*; 25 *(p 316)*.

31. Answer D

The concept of the proximal isovelocity surface area can be applied for calculating the area of a stenotic orifice. This method has been validated for the mitral valve area in patients with mitral stenosis. An angle correction factor is necessary for the angle between the mitral leaflets on the atrial side less than 180°. With the proximal isovelocity surface area method, the mitral valve area (MVA) is calculated according to the following equation:

$$\text{MVA} = 6.28 \times r^2 \times (\text{aliasing velocity}/\text{peak velocity}) \times (\alpha/180),$$

where α is the angle between the mitral leaflets on the atrial side. Using the information provided in this question, we can calculate the mitral valve area for this 56-year-old patient. The peak mitral inflow velocity needs to be converted from 2.3 m/s to 230 cm/s for this calculation. Thus,

$$\begin{aligned}\text{MVA} &= 6.28 \times 0.8^2 \times (56/230) \times (160/180)\\ &= 6.28 \times 0.64 \times (0.24) \times (0.89)\\ &= 0.86\ \text{cm}^2.\end{aligned}$$

Therefore, this patient has a mitral valve area of 0.86 cm^2, which indicates severe mitral stenosis. **References** 23 *(pp 68, 115)*; 26 *(p 253)*.

32. Answer D

When left ventricular systolic function is abnormal and cardiac output is reduced, aortic stenosis may be functionally severe because of the inability of the left ventricle to generate enough pressure to open a moderately stenotic valve fully. Gradual infusion of a low dose of dobutamine to increase stroke volume may be helpful in differentiating morphologically or anatomically severe aortic stenosis from functional or pseudo severe aortic stenosis.

In patients with functional or pseudo severe aortic stenosis, the aortic valve area is increased and the mean gradient is not changed because dobutamine infusion increases cardiac contractility and stroke volume, and hence, enough pressure may be generated by the left ventricle to open the aortic valve fully. In addition, an increase in the left ventricular outflow tract time velocity integral in these patients is far greater than the time velocity integral of the aortic valve, resulting in an increase in the ratio of the left ventricular outflow tract to the aortic valve time velocity integral.

In patients with anatomic or true severe aortic stenosis, dobutamine infusion increases not only the mean gradient and peak velocity, but also the left ventricular outflow tract time velocity integral and the aortic valve time velocity integral proportionally. Therefore, the ratio of the left ventricular outflow tract to the aortic valve time velocity integral remains unchanged in patients with true severe aortic stenosis. (See also Questions 19 and 20.) **Reference** 23 *(p 111)*.

33. Answer C

34. Answer D

In the continuous wave Doppler spectrum shown with Question 33, the aortic forward flow signal has a peak velocity (V) of 4.7 m/s. According to the simplified Bernoulli equation, the peak pressure gradient (P) can be calculated as the following:

$$
\begin{aligned}
P &= 4V^2 \\
&= 4 \times 4.7^2 \\
&= 88.36 \text{ mm Hg.}
\end{aligned}
$$

By tracing the velocity signal, the mean pressure gradient across the aortic valve is 60 mm Hg for this patient. Both peak velocity greater than 4.5 m/s and mean gradient greater than 50 mm Hg indicate severe aortic stenosis. **Reference** 23 *(pp 106–111)*.

35. Answer B

The Duke criteria have been proposed to improve the sensitivity and specificity of diagnostic criteria for infective endocarditis. They consist of two major criteria and six minor criteria.

The two major criteria are as follows:

1. positive blood culture for infective endocarditis
2. evidence of endocardial involvement, including the following:
   - A. positive echocardiogram for infective endocarditis showing
     - oscillating intracardiac mass on the valve or supporting structure or in the path of regurgitant jets or on iatrogenic devices, in the absence of an alternative anatomic explanation or
     - abscess or
     - new partial dehiscence of the prosthetic valve
   - B. new valvular regurgitation (worsening or changing of preexisting murmur not sufficient)

The six minor criteria are as follows:

1. predisposing heart condition or intravenous drug use;
2. temperature higher than 38.0°C;
3. vascular phenomena;
4. immunologic phenomena: glomerulonephritis, Osler nodes, Roth spots;
5. echocardiogram consistent with infective endocarditis but not meeting major criteria noted above; and
6. microbiologic evidence: positive blood culture but not meeting major criteria as noted above or serologic evidence of active infection with organism consistent with infective endocarditis.

The diagnosis of infective endocarditis is definite if a patient meets two major criteria, or one major criterion plus three minor criteria, or five minor criteria. **References** 23 *(pp 145–146)*; 25 *(pp 389–390)*.

36. Answer A

Typical microorganisms for infective endocarditis include *Streptococcus viridans, Streptococcus bovis*, the HACEK group of organisms, *Staphylococcus aureus*, and enterococci. The HACEK group consists of *Haemophilus* spp, *Actinobacillus actinomycetemcomitans, Cardiobacterium hominis, Eikenella* spp, and *Kingella kingae*. Parainfluenza is an RNA virus, which is not a typical microorganism for infective endocarditis. **Reference** 23 *(pp 145–146)*.

37. Answer C

Valvular vegetations typically occur on the regurgitant surfaces of the valve leaflets. Generally, vegetations tend to form on the atrial surfaces of the mitral or tricuspid valves and on the ventricular aspects of the aortic valve and pulmonary valves. **Reference** 23 *(pp 145–148)*.

38. Answer A

In patients with acute severe aortic regurgitation, left ventricular diastolic pressure increases rapidly because of the large regurgitant volume. This rapidly increased left ventricular diastolic pressure produces a restrictive diastolic filling pattern in mitral inflow, that is, increased early diastolic (E) velocity and decreased late diastolic (A) velocity with an increased E/A ratio. **References** 23 *(pp 119–122)*; 26 *(p 282)*.

39. Answer C

The deceleration time and pressure half-time of the aortic regurgitation signal is determined by the severity of aortic regurgitation. In patients with severe aortic regurgitation, the systemic diastolic pressure decreases quickly and left ventricular end-diastolic pressure rises rapidly. Therefore, the pressure difference between the aorta and the left ventricle diminishes rapidly, resulting in the Doppler signal of aortic regurgitation with shortened deceleration time and pressure half-time. **References** 23 *(pp 119–122)*; 26 *(pp 277–283)*.

40. Answer D

The pulsed wave Doppler spectral recording accompanying Question 40 shows systolic flow reversal in the pulmonary vein, which is an indicator of severe mitral regurgitation. Careful evaluation of pulmonary venous flow can provide important information on mitral regurgitation. Normally, pulmonary venous flow consists of the S wave during ventricular systole, the D wave during ventricular diastole, and the AR wave reflecting reversed flow in the pulmonary veins when the left atrium contracts (see the accompanying image of normal pulmonary venous flow). As the mitral regurgitant jet enters the left atrium, it displaces blood that was already in the chamber. With mitral regurgitation of increasing severity, the S wave becomes blunted and ultimately reversed, reflecting the rise in atrial pressure under the volume load of the regurgitation. Therefore, systolic flow reversal in the pulmonary veins is observed when severe mitral regurgitation is present. **References** 11 *(pp 208–211)*; 23 *(pp 123–124)*; 26 *(pp 285–293)*.

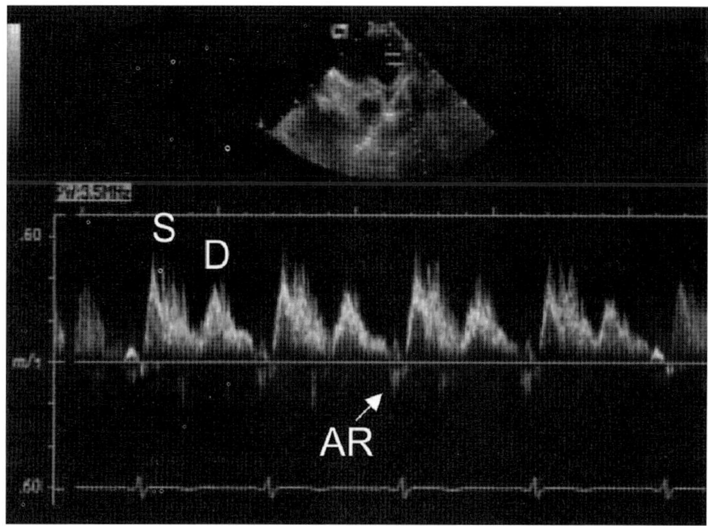

41. Answer E

42. Answer B

43. Answer C

The two-dimensional images accompanying Question 41 show that the tricuspid valve leaflets are thick and do not coapt. They are in a fixed position because of the sclerosing effect of carcinoid syndrome. Carcinoid heart disease is caused by a slow-growing metastatic carcinoid tumor, which usually originates in the ileum. Cardiac involvement occurs almost exclusively with hepatic metastases and is caused by substances released by the tumor, such as serotonin and bradykinin. Because the tumor substances are inactivated by the lung, carcinoid heart disease predominantly involves the right side of the heart, affecting both the tricuspid and pulmonic valves. In patients with a patent foramen ovale or pulmonary metastasis, carcinoid heart disease may involve the left side of the heart (about 7% of cases). The predominant tricuspid lesion of carcinoid heart disease is characteristic thickening (fibrosis) and restricted motion of the tricuspid valve, leading to incomplete coaptation and thus severe tricuspid regurgitation. In addition, tricuspid stenosis and varying degrees of pulmonic stenosis and regurgitation are usually present in patients with carcinoid heart disease. **Reference** 23 *(pp 172–174)*.

44. Answer C

In patients with tricuspid stenosis, the pressure half-time method can be used to evaluate the tricuspid valve area. However, the constant of 190 ms was proposed instead of the constant of 220 ms, which is used for calculation of the mitral valve area. Usually, tricuspid stenosis is considered severe when the mean gradient across the tricuspid valve is 7 mm Hg or higher and the pressure half-time exceeds 190 ms. Therefore, the pressure half-time of 200 ms indicates severe tricuspid stenosis. **Reference** 23 *(p 119)*.

45. Answer E

The ratio of aortic regurgitant jet width to left ventricular outflow tract diameter is used to estimate the severity of aortic regurgitation. Using color flow imaging, the minimal subvalvular regurgitant jet width is divided by the left ventricular outflow tract width in the aortic valve long axis view, and the ratio is used to classify the severity of aortic regurgitation in four grades. A ratio less than 25% is seen in mild aortic regurgitation. A ratio between 25% and 46% indicates moderate aortic regurgitation, and a ratio of 47% to 64% indicates moderately severe aortic regurgitation. A ratio of 65% or higher is a sign of severe aortic regurgitation. Semiquantitation of aortic regurgitation by such measurements is appropriate only with centrally directed jets in which the immediate subvalvular jet dimension can be well defined. **References** 11 *(pp 223–229)*; 23 *(pp 119–122)*.

46. Answer E

The following criteria suggest severe mitral regurgitation: a color flow area of 40% or more of the left atrial size; an eccentric mitral regurgitation jet reaching the posterior wall of the left atrium; a dense continuous wave Doppler signal; increased mitral early diastolic velocity of 1.5 m/s or more for a native mitral valve and 2 m/s or more for a prosthetic valve; left ventricular dimension 7 cm or more along with color flow evidence of mitral regurgitation; and left atrial size of 5.5 cm or more. **Reference** 23 *(pp 122–129)*.

47. Answer A

Normally, prosthetic valves (except stentless valves) are inherently stenotic in varying degrees compared with the respective native valves. Therefore, flow velocity across a normal prosthetic valve is higher than that expected for a native valve. An excellent correlation has been shown between Doppler and invasive dual-catheter pressure measurements made simultaneously across various prosthetic valves. The pressure gradient across a prosthetic valve can be determined by the modified Bernoulli equation, which states that pressure gradient is equal to four times the flow velocity squared. When the flow velocity is increased, the pressure gradient is increased. Therefore, the pressure gradient across a normal prosthetic valve is higher than that across the respective native valve. **Reference** 23 *(pp 133–139)*.

48. Answer A

The two-dimensional images accompanying Question 48 show the normal motion of a bileaflet mitral prosthesis. During diastole, the two disks are almost parallel. During systole, each disk moves about 85° toward the left atrium, resulting in closure of the disk. Color flow imaging shows multiple closing volume regurgitant jets. **Reference** 23 *(pp 140–141)*.

49. Answer A

Generally, the following criteria suggest severe tricuspid regurgitation: a color flow regurgitant jet area of 30% or more of the right atrial area; a dense continuous wave Doppler signal of tricuspid regurgitant jet; tricuspid anulus dilation with a diameter of 4 cm or more or inadequate cusp coaptation; an increased tricuspid inflow velocity ($\geq$1.0 m/s); and systolic flow reversals in the hepatic vein. Systolic flow reversals in the hepatic vein are seen in severe tricuspid regurgitation, and systolic flow reversals in the pulmonary veins are seen in severe mitral regurgitation. **Reference** 23 *(pp 129–130)*.

50. Answer C

The image accompanying Question 50 is a pulsed wave Doppler spectrum obtained with sample volume placed in the descending thoracic aorta. It demonstrates holodiastolic reversal flow in the descending thoracic aorta, which indicates severe aortic regurgitation. **References** 23 *(pp 120–122)*; 26 *(pp 282, 284)*.

51. Answer B

52. Answer C

53. Answer A

The mitral valve area can be calculated using the continuity equation—"what comes in must go out." According to this principle, the mitral inflow should be equal to the left ventricular outflow volume or the left ventricular stroke volume. Because flow volume is the product of cross-sectional area and the time velocity integral, the continuity equation can be rewritten as follows: MVA × MV TVI = LVOT CSA × LVOT TVI, where MVA stands for mitral valve area, MV TVI stands for mitral inflow time velocity integral, LVOT CSA is the left ventricular outflow tract cross-sectional area, and LVOT TVI is the left ventricular outflow tract time velocity integral. Mathematically, the cross-sectional area is calculated as follows:

$$\begin{aligned} \text{CSA} &= 3.14 \times (0.5\text{D})^2 \\ &= 3.14 \times 0.25 \times \text{D}^2 \\ &= 0.785 \times \text{D}^2, \end{aligned}$$

where D stands for the diameter. Thus, the continuity equation can also be expressed as follows: MVA × MV TVI = (0.785 × LVOT D^2) × LVOT TVI. Rearranging the equation yields a new equation to calculate the mitral valve area by the continuity principle: MVA = (0.785 × LVOT D^2 × LVOT TVI)/MV TVI. In this 76-year-old patient, MV TVI is 66 cm, LVOT TVI is 23 cm, and LVOT D is 2.1 cm. According to the continuity equation, the patient's MVA can be calculated as follows: MVA = $[0.785 \times (2.1)^2 \times 23]/66 = 79.6/66 = 1.2$ cm^2.

The severity of mitral stenosis is categorized according to mitral valve area: no mitral stenosis (normal valve area), 4 to 6 cm^2; mild, 1.6 to 2.0 cm^2; moderate, 1.1 to 1.5 cm^2;

and severe, less than 1.0 cm^2. Therefore, this patient had MVA 1.2 cm^2, which indicates moderate mitral stenosis.

In patients with mitral stenosis and concomitant severe aortic regurgitation, the continuity equation underestimates the severity of mitral stenosis. In such patients, the LVOT stroke volume, the aortic forward volume, the aortic regurgitant volume, and the mitral inflow volume have the following relationship: Mitral inflow volume = aortic forward volume = LVOT outflow volume−AR volume. Because the mitral inflow volume equals MVA × MV TVI, this equation can also be written as follows: MVA × MV TVI = aortic forward volume = LVOT outflow volume−AR volume.

In patients with concomitant aortic regurgitation, the correct continuity equation to calculate the MVA is the following: MVA = aortic forward volume/MV TVI = (LVOT outflow volume−AR volume)/MV TVI. Comparing the above equation with the continuity equation used to calculate the MVA in Question 51 (MVA = LVOT outflow volume/MV TVI), the numerator LVOT outflow volume is greater than the actual aortic forward volume in patients with aortic regurgitation, which is equal to the LVOT outflow volume minus the aortic regurgitant volume. Therefore, if the continuity equation MVA = LVOT outflow volume/MV TVI is used to calculate the mitral valve area in patients with severe aortic regurgitation, the calculated MVA will be increased falsely, leading to underestimation of the severity of mitral stenosis. **Reference** 23 *(pp 65–68, 115–118)*.

54. Answer D

Normally, mechanical prosthetic valves may have "built-in" regurgitant jet or jets known as "closing volume," depending on the types of the mechanical prostheses. However, a normal mechanical prosthetic valve usually should not have perivalvular regurgitation. Generally, perivalvular regurgitation is an abnormal finding in patients with mechanical prostheses, frequently due to perivalvular abscess and sewing ring dehiscence. **References** 23 *(pp 133–143)*; 25 *(p 804)*.

55. Answer A

On the basis of the Doppler echocardiography and color flow imaging, the severity of aortic regurgitation (AR) is determined as follows:

SEVERITY CRITERIA	MILD AR	SEVERE AR
Aortic regurgitation pressure half-time	≥400 ms	≤250 ms
Left ventricular diastolic dimension (in patients with chronic aortic regurgitation)	≤6.0 cm	≥7.5 cm
Continuous wave Doppler signal of AR jet	Faint	Dense
Regurgitant jet area/left ventricular outflow tract area ratio	≤30%	≥60%

Because the 90-year-old patient has an aortic regurgitation pressure half-time greater than 400 ms, this patient most likely has mild aortic regurgitation. In contrast, the other three patients most likely have severe aortic regurgitation because they have a dense continuous wave Doppler signal of aortic regurgitant jet, left ventricular diastolic dimension greater than 7.5 cm, and a ratio of regurgitant jet area to left ventricular outflow tract area greater than 60%, respectively. **Reference** 23 *(pp 119–122)*.

56. Answer B

57. Answer C

On the basis of the Doppler information shown in the image accompanying Question 56, the mitral valve area can be calculated by the pressure half-time method. The continuous wave Doppler recording of mitral inflow revealed a deceleration time of 520 ms. The pressure half-time is always 29% of deceleration time. Thus, pressure half-time = 520 × 0.29 = 150 ms. Then, the mitral valve area (MVA) can be calculated by the pressure half-time method:

$$\begin{aligned} \text{MVA} &= 220/\text{pressure half-time} \\ &= 220/150 \\ &= 1.47\ \text{cm}^2. \end{aligned}$$

Therefore, the mitral valve area is 1.47 cm^2 or approximately 1.5 cm^2, which is consistent with moderate mitral stenosis. **Reference** 23 *(pp 67–68, 115)*.

58. Answer B

For this 72-year-old patient, both color flow imaging and Doppler echocardiography are consistent with the patient's worsening mitral regurgitation. Generally, color flow imaging may overestimate a regurgitant jet at a low aliasing velocity. The regurgitant jet becomes smaller as the aliasing velocity increases. At an aliasing velocity of 70 cm/s, the mitral regurgitant jet is not overestimated. Hence, the larger mitral regurgitant jet detected by color flow imaging indicated that the patient's mitral regurgitation became more severe over time. When mitral regurgitation becomes more severe, the velocity of mitral regurgitation tends to become slower because the increase in left atrial pressure reduces the transmitral systolic gradient, unless the left ventricular pressure is markedly increased, as in patients with aortic stenosis or hypertrophic obstructive cardiomyopathy. In addition, Doppler echocardiography may reveal a higher velocity of antegrade mitral inflow due to increased volume through the mitral orifice during diastole. **References** 23 *(pp 123–124)*; 25 *(pp 291–303)*.

59. Answer A

In patients with mild aortic prosthetic regurgitation, the following echocardiographic features are observed from transesophageal echocardiography: pressure half-time of the regurgitant jet of 400 ms or greater; a faint continuous wave Doppler signal of aortic regurgitation; mild early diastolic flow reversal in the descending thoracic aorta; and a regurgitant fraction less than 30%. **Reference** 23 *(pp 139–140)*.

60. Answer D

The continuous wave Doppler spectrum, as shown in the image accompanying Question 60, demonstrates the aortic regurgitant jet with peak velocity of 4 m/s and pressure half-time of 240 ms. Aortic regurgitation is considered severe when the pressure half-time of the aortic regurgitant jet is 250 ms or less. In addition, the pulsed wave Doppler spectrum shown with Question 60 shows a restrictive diastolic filling pattern in mitral inflow, with the ratio of early (E) to late (A) filling (E/A ratio) about 4 and deceleration time of 120 ms. When severe aortic regurgitation develops acutely, the left ventricular diastolic pressure increases rapidly and produces a restrictive mitral inflow pattern with high E velocity, low A velocity, and increased E/A ratio. Normal deceleration time is 160 to 240 ms. In a restrictive mitral inflow pattern, the deceleration time is decreased. Therefore, on the basis of the Doppler information, the patient had acute severe aortic regurgitation. After aortic valve replacement, transesophageal echocardiography shows that the restrictive pattern usually normalizes. **Reference** 23 *(pp 119–122)*.

61. Answer A

The complications of prosthetic valves include endocarditis, ring abscess, dehiscence, intracardiac thrombi, and hemolysis. Although hemolysis is uncommon, it is an alarming complication of mitral valve replacement. Usually, hemolysis is associated with distinct patterns of mitral regurgitant flow disturbance. Collision of the mitral regurgitation jet against a cardiac structure with rapid deceleration is the most common reason for hemolysis. Transesophageal echocardiography has demonstrated that regurgitation through a small orifice is associated with greater hemolysis. **Reference** 23 *(pp 133–143)*.

62. Answer E

In patients with severe aortic stenosis and low cardiac output, the aortic flow velocity can be deceptively low (<4.5 m/s), as in this patient. Generally, the peak velocity and the mean pressure gradient across the aortic valve vary with changes in left ventricular contractility and stroke volume. Although the peak velocity is less than 4.5 m/s and the mean pressure gradient is less than 50 mm Hg, severe aortic stenosis cannot be excluded in this patient because of the decreased left ventricular function (left ventricular ejection fraction, 30%) and low cardiac output. In addition, the left ventricular outflow tract velocity is usually about 1 m/s in patients with normal left ventricular function and decreases when stroke volume is reduced. The ratio of the left ventricular outflow tract to the aortic valve time velocity integral is independent of any change in stroke volume. Since this patient has left ventricular outflow tract velocity of 43 cm/s, which is equal to 0.43 m/s, and aortic valve velocity of 4.3 m/s, the ratio of the left ventricular outflow tract (LVOT) to the aortic valve (AoV) time velocity integral is as follows: (LVOT velocity/AoV velocity) = (0.43/4.3) = 0.1.

When left ventricular systolic function is abnormal and cardiac output is reduced, the ratio of the left ventricular outflow tract to the aortic valve time velocity integral of 0.25 or less indicates severe aortic stenosis. Because the above-calculated ratio is 0.1, this patient with a low left ventricular ejection fraction most likely has severe aortic stenosis even though the peak velocity is less than 4.5 m/s and the mean gradient is less than 50 mm Hg. **Reference** 23 *(pp 104–113)*.

63. Answer E

The intervalvular fibrosa is the connective tissue between the aortic valve and the anterior leaflet of the mitral valve. The transesophageal echocardiographic long axis view accompanying Question 63 shows an abscess cavity at the aortic and mitral valve intervalvular fibrosa. **Reference** 23 *(pp 148–150)*.

64. Answer E

Perivalvular regurgitation, as shown in the accompanying images, occurs between the sewing ring (SW) and the surrounding valve anulus. (MV indicates mitral valve.) It results from failure of complete fixation of the valve along the suture line and may range from a pinhole leak to partial or complete valve dehiscence. In patients with a history of valvular replacement, perivalvular regurgitation is usually pathologic. Color flow imaging is useful in detecting perivalvular regurgitation. Typically, perivalvular regurgitation appears on color flow imaging as regurgitation originating outside the sewing ring, i.e., flow occurring around, rather than through, the prosthetic valve. Although a low aliasing velocity may overestimate the turbulent regurgitant jet, overestimation is unlikely to occur at an aliasing velocity of 65 cm/s on the color map. **References** 25 *(pp 1213–1214)*; 26 *(p 306)*.

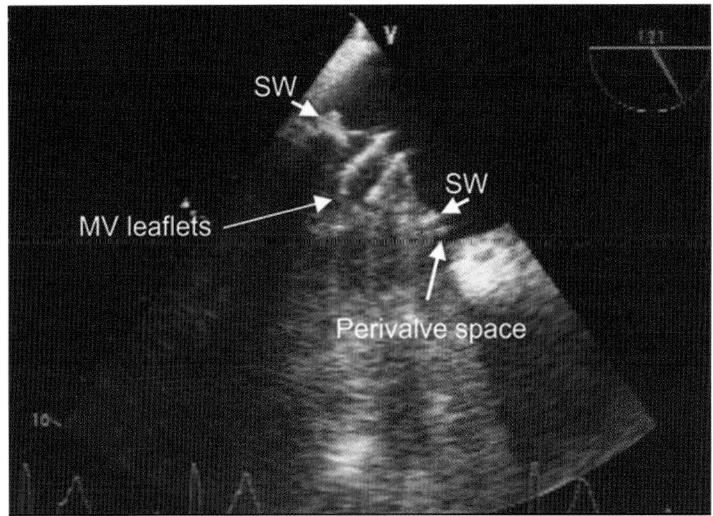

A

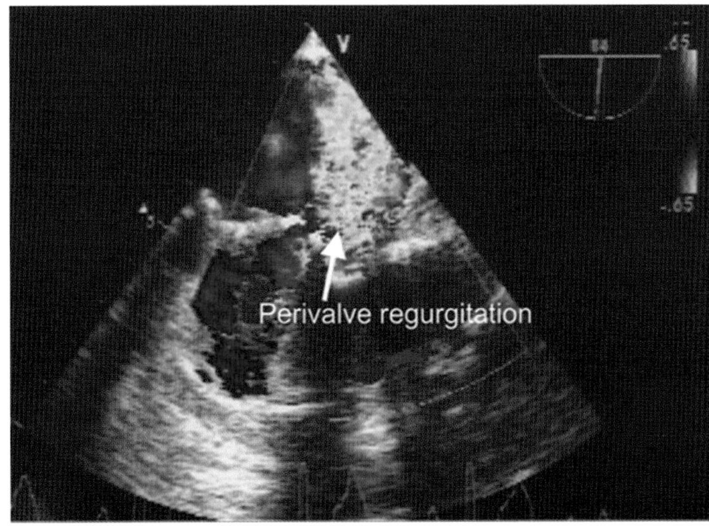

B

65. Answer E

66. Answer C

Immediately after coming off cardiopulmonary bypass, small perivalvular regurgitation with low flow velocity has been observed by intraoperative transesophageal echocardiography examination in patients undergoing valvular replacement, especially before the administration of protamine. In such a situation, the small perivalvular regurgitation with low flow velocity is frequently caused by the needle holes. It usually disappears after administration of protamine. Therefore, the next step of management for this patient is administration of protamine.

67. Answer C

The primary Doppler method for calculating a mechanical prosthetic valve area is based on the continuity principle, which states that, in the absence of regurgitation or shunts, flow through the prosthetic valve must equal flow through other areas of the heart. According to the continuity equation, mitral inflow equals left ventricular outflow tract outflow. Because flow volume equals the product of the mitral valve area (MVA) and the time velocity integral (TVI), the continuity equation can be written as follows: MVA × mitral TVI = LVOT area × LVOT TVI. Rearranging the above equation yields calculation of the mitral valve area: MVA = (LVOT area × LVOT TVI)/mitral TVI. This continuity equation measures the effective orifice area rather than the physical boundaries of an orifice.

The pressure half-time method was originally derived for native rheumatic mitral stenosis, and the empiric constant 220 ms in the half-time equation implicitly reflects, among other factors, the geometry and discharge coefficient of this type of stenosis. Application of this general equation and the cited constant to the wide range of available prostheses cannot be expected to yield accurate results. Not surprisingly, considerable overestimation by the pressure half-time method has been reported. Planimetry cannot be used to measure the area of a mechanical prosthesis. **Reference** 23 *(pp 65, 67, 115)*.

68. Answer A

Normally, mechanical prosthetic valves have closing volume or built-in regurgitant jets. Typically, the closing volume is seen in either early systole (at the mitral position) or early diastole (with aortic valve regurgitation). The normal prosthetic closing volume is low-velocity regurgitant flow with the following features:

	IN THE MITRAL POSITION	IN THE AORTIC POSITION
Regurgitant jet area	$<2\ cm^2$	$<1\ cm^2$
Jet length	<2.5 cm	<1.5 cm

Each mechanical prosthesis has a characteristic flow pattern. For example, the commonly used St. Jude prosthesis is a bileaflet mechanical valve with a minor central orifice and two lateral major flow orifices. The structure of this mechanical prosthesis gives rise to one central and two side built-in regurgitant jets or closing volume. The

Bjork-Shiley prosthesis is a tilting-disk prosthesis and has two unequal side jets. The Medtronic-Hall prosthesis is also a tilting-disk prosthesis, but it has a large central jet. The Starr-Edwards prosthesis is a ball-cage mechanical prosthesis and has two curved side jets. **References** 23 *(pp 133–143)*; 26 *(p 305)*.

69. Answer C

The Doppler color flow imaging technique is so sensitive that it detects trivial to mild degrees of valvular regurgitation that are not detected even with careful auscultation. Studies have shown that trivial to mild degrees of valvular regurgitation are common in the clinically normal population, and its prevalence increases with age. However, the age-related prevalence of valvular regurgitation in normal volunteers demonstrated that aortic regurgitation was not present in persons younger than 50 years. Therefore, a 40-year-old man normally should not have aortic regurgitation. **Reference** 23 *(p 130)*.

70. Answer D

71. Answer D

72. Answer E

The amount of blood flow across a regurgitant orifice can be estimated with the proximal isovelocity surface area (PISA) method, which is based on the principle of conservation of flow and the continuity equation. As blood in the left ventricle converges toward the mitral regurgitant orifice, blood flow velocity increases and forms a series of hemispheric waves, whose surface has the same velocity (isovelocity). Because the flow velocity at the PISA is the same as the aliasing velocity, the flow rate at the surface of a hemispheric PISA is calculated as the area of the hemisphere times the aliasing velocity. Mathematically, the area of the hemisphere is equal to $2 \times 3.14 \times r^2$. Therefore, flow rate at PISA $= 2 \times 3.14 \times r^2 \times$ aliasing velocity. Based on the principle of flow conservation, the flow rate at PISA is equal to the flow rate across the regurgitant orifice. Thus, $2 \times 3.14 \times r^2 \times$ aliasing velocity = ERO × MR velocity, where ERO is the effective regurgitant orifice. Rearranging the equation yields calculation of the ERO as follows:

$$\begin{aligned} \text{ERO} &= (2 \times 3.14 \times r^2 \times \text{ aliasing velocity})/\text{MR velocity} \\ &= (6.28 \times 1 \times 36)/450 \\ &= 0.5\ \text{cm}^2. \end{aligned}$$

The regurgitant volume is the product of the ERO and the MR time velocity integral (TVI). This patient's MR volume can be calculated as follows:

$$\begin{aligned} \text{RV} &= \text{ERO} \times \text{MR TVI} \\ &= 0.5 \times 200 \\ &= 100\ \text{mL}. \end{aligned}$$

The severity of mitral regurgitation is categorized according to the effective regurgitant orifice (ERO), regurgitant volume (RV), and regurgitant fraction (RF).

MITRAL REGURGITATION	ERO (mm^2)	RV (mL)	RF (%)
Grade I (mild)	<20	<30	<30
Grade II (moderate)	20–29	30–44	30–39
Grade III (moderately severe)	30–39	45–59	40–49
Grade IV (severe)	>40	>60	>50

This patient had ERO of 0.5 cm^2 or 50 mm^2 and RV of 100 mL, which are consistent with severe mitral regurgitation. **Reference** 23 *(pp 62–63, 120–129)*.

73. Answer B

This patient had mitral valve replacement with a bioprosthesis. As seen in the accompanying image, the stents of the prosthesis are well visualized (arrows). Generally, bioprostheses are made of pericardium or porcine heterograft. During transesophageal echocardiography, the leaflets appear delicate and thin. In comparison with mechanical prosthesis, the major advantage of bioprosthesis is the freedom from life-long anticoagulation therapy; however, a bioprosthesis is less durable than a mechanical prosthesis. Degeneration of the bioprosthesis occurs with time. **Reference** 11 *(pp 275, 278)*.

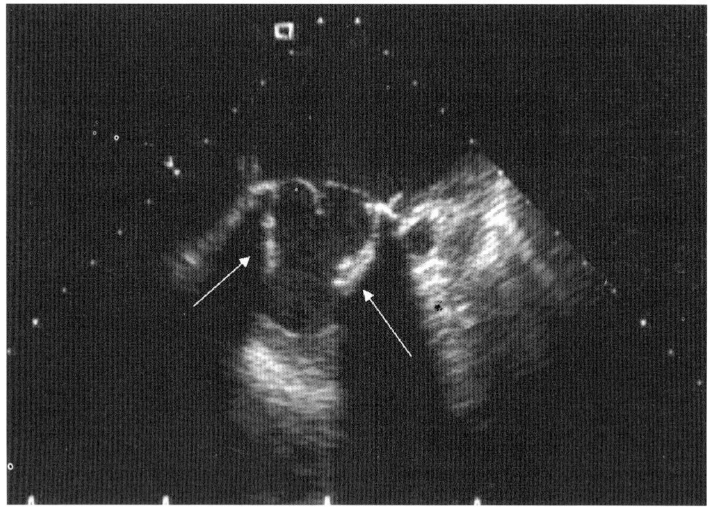

74. Answer E

In comparison to a stented bioprosthesis of the same size, the stentless design of the freestyle bioprosthesis offers much better hydrodynamic performance because it provides a larger effective orifice area while a stent and suture ring can obstruct flow. Due to its large effective orifice area, the freestyle bioprosthesis has low transvalvular gradients and laminar flow similar to a native valve. Postoperatively, the stentless valve has excellent gradients and an effective orifice area. Its hemodynamic performance often continues to improve over time.

75. Answer E

76. Answer D

77. Answer C

Based on the color flow image accompanying Question 75, the regurgitant jet is outside the sewing ring of the St. Jude mitral prosthesis. Therefore, this is a perivalvular regurgitation due to the gap between the sewing ring and the surrounding mitral anulus. Normally, the sewing ring and anulus should move as a unit. When there is unusual rocking movement of the prosthesis with perivalvular regurgitation, it is a sign of dehiscence of the prosthesis. If this occurs in a febrile patient, infective endocarditis should be considered. **Reference** 23 *(p 142)*.

78. Answer D

79. Answer E

The two-dimensional image accompanying Question 78 shows systolic anterior motion of the mitral valve. When this occurs after mitral valve repair, contributing factors include an elongated anterior mitral leaflet, anterior displacement of coaptation points, and a smaller postrepair mitral anulus. In such a situation, intraoperative transesophageal echocardiography reveals that the elongated anterior mitral leaflet has its coaptation point in the body of the leaflet with its distal portion moving toward the interventricular septum, resulting in leaflet-septal contact with dynamic left ventricular outflow tract obstruction in early systole and incomplete mitral leaflet coaptation in midsystole. Color flow imaging demonstrates the associated mitral regurgitation and the accelerated left ventricular outflow tract flow velocity. Systolic anterior motion is accentuated when the left ventricle is underfilled and hyperdynamic. An increase in volume and decrease in an inotropic agent such as dopamine can reduce systolic anterior motion or even make it disappear. (See also Questions 13 and 101.) **References** 11 *(pp 514–515)*; 23 *(pp 238–240)*; 24 *(p 42)*.

80. Answer D

In the right heart view accompanying Question 80, the globular masses involving the tricuspid leaflets are vegetations due to infective endocarditis. Although right-sided endocarditis is much less common, it has been associated with intravenous drug use, right heart instrumentation, and immunocompromise. **Reference** 11 *(p 313)*.

81. Answer C

82. Answer D

The bypass transesophageal echocardiography image accompanying Question 81, taken before bypass, was obtained with the probe in mid esophagus at about 50°. It shows a severely calcified aortic valve with three cusps. Generally, degenerative calcification of the aortic valve is the most common cause of aortic stenosis, especially in the elderly. The transesophageal echocardiographic images accompanying Question 82, taken after bypass, show a bioprosthesis at the aortic position. The mid-esophageal aortic valve short axis view clearly reveals three stents of the tissue valve, with the thin, delicate leaflets. Therefore, this 80-year-old patient has severe aortic stenosis because of degenerative calcification and undergoes aortic valve replacement with a bioprosthesis.

83. Answer A

The dimensionless obstructive index (DOI) is used to evaluate an aortic prosthetic valve. It is calculated as follows: DOI = LVOT velocity/aortic prosthesis velocity, where LVOT is left ventricular outflow tract.

The LVOT velocity can be measured by pulsed wave Doppler and the aortic prosthesis velocity by continuous Doppler. The normal value of the DOI is 0.3 or higher. As the velocity across the aortic prosthesis increases, the DOI decreases. In patients with prosthetic obstruction, the LVOT to aortic prosthesis velocity ratio is 0.2 or less.

If an aortic prosthesis is obstructed, flow velocity increases unless cardiac output decreases. Increased flow velocity across an aortic prosthesis is seen in patients with severe aortic prosthetic regurgitation because of increased flow through the aortic prosthesis. The LVOT flow velocity is normal to slightly decreased in patients with aortic obstruction and increased in patients with severe aortic regurgitation. Therefore, the LVOT to aortic prosthesis velocity ratio or time velocity integral ratio is helpful in differentiating increased flow velocity across an aortic prosthesis due to a prosthetic obstruction (the ratio ≤ 0.2) from increased velocity due to regurgitation (the ratio remains normal, ≥ 0.3). **References** 23 *(pp 136, 138)*; 25 *(p 805)*.

84. Answer E

Normally, a small amount of built-in regurgitation is present for all types of mechanical prostheses. This is known as closing volume, which varies depending on the types of the mechanical prostheses. The St. Jude prosthesis is a bileaflet mechanical valve. It has three built-in regurgitant jets: one central and two side jets, as shown in the accompanying transesophageal echocardiographic images during systole without (A) and with (B) color flow imaging. Therefore, this is a normal St. Jude prosthetic valve with a normal regurgitant flow pattern (arrows indicate closing volume). **Reference** 23 *(pp 139–140)*.

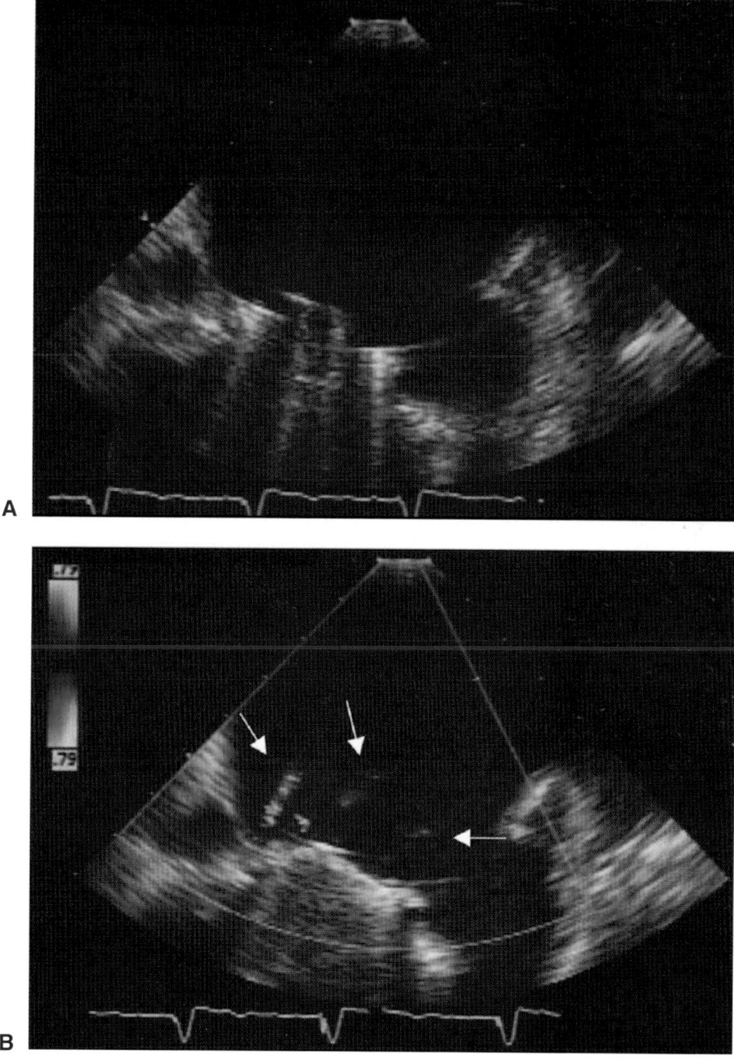

85. Answer D

The mitral prosthetic valve shown in the image accompanying Question 85 is a bileaflet mechanical prosthesis. The most commonly used bileaflet mechanical valve is the St. Jude prosthesis. From the transesophageal echocardiographic image obtained during diastole, it is clear that both leaflets are opened. However, one of the leaflets did not close during systole. **Reference** 23 *(p 141)*.

86. Answer E

The image accompanying Question 86 is a transverse plane, focused on the left ventricular outflow tract view of the aortic valve. Two vegetations are attached to the ventricular aspect of the aortic valve. Because the patient is also febrile, infective endocarditis is the most likely diagnosis. The location and the morphology of the vegetation are different from subaortic stenosis or flail aortic cusp. In a patient with normal left ventricular function, thrombus formation on the aortic valve is unlikely. **Reference** 11 *(p 311)*.

87. Answer D

With a deep transgastric view, the ultrasound beam parallels the blood flow through the aortic prosthesis, and hence, the measured Doppler information is more accurate. If the ultrasound beam is not parallel to blood flow through the aortic prosthesis, the measured mean gradient through the aortic prosthesis is underestimated, depending on the angle between the ultrasound beam and the blood flow (overestimation usually does not occur). All types of mechanical prosthetic valves, including the St. Jude prosthesis, are inherently stenotic. According to the normal Doppler values from the Mayo Clinic echocardiography laboratory, the St. Jude aortic prostheses have a mean pressure gradient of 14.4 ± 7.7 mm Hg. The mean gradient of 20 mm Hg for a St. Jude prosthetic valve in the aortic position is considered normal, especially with the small (19-mm) St. Jude prosthesis in this patient. **Reference** 23 *(pp 133–136)*.

88. Answer D

89. Answer D

90. Answer D

When the mitral regurgitant jet is eccentric with a distorted proximal isovelocity surface area, the continuity equation should be used to calculate the regurgitant volume and fraction. According to the continuity equation, what goes into the left ventricle during diastole (mitral inflow) must come out of the left ventricle during systole. Therefore, the mitral inflow volume is equal to the left ventricular outflow plus the mitral regurgitant volume, that is, mitral inflow = left ventricular outflow + mitral regurgitant volume. Rearranging the equation, the mitral regurgitant volume can be calculated as mitral regurgitant volume = mitral inflow−left ventricular outflow. Because flow volume is equal to the product of the cross-sectional area (CSA) and the time velocity integral (TVI), we can calculate the mitral regurgitant volume as follows:

$$\begin{aligned}
\text{Mitral RV} &= \text{MVA} \times \text{mitral TVI} - \text{LVOT CSA} \times \text{LVOT TVI} \\
&= (0.785 \times \text{mitral D}^2) \times \text{mitral TVI} - (0.785 \times \text{LVOT D}^2) \times \text{LVOT TVI} \\
&= 0.785 \times (3.8)^2 \times 18 - 0.785 \times (2.1)^2 \times 22 \\
&= 204 - 76 \\
&= 128 \text{ mL.}
\end{aligned}$$

By definition, the mitral regurgitant fraction is the percentage of mitral regurgitant volume compared with the total mitral inflow volume: Mitral RF = mitral RV/mitral inflow = (128/204) × 100% = 62%. Both a mitral regurgitant volume of 128 mL and a regurgitant fraction of 62% are consistent with severe mitral regurgitation. **Reference** 23 *(pp 123–129)*.

91. Answer E

92. Answer D

93. Answer D

In this 56-year-old patient, the accompanying prebypass two-dimensional image demonstrates a flail posterior mitral leaflet (arrow) caused by the ruptured chordae tendineae (part A) (LA, left atrium; LV, left ventricle). The color flow imaging (part B) shows an eccentric mitral regurgitation jet (arrow) directed toward the anterior mitral leaflet and the atrial septum. The two-dimensional echocardiographic evidence of disruption of the mitral valve apparatus, such as flail mitral leaflet caused by ruptured chordae tendineae in this patient, indicates or suggests severe mitral regurgitation. It should be remembered that the eccentric regurgitant jet area usually underestimates the severity of mitral regurgitation.

The scallop involved can be identified by starting at 0° where the anterior versus the posterior leaflet is first identified (part C), then scanning off axis to between 40° and 70°, i.e., the commissural view, where P3 is on the left, A2 in the middle, and P1 on the right, a flail or prolapsed P2 is seen across from A2 (part D).

Because the commissural view (part D) showed the flail leaflet in the middle, the conclusion is the middle scallop of the posterior mitral leaflet is flail. This patient underwent mitral valve repair with anuloplasty and did well postoperatively. Part E of the accompanying figure shows a schematic of each possible flail posterior scallop. **Reference** 6 *(p 374)*

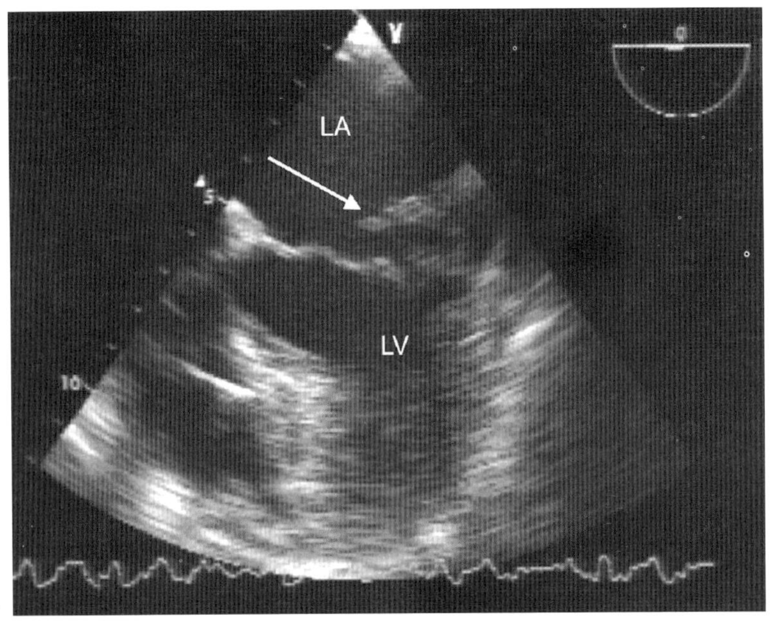

A

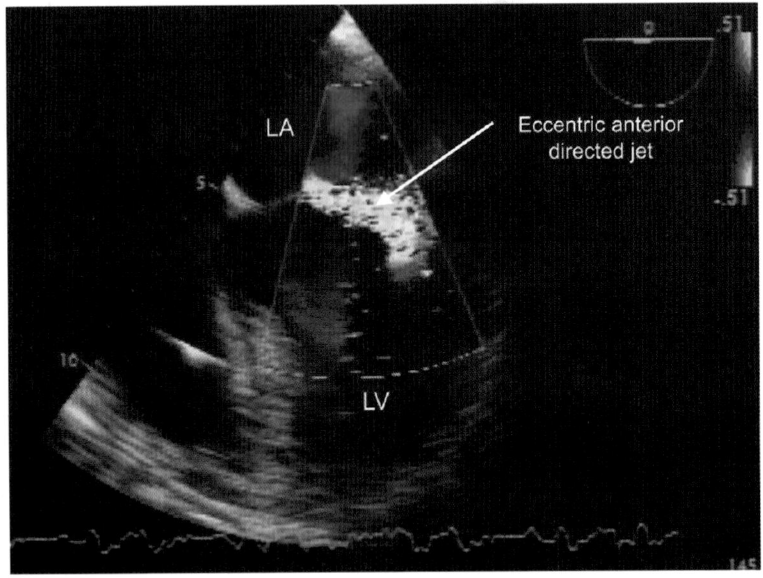

B

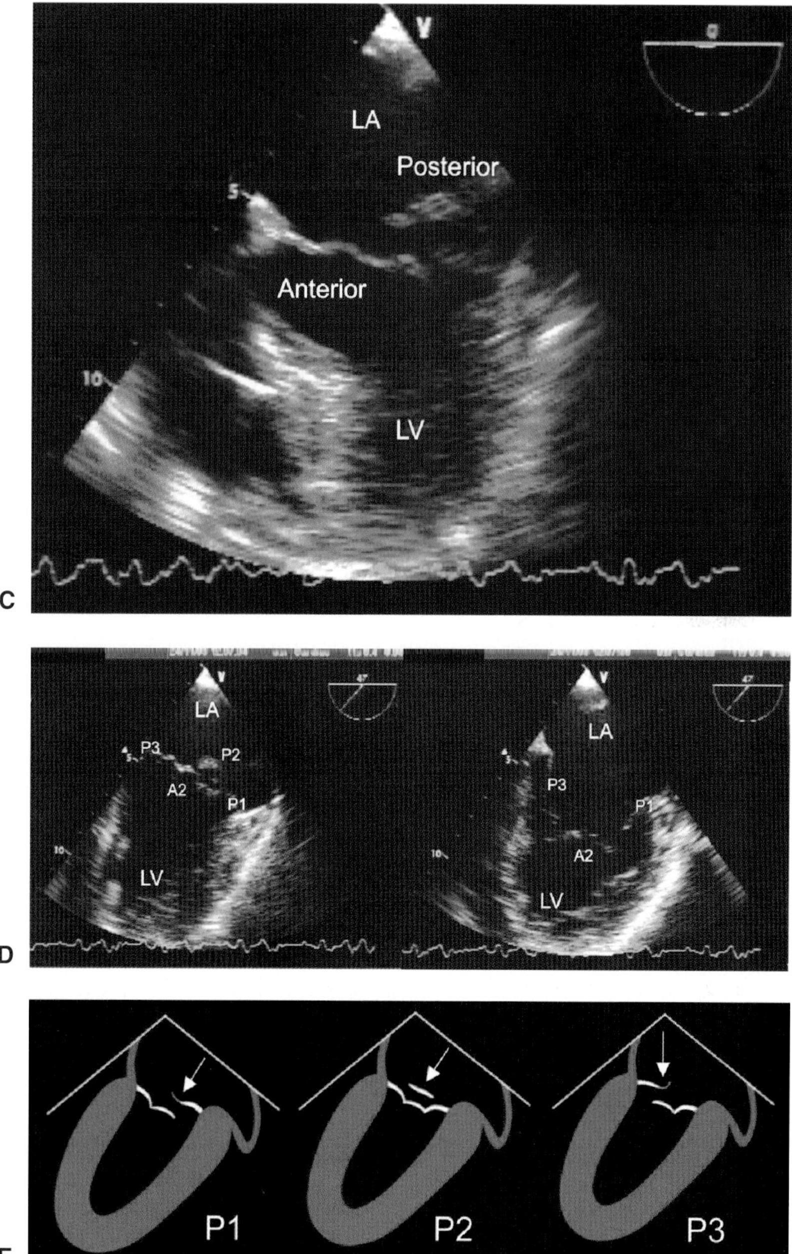

Figure from Click and Oh (6). Used with permission of Mayo Foundation for Medical Education and Research.

94. Answer B

The accompanying image on the left at 0° shows a flail posterior leaflet with ruptured chordae (arrow), and the image on the right at 55° shows ruptured chordae to the P1 scallop (arrow). LA indicates left atrium; LV, left ventricle.

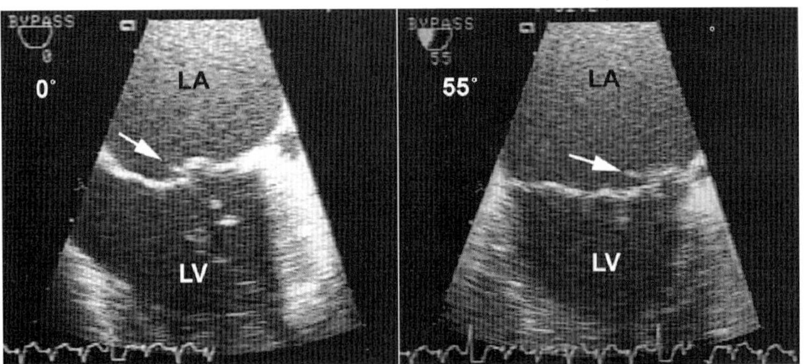

95. Answer E

In patients with severe chronic anemia, the cardiac output increases to compensate for the oxygen carrying capacity. Increased cardiac output leads to an increase in the peak velocity and the mean pressure gradient across the aortic valve. Therefore, in the settings of increased cardiac output across the aortic valve, aortic stenosis may not be severe even when the peak velocity is 4.5 m/s or more and the mean pressure gradient is 50 mm Hg or more. Because the ratio of the left ventricular outflow tract to the aortic valve time velocity integral or velocity is independent of stroke volume, it is more helpful in determining the severity of aortic stenosis in patients with an increased cardiac output. When cardiac output is increased, the left ventricular outflow tract velocity or time velocity integral increases in proportion to the peak aortic velocity or time velocity integral, resulting in an unchanged ratio of the left ventricular outflow tract to the aortic valve time velocity integral. Generally, the ratio of the left ventricular outflow tract to the aortic valve time velocity integral or a time velocity integral ratio of less than 0.2 indicates severe aortic stenosis. Because the patient has a ratio of left ventricular outflow tract to aortic valve time velocity integral of 0.3 and does not have severe aortic stenosis based on two-dimensional echocardiography, the increased mean gradient across the aortic valve could be explained by increased cardiac output secondary to severe anemia. It should be emphasized that the severity of valvular lesions must be determined by an integrated approach, especially when there is a discrepancy between the clinical, two-dimensional, and Doppler echocardiographic findings. **Reference** 23 *(pp 104–113)*.

96. Answer A

97. Answer E

The Medtronic-Hall prosthesis is a tilting mechanical disk valve, which rotates around a central strut. Normally, the Medtronic-Hall prosthesis produces a characteristic flow pattern of closing volume, which has the appearance of a large central regurgitant jet on color flow imaging. Therefore, the image accompanying Question 96 is the normal flow pattern for the Medtronic-Hall prosthesis, and the elective surgery for the patient should proceed as scheduled. **Reference** 23 *(pp 139–140)*.

98. Answer D

The severity of this patient's mitral regurgitation can be determined according to the simplified proximal isovelocity surface area (PISA) method. If the aliasing velocity is about 30 cm/s and the mitral regurgitation peak velocity is assumed to be about 500 cm/s, the PISA method for effective regurgitant orifice (ERO) calculation can be simplified as follows:

$$\begin{aligned} \text{ERO} &= (6.28 \times r^2 \times \text{aliasing velocity})/\text{MR peak velocity} \\ &= (6.28 \times r^2 \times 30\ \text{cm/s})/(500\ \text{cm/s}) \\ &= 0.38 \times r^2. \end{aligned}$$

Therefore, the ERO becomes 0.38 cm^2 when the PISA radius is 1 cm. Since an ERO of 0.4 cm^2 or more defines severe mitral regurgitation, a PISA radius of 1 cm or more indicates severe mitral regurgitation when the aliasing velocity is 30 cm/s or more. Because the peak mitral regurgitation velocity is assumed to be 500 cm/s, this simplification overestimates the ERO if the systemic blood pressure is increased, which would result in a mitral regurgitation peak velocity much higher than 500 cm/s. This 65-year-old man with normal blood pressure has a PISA radius greater than 1 cm at an aliasing velocity of 32 cm/s. According to the simplified PISA method, his mitral regurgitation is severe. **Reference** 23 *(pp 126–127)*.

99. Answer C

100. Answer E

Pressure half-time is the time interval for the peak pressure gradient to reach its half level. It is equal to 29% of the deceleration time. Because the deceleration time of the aortic regurgitant flow is 800 ms in the image accompanying Question 99, the pressure half-time can be calculated as follows:

$$\begin{aligned} \text{Pressure half-time} &= 0.29 \times 800 \\ &= 232\ \text{ms}. \end{aligned}$$

The pressure half-time of the aortic regurgitant jet is used to estimate the severity of aortic regurgitation. When the pressure half-time is 250 ms or less, the aortic regurgitation is usually severe. **Reference** 23 *(pp 67–68, 119–122)*.

101. Answer E

The systolic anterior motion of a mitral valve after repair is frequently caused by a reversible hyperdynamic state and accentuated by a small or underfilled left ventricle. A hyperdynamic left ventricle with increased contractility decreases the size of the left ventricle, leading to worsening systolic anterior motion. The appropriate management for such a situation is to increase the preload, decrease left ventricular contractility, and increase the afterload, especially if the patient is hypotensive. Among the choices listed in the question, the best pharmacologic management for this hypotensive patient with systolic anterior motion is phenylephrine, an α-agonist that increases systemic vascular resistance with an increase in systemic blood pressure. All the other choices are actually contraindicated in this clinical scenario because they increase the left ventricular contractility and make the systolic anterior motion worse with further decrease in systemic blood pressure. **References** 11 *(pp 514–515)*; 23 *(pp 238–240)*; 24 *(p 42)*.

102. Answer C

According to the American Society of Echocardiography/Society of Cardiovascular Anesthesiologists guidelines for performing comprehensive intraoperative multiplane transesophageal echocardiography, the image accompanying Question 102 is an upper esophageal aortic arch short axis view. The aorta is located posteriorly, near the transducer. On the left side of the image, the right ventricular outflow tract, the pulmonic valve, and the pulmonary artery can be observed. The color flow imaging demonstrates a small flow jet through the pulmonic valve, away from the transducer, during diastole. This finding is consistent with mild pulmonary regurgitation. **Reference** 37.

103. Answer A

The M-mode echocardiogram accompanying Question 103 demonstrates the fluttering motion of the anterior mitral leaflets (arrows) caused by severe aortic regurgitation. Also, M-mode echocardiography is helpful in demonstrating premature mitral valve closure or diastolic opening of the aortic valve as a sign of severe, usually acute aortic regurgitation and a marked increase in left ventricular diastolic pressure. In patients with aortic stenosis and a calcified aortic valve, M-mode echocardiography shows a decreased aortic valve opening (arrow, part A of the accompanying figure) with thickened cusps as well as multiple dense echoes in the aortic root during systole and diastole. Ao indicates aorta; LA, left atrium.

In patients with mitral stenosis, M-mode echocardiography typically shows thickened mitral leaflets and prolonged E-F slope. (See also Question 14 for M-mode echocardiography in a patient with mitral stenosis.) In patients with mitral valve prolapse, M-mode echocardiography demonstrates systolic bowing (arrows) of the posterior mitral leaflet below the C-D line (part B of the accompanying figure). LV indicates left ventricle; RV, right ventricle. **Reference** 23 *(pp 105, 119, 123)*.

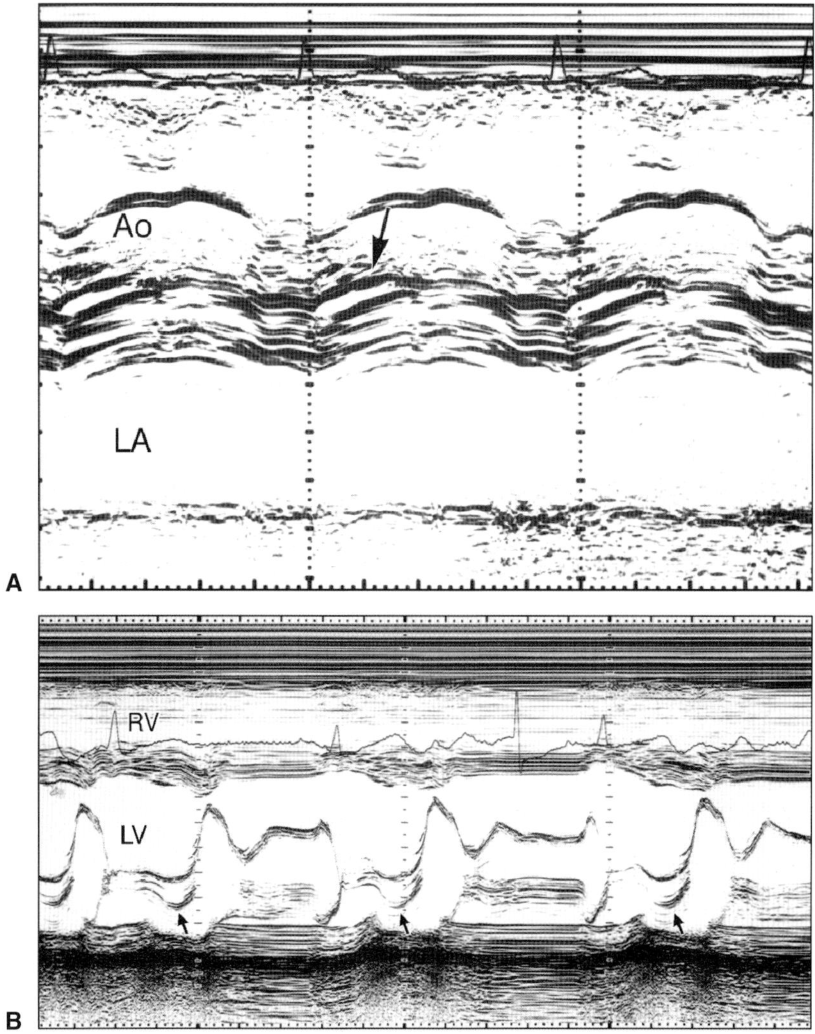

Figure from Oh et al. (23). Used with permission of Mayo Foundation for Medical Education and Research.

Chapter 11

Echocardiographic Manifestations of Congenital Heart Disease in Adult Patients

Questions

Multiple choice (choose the *one* best answer):

1. Which one of the following patients has mitral and tricuspid valves inserted at the same level?
   A. A patient with a normal heart.
   B. A patient with Ebstein's anomaly.
   C. A patient with ostium primum atrial septal defect.
   D. A patient with complete atrioventricular canal defect.
   E. C and D.

2. The aortic valve shown in the accompanying transesophageal echocardiographic image is
A. a unicuspid aortic valve.
B. a bicuspid aortic valve.
C. a normal aortic valve with three cusps.
D. an abnormal aortic valve with three cusps.
E. a quadricuspid aortic valve.

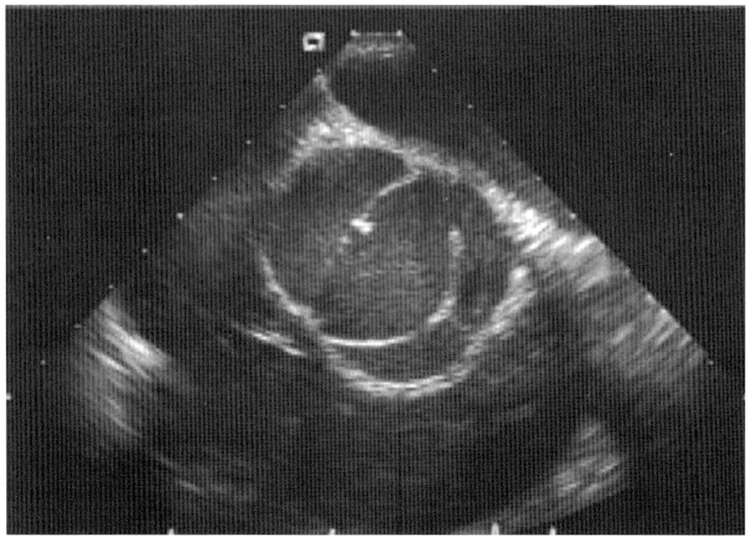

3. The etiology of the aortic valve abnormality shown in Question 2 is
A. rheumatic.
B. congenital.
C. degenerative.
D. traumatic.
E. ischemic.

4. Frequently, patients with this type of aortic valve abnormality also have
A. mitral stenosis.
B. tricuspid stenosis.
C. pulmonary stenosis.
D. papillary muscle dysfunction.
E. coarctation of the aorta.

5. The congenital cardiac lesion shown in the accompanying image is
A. tetralogy of Fallot.
B. Ebstein's anomaly.
C. partial atrioventricular canal.
D. secundum atrial septal defect.
E. sinus venosus atrial septal defect.

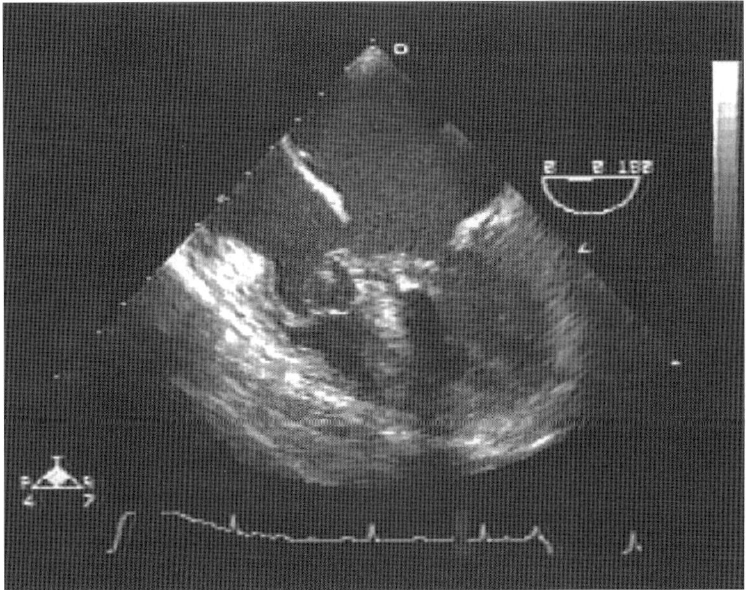

6. Patients with the congenital cardiac lesion shown in Question 5 also have
A. pulmonary stenosis.
B. supravalvular aortic stenosis.
C. aortic regurgitation.
D. cleft mitral valve.
E. parachute mitral valve.

7. The accompanying two-dimensional image was obtained in a patient with congenital heart disease. The diagnosis is
   A. hypoplastic left ventricle.
   B. Ebstein's anomaly.
   C. transposition of the great arteries.
   D. tetralogy of Fallot.
   E. ventricular septal defect.

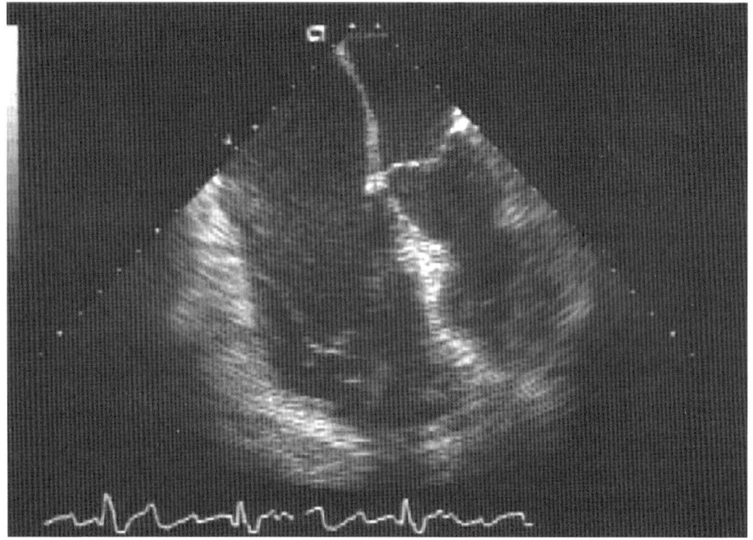

8. Which one of the following is the anomaly most commonly associated with the congenital lesion shown in the image accompanying Question 7?
   A. Atrial septal defect.
   B. Membranous ventricular septal defect.
   C. Muscular ventricular septal defect.
   D. Supracristal ventricular septal defect.
   E. Coarctation of aorta.

9. The accompanying transesophageal echocardiographic image (AV, atrioventricular valve; LA, left atrium; LV, left ventricle; MV, mitral valve; RA, right atrium; RV, right ventricle) shows

A. a normal heart.

B. supra-aortic stenosis.

C. subaortic stenosis.

D. moderator band.

E. congenital cor triatriatum.

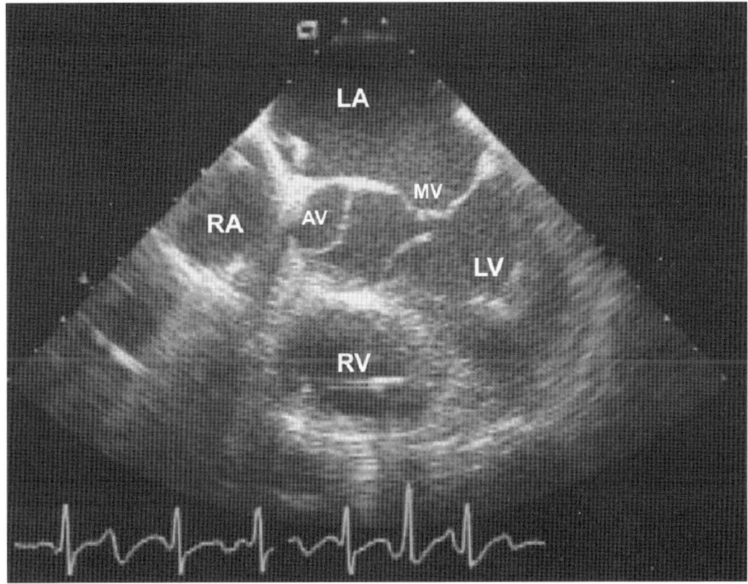

10. A patient with a congenital anomaly of the atrial septum undergoes transesophageal echocardiography. Based on the accompanying image, the diagnosis is
   A. patent foramen ovale.
   B. primum atrial septal defect.
   C. secundum atrial septal defect.
   D. sinus venosus atrial septal defect.
   E. coronary sinus atrial septal defect.

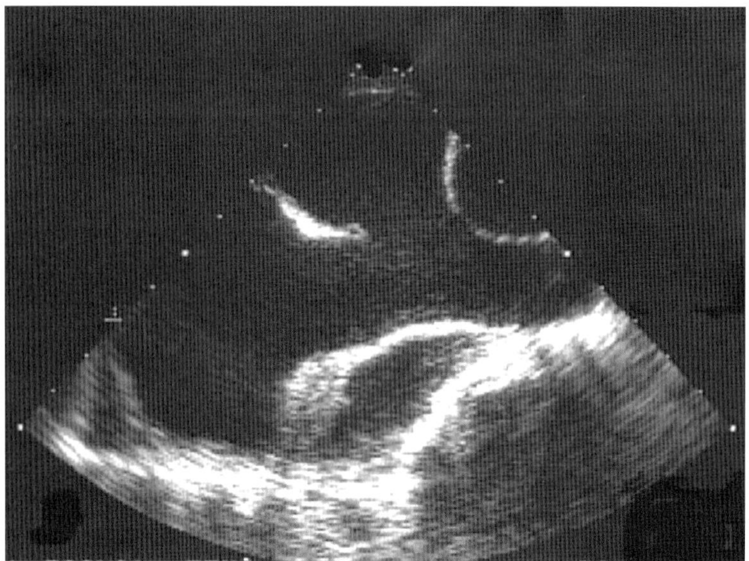

11. The abnormality shown in Question 10 is associated with a high incidence of
   A. partial anomalous pulmonary venous connection.
   B. persistent left superior vena cava.
   C. subaortic stenosis.
   D. cleft mitral valve.
   E. parachute mitral valve.

12. After an upper extremity venous injection of echocontrast material in a patient with persistent left superior vena cava, the echocontrast material is most likely visible in
   A. the left atrium, then the left ventricle.
   B. the left ventricle, then the left atrium.
   C. the left atrium, then the right atrium.
   D. the right atrium, then the coronary sinus.
   E. the coronary sinus, then the right atrium.

13. The accompanying two-dimensional and color flow images show

A. normal superior vena cava, pulmonary artery, and veins.

B. normal ascending aorta, superior vena cava, and right upper pulmonary vein.

C. partial anomalous pulmonary venous connection.

D. persistent left superior vena cava.

E. patent ductus arteriosus.

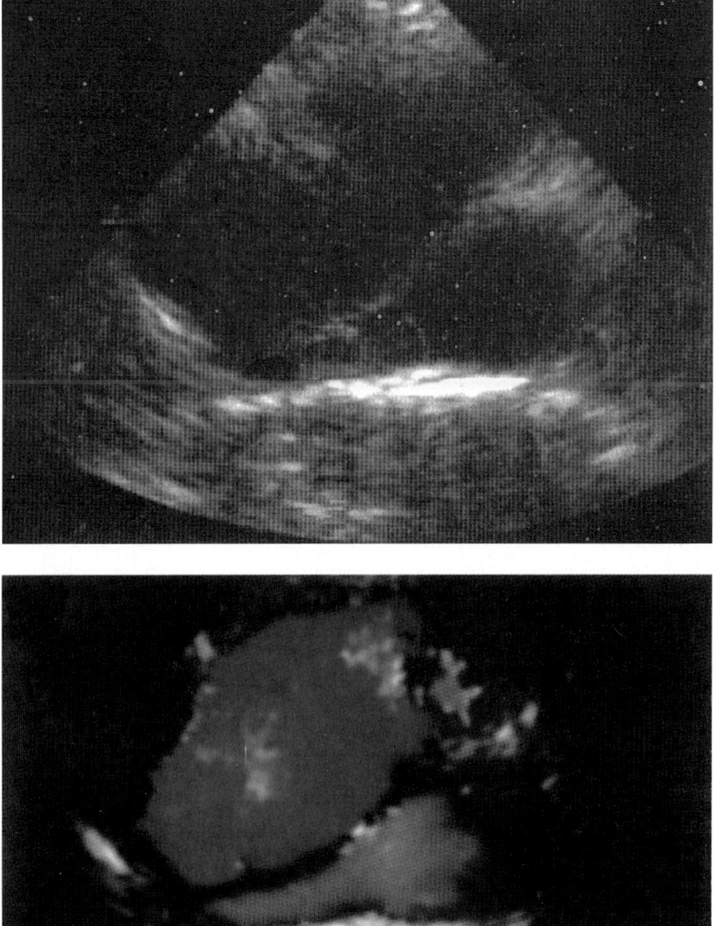

Figure from Ammash et al. (1). Used with permission.

14. Which one of the following ventricular septal defects is commonly associated with aortic regurgitation?

A. Membranous ventricular septal defect.
B. Supracristal ventricular septal defect.
C. Inflow ventricular septal defect.
D. Muscular ventricular septal defect.
E. None of the above.

15. The accompanying color flow image shows

A. pulmonary stenosis.
B. pulmonary regurgitation.
C. persistent left superior vena cava.
D. anomalous pulmonary venous connection.
E. patent ductus arteriosus.

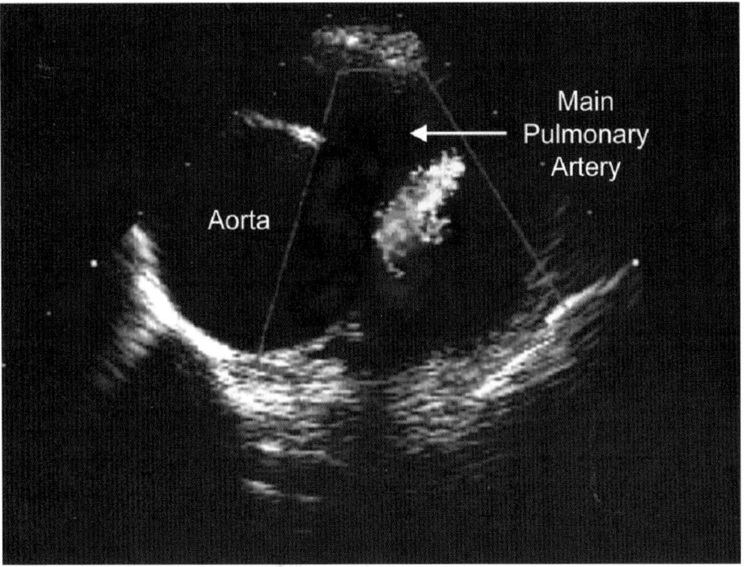

16. In patients with corrected transposition of the great arteries, the systemic ventricle is best identified by

A. the eustachian valve.
B. atrioventricular valve morphology.
C. the inferior vena cava.
D. the superior vena cava.
E. the flap valve of fossa ovale.

17. The accompanying transesophageal echocardiographic images show a mid-esophageal bicaval view, without (A) and with (B) color flow. Most likely, the patient has

A. patent foramen ovale.
B. primum atrial septal defect.
C. secundum atrial septal defect.
D. an atrial septal aneurysm.
E. C and D.

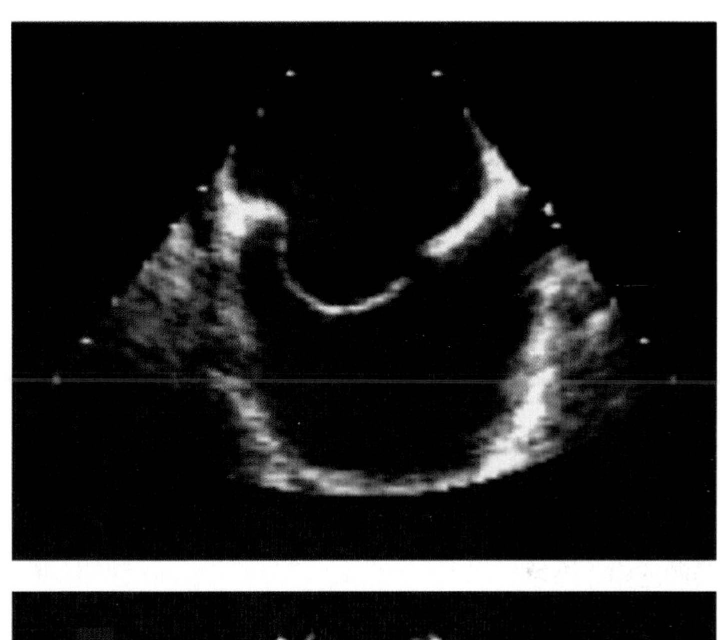

A

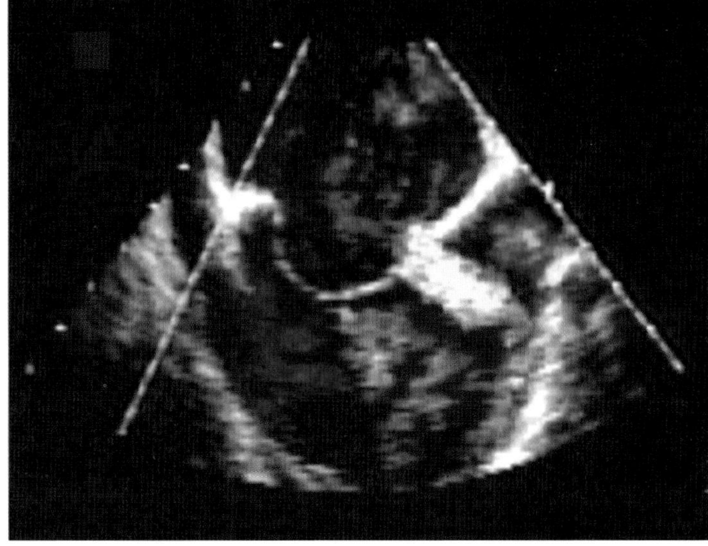

B

18. The congenital abnormality seen in the accompanying transesophageal echocardiographic image is best described as

A. a dilated ascending aorta.

B. corrected transposition of great arteries.

C. a congenital aneurysm of ascending aorta.

D. Marfan's syndrome.

E. tetralogy of Fallot.

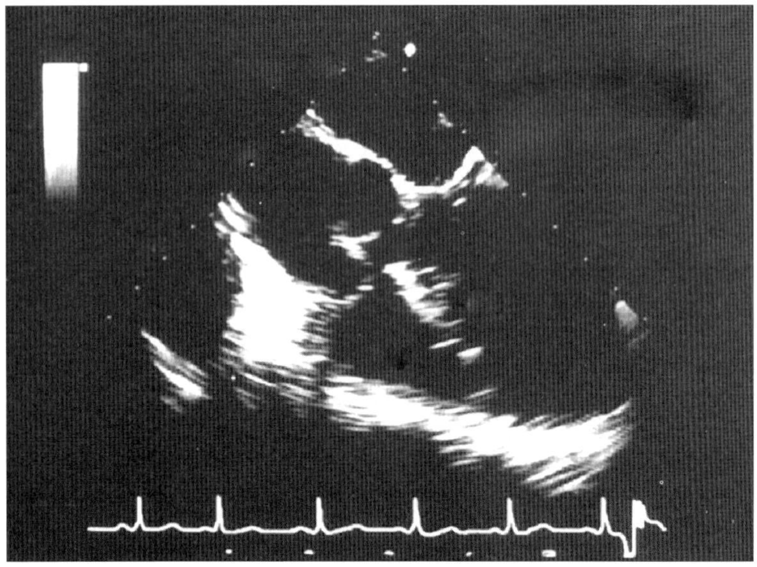

Figure from Nanda and Domanski (20). Used with permission.

19. The accompanying transesophageal echocardiographic image (LA, left atrium; RA, right atrium) is obtained in a 34-year-old patient before bypass. The intraoperative image also reveals a prominent eustachian valve. Based on this two-dimensional image, the patient has

A. a large patent foramen ovale.
B. primum atrial septal defect.
C. secundum atrial septal defect.
D. coronary sinus atrial septal defect.
E. sinus venosus atrial septal defect.

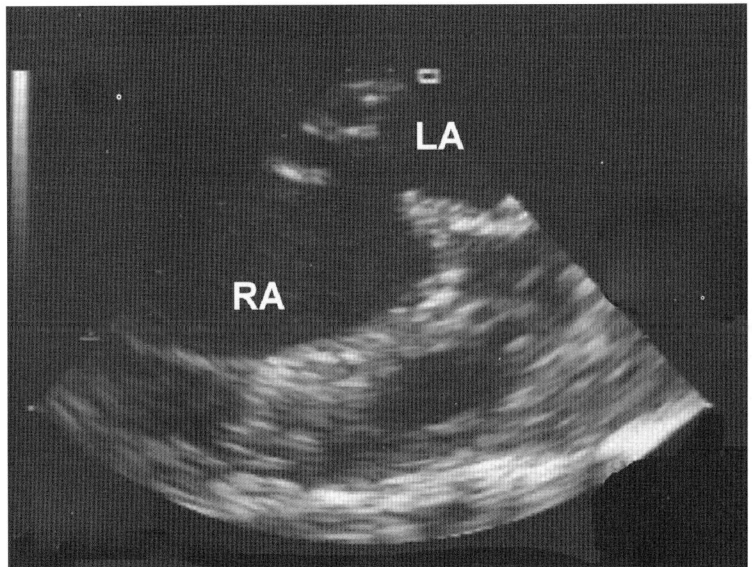

20. The patient described in Question 19 has repair of the atrial septal defect and is taken off cardiopulmonary bypass, intraoperative transesophageal echocardiography (LA, left atrium; RA, right atrium) reveals the accompanying image. A mobile structure is seen in the left atrium (arrow), and the blood flow from the inferior vena cava is found entering the left atrium. The cardiologist should tell the surgeon

A. to put the patient back on bypass because the patch is sewed to the wrong structure.

B. the postbypass transesophageal echocardiographic findings are expected and normal for this type of surgery.

C. the patient also has congenital cor triatriatum in the left atrium.

D. a linear thrombus is found in the left atrium.

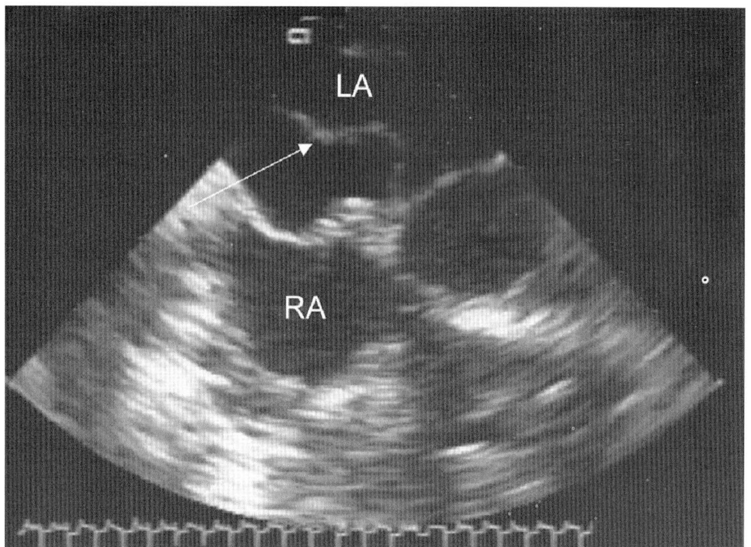

Answers & Discussion

1. Answer E

The internal cardiac crux is an important echocardiographic anatomic landmark used in the evaluation of many congenital cardiac anomalies. The components of the internal cardiac crux include the atrial septum, ventricular septum, and septal portions of the mitral and tricuspid valves. Normally, the tricuspid valve originates from the crest of the ventricular septum, and the septal portion of the mitral valve inserts at a higher level off the lower atrial septum. The portion of the ventricular septum between the two valves represents the atrioventricular septum, which is a potential communication between the left ventricle and the right atrium.

In the accompanying mid-esophageal four-chamber illustration, the normal internal cardiac crux is characterized by an apparent lower insertion of the septal leaflet of the morphologic tricuspid valve. In patients with partial (i.e., ostium primum atrial septal defect) and complete (i.e., ostium primum atrial septal defect and inlet ventricular septal defect) atrioventricular canal defects, the mitral valve is characteristically displaced downward, resulting in insertion of the septal portions of the mitral and tricuspid valves at the same level. (See also Questions 5 and 6.) **References** 11 *(p 386)*; 23 *(pp 229–230)*; 42 *(pp 986–987)*.

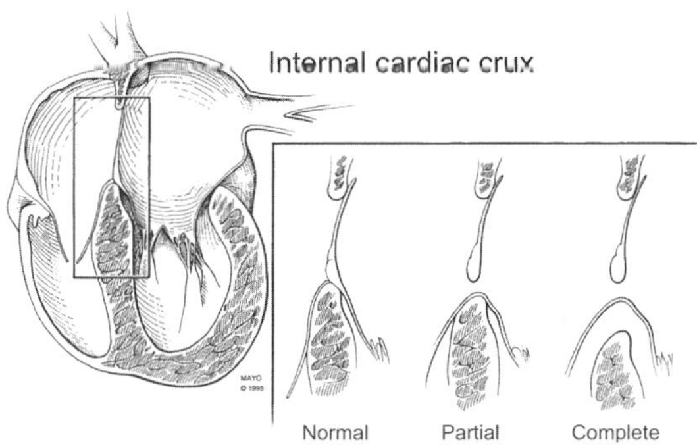

Figure from Oh et al. (23). Used with permission of Mayo Foundation for Medical Education and Research.

2. Answer B

3. Answer B

4. Answer E

The two-dimensional images accompanying this question are the transesophageal echocardiograms of short axis (A) and long axis (B) views of a bicuspid aortic valve in a systolic frame. In the short axis view, the commissures are seen at the 2- and 8-o'clock positions, with the raphe at the 4- to 5-o'clock position (arrow). In the long axis view, the arrow points to the doming of the anterior aortic cusp. The surgical view is seen in part C.

A bicuspid aortic valve is the most common congenital cardiac anomaly and is found in 0.9% to 2.5% of patients in autopsy series. Bicuspid aortic valves are clinically important because they can be associated with hemodynamically important aortic stenosis or may undergo progressive thickening, fibrosis, and, eventually, calcification, leading to critical obstruction. Symptomatic aortic stenosis caused by a bicuspid aortic

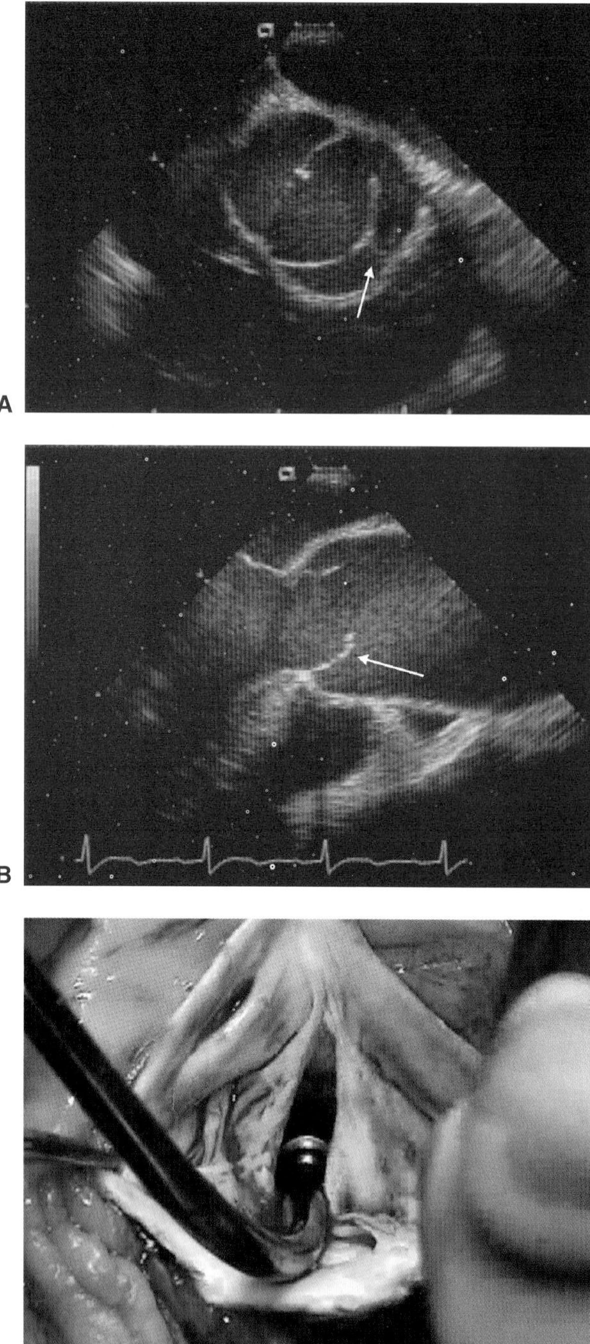
A
B
C

valve usually occurs before the age of 65 years. In addition, bicuspid valves are frequently insufficient, are a common site of infection in bacterial endocarditis, and may be associated with a variety of other congenital disorders of the heart. Patients with a bicuspid aortic valve have a higher incidence of coarctation of the aorta. About 50% of patients with coarctation of the aorta also have a bicuspid aortic valve. Therefore, coarctation of the aorta should always be looked for in patients with a bicuspid aortic valve and vice versa. **References** 10 *(pp 368–369, 372–373)*; 11 *(pp 122, 416)*; 23 *(pp 226–228)*; 26 *(p 400)*; 39 *(pp 422–425)*; 42 *(pp 506–508)*.

5. Answer C

6. Answer D

The congenital cardiac lesion (arrow) shown in the accompanying mid-esophageal four-chamber view is a partial atrioventricular canal defect. (LA indicates left atrium; LV, left ventricle; RA, right atrium.) An atrioventricular canal defect is also called an atrioventricular septal defect or an endocardial cushion defect. Atrioventricular canal defects occur from a failure of the embryonic endocardial cushions to meet and partition the heart. The result is a defect in the center of the heart, which affects the septa and the support apparatus of the atrioventricular valves. The most severe form is the complete atrioventricular canal defect, which has an ostium primum atrial septal defect, an inlet ventricular septal defect, and a common atrioventricular valve that is markedly abnormal. In the absence of the inlet ventricular septal defect, a partial atrioventricular canal is present. In patients with a partial atrioventricular canal defect, the mid-esophageal four-chamber view characteristically shows the ostium primum atrial septal defect and the apical displacement of the left atrioventricular valve. In addition, these patients also have so-called cleft mitral valve, which is commonly described as an abnormal left atrioventricular valve with the anterior leaflet divided into a superior and inferior portion by a cleft. **References** 39 *(pp 277–289)*; 42 *(pp 1018–1022)*.

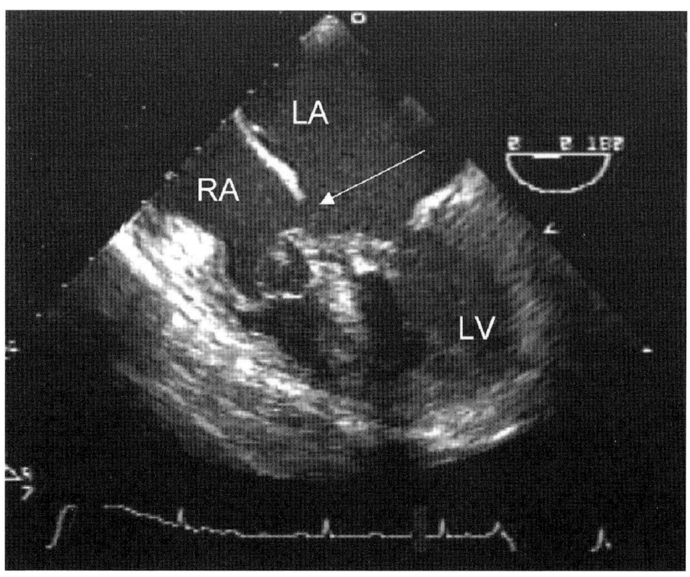

7. Answer B

8. Answer A

The mid-esophageal four-chamber view accompanying this question (LA, left atrium; LV, left ventricle; RA, right atrium; RV, right ventricle) shows the apical displacement of the tricuspid valve (arrow) with the atrialized right ventricle, which is characteristic of Ebstein's anomaly. Ebstein's anomaly is a severe deformity of the tricuspid valve, which results from failure of the normal development of the septal and posterior leaflets. The leaflets become displaced apically and adhere to the wall of the right ventricle and septum, creating the atrialized right ventricle. The anterior leaflet enlarges and becomes "sail-like," with variable attachments to the trabecular portion of the right ventricle and outflow area. Tethering of the tricuspid leaflets to the underlying myocardium can be seen in both transverse and longitudinal planes.

In addition to the morphologic abnormalities of the tricuspid valve, the right atrium is dilated in Ebstein's anomaly, reflecting the presence of tricuspid regurgitation since the fetal period. Doppler ultrasound demonstrates tricuspid regurgitation in almost all patients with the lesion. In fact, tricuspid regurgitation and right atrial enlargement are characteristic features of Ebstein's anomaly that can be detected in the fetus before displacement of valve leaflets is seen. Usually, the diagnosis of Ebstein's anomaly is made by echocardiography, and other tests are not needed. An atrial septal defect is present in 40% to 60% of patients with Ebstein's anomaly, but ventricular septal defects are occasionally present. In addition, patients with Ebstein's anomaly have a higher incidence of the Wolff-Parkinson-White syndrome and resultant supraventricular tachycardia. **References** 26 *(pp 406–407)*; 39 *(pp 389–394)*; 40 *(p 92)*; 42 *(pp 840–842)*.

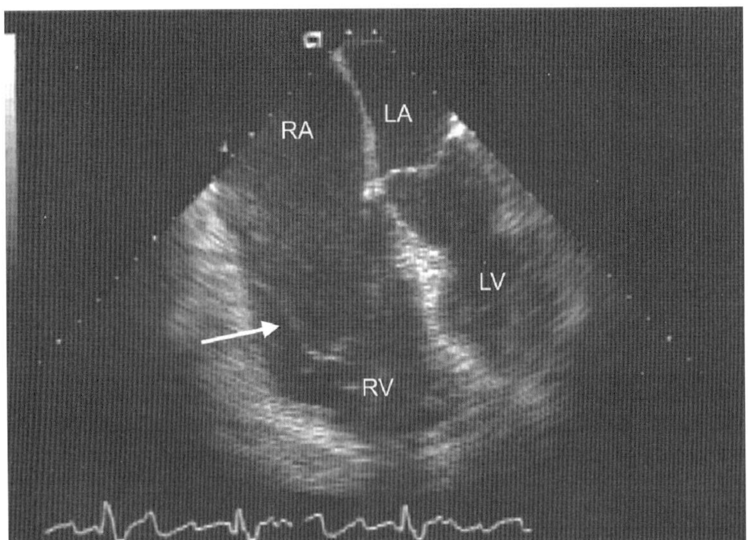

9. Answer C

The transesophageal echocardiographic image accompanying Question 9 reveals discrete membranous subaortic stenosis. The arrow in the accompanying two-dimensional image points to the thin membrane below the aortic valve in the left ventricular outflow tract, which is the cause of subaortic stenosis in this patient. (Also in this image, AV, aortic valve; LA, left atrium; LV, left ventricle; MV, mitral valve; RA, right atrium; RV, right ventricle.)

Congenital subaortic obstruction can range anatomically from a muscular ridge to a thin membrane. Typically, the thin, fibrous membrane or ridge forms a barrier within the left ventricular outflow tract, about 1 to 1.5 cm below the aortic valve. Sometimes it is located immediately adjacent to the aortic valve. The membrane usually extends from the anterior septum to the anterior mitral leaflet. The degree of obstruction to flow is variable. The possibility of a subaortic membrane should be considered when high-velocity flow is recorded in the left ventricular outflow tract, but the aortic valve leaflets appear normal. Transesophageal echocardiography may allow direct imaging of the subaortic membrane, especially if multiple image planes are used to identify this thin structure. With a two-dimensional image, the membrane is seen as a discrete linear echo in the left ventricular outflow tract perpendicular to the interventricular septum. The associated abnormalities include aortic regurgitation, which may be present because of chronic exposure of the aortic valve leaflets to the high-velocity subaortic flow, resulting in a "jet lesion" on the aortic valve. Rarely, the coexisting aortic regurgitation is caused by fibrous attachments from the subaortic membrane to the aortic valve leaflets.

Supra-aortic stenosis most commonly presents as a fusiform fibrous thickening of the ascending aortic wall. The moderator band is the prominent septoparietal muscle bundle found in the morphologic right ventricle. Cor triatriatum is characterized by partition of the left atrium into two discrete chambers by a fibrous or fibromuscular diaphragm. This diaphragm typically divides the left atrium above the atrial appendage and fossa ovalis. One or more openings in the fibrous membrane permit the flow of blood from the pulmonary venous system into the true left atrium. The size of these openings determines the degree of left atrial obstruction. **References** 23 *(pp 226–228)*; 42 *(pp 564–568)*.

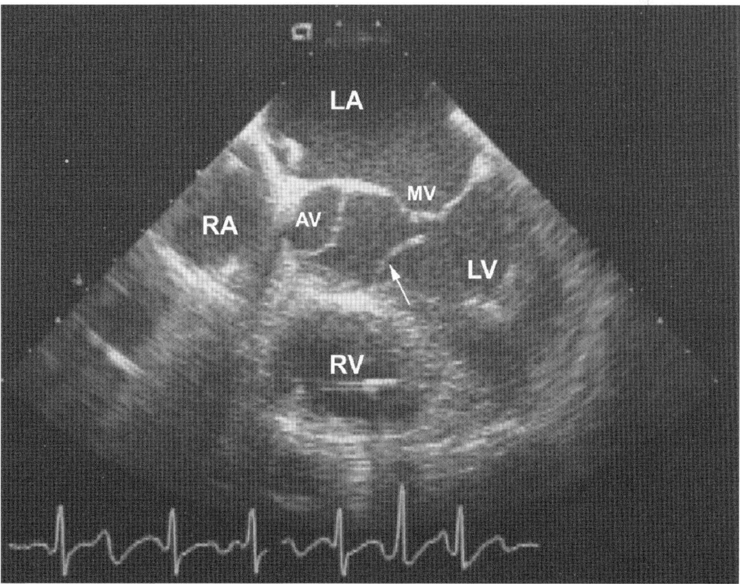

10. Answer D

11. Answer A

The accompanying two-dimensional transesophageal echocardiographic image (LA, left atrium; RA, right atrium; SVC, superior vena cava) shows the sinus venosus atrial septal defect. In this long axis image, the large atrial septal defect (arrows) is just next to the superior vena cava, where this vessel enters the right atrium. There is an absence of the superior limbus of the atrial septum. Sinus venosus atrial septal defect is associated with a high incidence of partial anomalous pulmonary venous connection. **References** 11 *(p 395)*; 23 *(pp 225, 227)*; 26 *(pp 407–410)*.

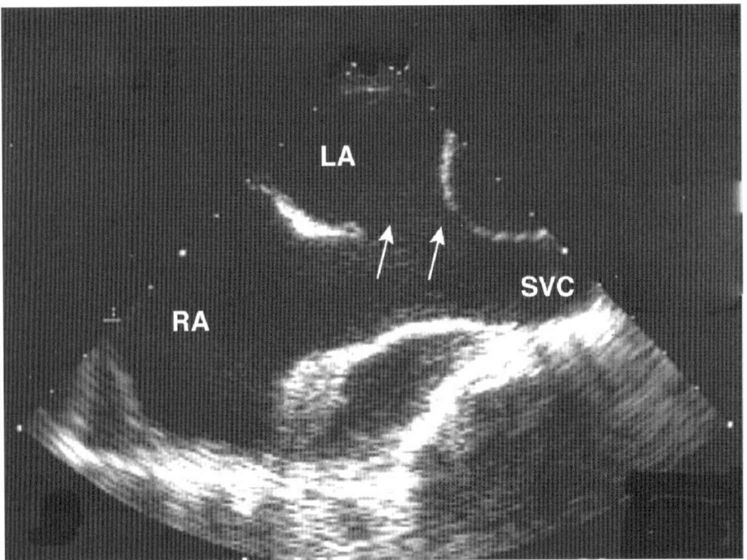

12. Answer E

A persistent left superior vena cava is the most common congenital anomaly involving the systemic veins. It occurs in approximately 0.5% of the general population and 3% to 10% of patients with congenital heart disease. In more than 90% of cases, the left superior vena cava drains into the right atrium by way of the coronary sinus, resulting in a dilated coronary sinus. As in the accompanying figure (part A) (LA, left atrium; LV, left ventricle), the finding of an enlarged coronary sinus (arrow) should alert the clinician to the possibility of a persistent left superior vena cava connecting to the coronary sinus. The presence of the left superior vena cava draining to the coronary sinus can be confirmed by intravenous contrast injections into the left arm. After a left arm intravenous injection, contrast echoes usually are seen first in the coronary sinus (arrow), with shadowing (block arrows), as seen in the accompanying figure (part B), and subsequently, in the right atrium. Less often, the persistent left superior vena cava drains into the left atrium or a pulmonary vein, resulting in a right-to-left shunt. **References** 10 *(pp 339–401)*; 11 *(pp 386, 388)*.

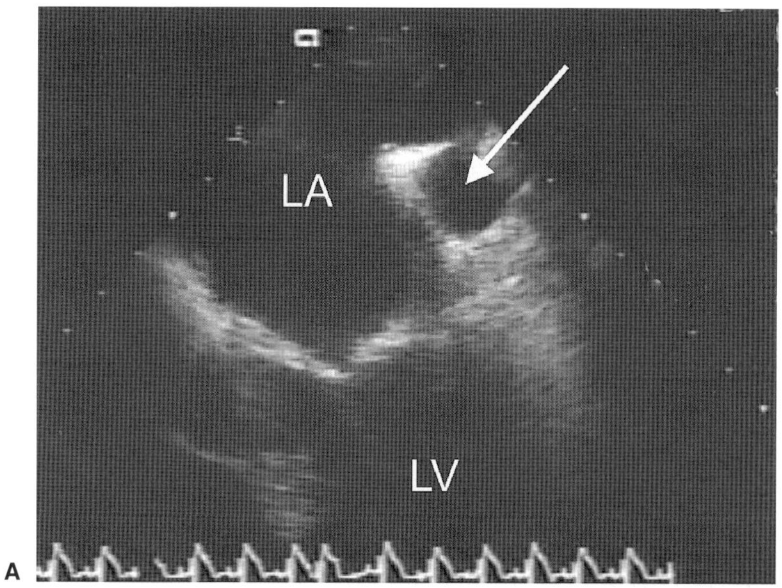

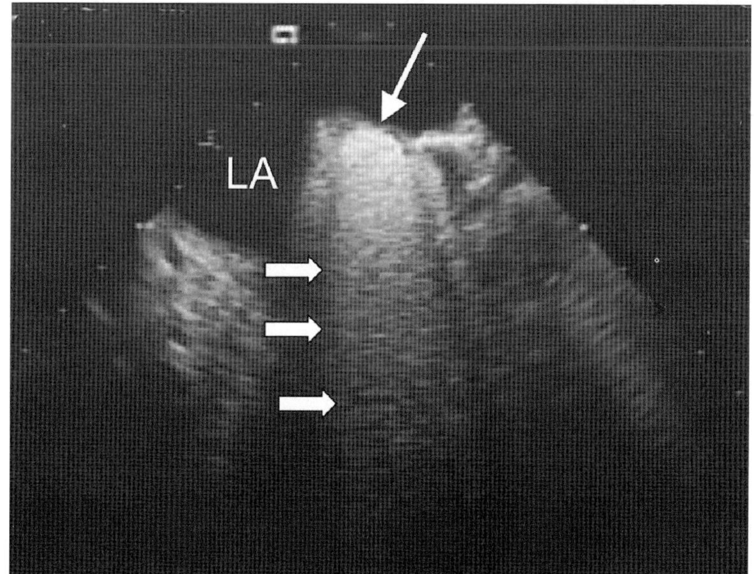

13. Answer C

Partial anomalous pulmonary venous connection is a relatively uncommon congenital anomaly. It represents persistence of the embryonic anastomosis between the systemic and pulmonary vein plexus, resulting in one or more anomalously connected pulmonary veins. The most common form of partial anomalous pulmonary venous connection is commitment of the right upper pulmonary vein to the right superior vena cava (accounting for more than 90% of cases, often in association with a sinus venosus atrial

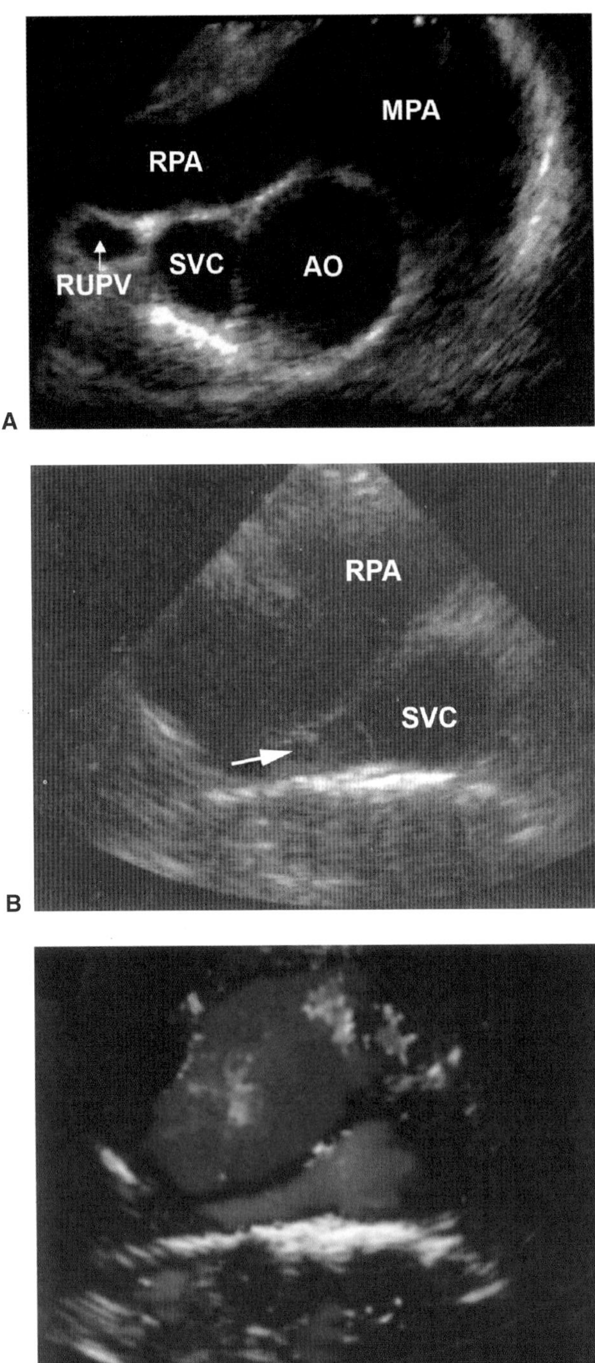

Figure from Ammash et al. (1). Used with permission.

septal defect). This anomaly is best visualized by use of the horizontal transducer plane at the level of right pulmonary artery. Normally, the accompanying transesophageal echocardiographic view (part A) shows the right pulmonary artery in its long axis. Anterior to the right pulmonary artery are three ovoid-appearing vessels—the furthest rightward (leftward of the image display screen) is the distal right upper pulmonary vein lying immediately adjacent to the superior vena cava. (AO represents aorta; MPA, main pulmonary artery; RPA, right pulmonary artery; RUPV, right upper pulmonary vein; SVC, superior vena cava.)

A typical partial anomalous pulmonary venous connection is for the right upper pulmonary vein to join the superior vena cava at this level. The anomalous vein appears as a vessel entering the medial wall of the superior vena cava. The conjoined structures would then form a "teardrop" appearance. Color flow Doppler examination is helpful in confirming the entry of turbulent blood into the medial superior vena cava.

In the two-dimensional and color flow images accompanying Question 13 (parts B and C shown here), the superior vena cava has the "teardrop" appearance (arrow in part B of image shown here), which is caused by the entry of the right upper pulmonary vein into the medial aspect of the superior vena cava. **References** 1; 10 *(pp 402–404)*; 11 *(pp 388–392)*; 23 *(p 227)*.

14. Answer B

A ventricular septal defect is an abnormal opening in the ventricular septum, which allows communication between the right and left ventricles. It is the most common form of congenital heart disease, accounting for about 25% of defects. Depending on the anatomic location of the defect, a ventricular septal defect can be categorized as perimembranous, supracristal (infundibular or subpulmonary), muscular, or inlet ventricular septal defect.

The most common form of ventricular septal defect is a perimembranous ventricular septal defect, which is also called a membranous ventricular septal defect. It involves or is adjacent to the membranous septum. A supracristal ventricular septal defect is also called an infundibular, subpulmonary, outlet, or subarterial ventricular septal defect. A supracristal ventricular septal defect accounts for about 5% to 7% of all ventricular septal defects and is more common in Asian patients. Commonly associated with a supracristal ventricular septal defect are aneurysmal enlargement of the aortic sinus and aortic regurgitation caused by prolapse of the aortic valve leaflets. A muscular ventricular septal defect may be either single or multiple. An inlet ventricular septal defect involves the inflow portion of the ventricular septum. Usually, an inlet ventricular septal defect is associated with atrioventricular valvular abnormalities and is one of the components of the complete atrioventricular canal. **References** 10 *(pp 384–392)*; 11 *(p 229)*; 23 *(pp 225–226)*; 26 *(pp 411–414)*; 42 *(pp 946–951)*.

15. Answer E

The image accompanying Question 15 is a mid-esophageal ascending aorta short axis view with main pulmonary artery. A turbulent jet is observed in the main pulmonary artery. This turbulent jet is produced by a patent ductus arteriosus, which is the persistent patency of a normal structure, the ductus arteriosus, during intrauterine life. The complex cascade of events that occurs during the transition from fetal to neonatal circulation results in the constriction of medial smooth muscle and the functional closure of the ductus arteriosus 1 to 4 days after birth. Usually, the ductus arteriosus undergoes complete anatomic closure and fibrosis within 3 weeks after delivery of term infants. The incidence of patent ductus arteriosus is much higher in premature infants and is related to the degree of prematurity. Anatomically, the patent ductus arteriosus arises from the descending thoracic aorta, near the origin of the left subclavian artery, and enters the anterior surface of the main pulmonary artery. Because pulmonary vascular resistance is less than systemic vascular resistance, a left-to-right shunt usually occurs in patients with patent ductus arteriosus; that is, blood flows from the descending thoracic aorta into the main pulmonary artery, resulting in the turbulent jet seen in the main pulmonary artery during transesophageal echocardiography. **References** 20 *(p 332)*; 39 *(pp 452–453)*; 42 *(pp 894–898)*.

16. Answer B

Corrected transposition of the great arteries is also called *l*-transposition, ventricular inversion, and a number of other names that attempt to identify the complexity of the problem. It is a condition in which both atrioventricular discordance and ventriculoarterial discordance occur. On the patient's right, the morphologic right atrium is connected to the morphologic left ventricle, which is, in turn, connected to the pulmonary artery. On the patient's left, the morphologic left atrium is connected to the morphologic right ventricle, which is connected to the aorta. Because discordant connections are present at both atrioventricular and ventriculoarterial levels, the circulation is hemodynamically correct; that is, systemic venous blood flows to the pulmonary artery and pulmonary venous blood flows to the aorta.

In patients with corrected transposition of the great arteries, the functional left ventricle or the systemic ventricle is the morphologic right ventricle. The atrioventricular valve morphology is useful in identifying the cardiac chambers because the atrioventricular valve always belongs to the appropriate ventricle; that is, the tricuspid valve is always found in the morphologic right ventricle even though the right ventricle is on the left in patients with corrected transposition of the great arteries, and the mitral valve is always found in the morphologic left ventricle. The tricuspid valve is inserted closer to the cardiac apex, has three leaflets, and has chordal insertions into the ventricular septum. In contrast, the mitral valve is inserted at a higher level and farther from the cardiac apex. It is a fish-mouth bicuspid valve and has chordal insertions into the two papillary muscles in the left ventricle. Therefore, in patients with corrected transposition of the great arteries, the functional left ventricle or systemic ventricle is the morphologic right ventricle that can be identified by the presence of the tricuspid valve.

Both the superior vena cava and the inferior vena cava enter the right atrium and cannot identify the functional left ventricle. The eustachian valve originates from the orifice of the inferior vena cava and is seen in the right atrium. Therefore, it is the morphologic right atrium (not the morphologic right ventricle) that can be identified by the presence of the eustachian valve. Besides the eustachian valve, the limbus of the fossa ovalis is another anatomic landmark for the morphologic right atrium. The flap valve of the fossa ovalis is the anatomic landmark for the morphologic left atrium. **References** 10 *(p 415)*; 39 *(pp 297–300, 556–558)*; 40 *(pp 78–81)*.

17. Answer E

The accompanying transesophageal echocardiographic bicaval view (LA, left atrium; RA, right atrium) shows an atrial septal aneurysm protruding into the right atrium (arrows) and associated secundum atrial septal defect (block arrow) (A). Left-to-right shunting (B, arrow) is also seen with color flow Doppler. An atrial septal aneurysm can involve the region of the fossa ovalis or the entire atrial septum. Echocardiographically, an atrial septal aneurysm is defined as the atrial septum or part of it exhibiting aneurysmal dilation and protruding at least 1.5 cm beyond the plane of the atrial septum. The

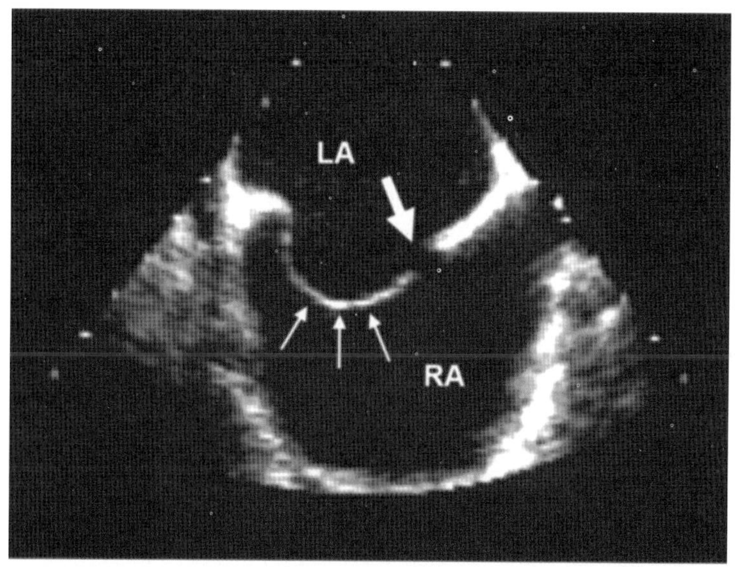

A

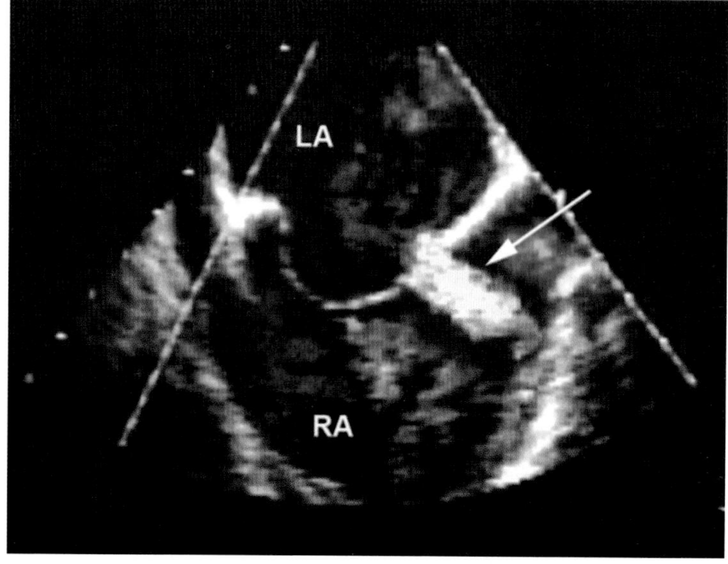

B

atrial septum may exhibit phasic excursion during the cardiorespiratory cycle exceeding 1.5 cm, and the base of the aneurysm protrusion may be at least 1.5 cm in diameter.

Atrial septal aneurysms are divided into two distinct groups: those in which the aneurysm involves only the region of the fossa ovalis and those in which the entire atrial septum is involved. Fossa ovalis aneurysms are further subdivided according to the direction of their maximal excursion during the cardiorespiratory cycle: type 1 into the right atrium and type 2 into the left atrium. Although atrial septal aneurysm formation can be secondary to interatrial pressure differences, an atrial septal aneurysm most likely represents congenital malformations of the atrial septum because atrial septal aneurysms are rare in patients with chronically elevated atrial pressures (e.g., mitral stenosis), and hence, an acquired origin of atrial septal aneurysm is unlikely. Atrial septal defects or patent foramen ovale have been found in 32% of patients with a fossa ovalis aneurysm. In addition, an atrial septal aneurysm was much more common in patients with a stroke than in patients without stroke. The mechanisms for cardioembolic stroke in patients with an atrial septal aneurysm include right-to-left atrial shunting and thrombogenic properties of the aneurysm itself. **References** 10 *(pp 594–598)*; 11 *(pp 485–488)*; 26 *(p 369)*; 39 *(pp 244–246)*; 42 *(pp 931–933)*.

18. Answer E

The two-dimensional transesophageal echocardiographic image accompanying Question 18 reveals the outlet ventricular septal defect and overriding aorta. (In the image shown here, AO indicates aorta; LA, left atrium; LV, left ventricle; MV, mitral valve; RA, right atrium; RV, right ventricle; TOF, tetralogy of Fallot; VS, ventricular septum; small block arrow, ventricular septal defect.) Only patients with tetralogy of Fallot have outlet ventricular septal defect and overriding aorta. Tetralogy of Fallot is classically defined

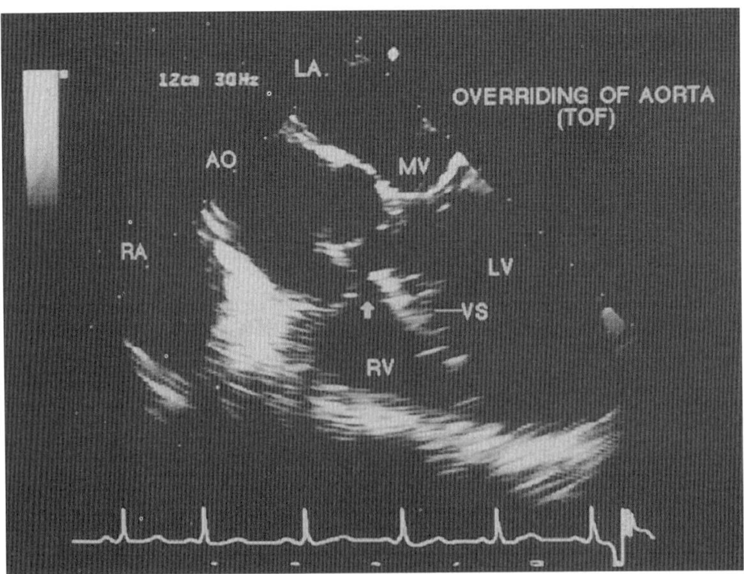

Figure from Nanda and Domanski (20). Used with permission.

as 1) ventricular septal defect, 2) pulmonary stenosis, 3) overriding aorta, and 4) right ventricular hypertrophy. The ventricular septal defect in tetralogy of Fallot results from anterior and cephalad displacement of the infundibular septum and is always large and nonrestrictive. Several types of ventricular septal defects have been reported to occur in tetralogy of Fallot. The most usual type of defect is a perimembranous outlet defect, which accounts for 74% of all ventricular septal defects occurring in tetralogy of Fallot. The pulmonary stenosis in tetralogy of Fallot is highly variable but usually increases in severity with age. In tetralogy of Fallot, right ventricular outflow tract narrowing is nearly always a consequence of anterior and cephalad deviation of the outlet septum. Hypertrophy of the septoparietal trabeculations exacerbates the subpulmonary stenosis in most cases. The pulmonary valve is bicuspid in about 50% of patients with tetralogy of Fallot with a high incidence of stenosis. In patients with a tricuspid pulmonary valve, one-third have thickening or doming of the leaflets, leading to pulmonary stenosis. In the most extreme form of pulmonary stenosis, the pulmonary valve is atretic (3%) with a blind-ending infundibulum. The degree of overriding of the aortic valve varies between 10% and 95%. The aortic and mitral valves remain in fibrous continuity. **References** 10 *(pp 406–407)*; 20 *(p 370)*; 39 *(pp 265–277)*; 40 *(pp 134–135)*; 42 *(pp 1025–1031)*.

19. Answer C

20. Answer A

The accompanying transesophageal echocardiographic image taken before bypass (part A) (ASD, atrial septal defect; EV, eustachian valve; LA, left atrium; RA, right atrium) is a mid-esophageal bicaval view that reveals a secundum atrial septal defect (long thin arrow). Sometimes, the prominent eustachian valve (shorter arrow) may complicate the surgical closure of the atrial septal defect. Part B is the image after repair/bypass. In this case, the patch used to close the atrial septal defect is inadvertently sewed (long thin arrow) to the eustachian valve. After bypass, the upper portion of the atrial septum is a mobile structure in the left atrium. The blood flow from the inferior vena cava (block arrow) was found entering the left atrium because the eustachian valve was sewed to the inferior limbus of the atrial septum by the patch, which directed the blood flow from the inferior vena cava into the left atrium through the secundum atrial septal defect. The surgeon should return the patient to bypass for surgical closure of the secundum atrial septal defect with the patch in the correct position, i.e., between the superior and inferior portions of the atrial septum.

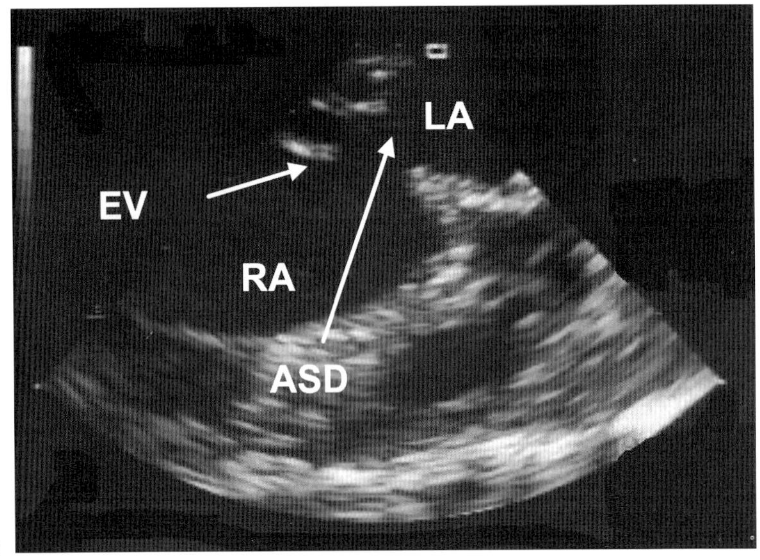

A

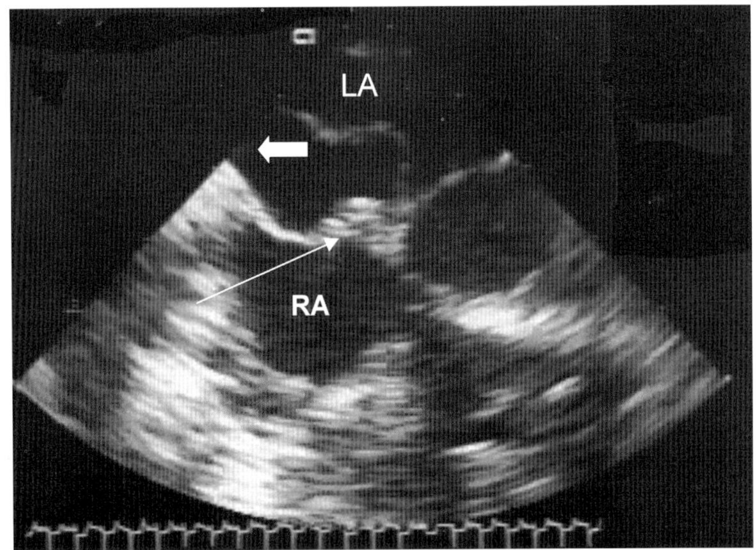

B

Chapter 12

Echocardiography of the Aorta and Pericardium

Questions

Multiple choice (choose the *one* best answer):

1. The accompanying two-dimensional image is obtained during transesophageal echocardiography examination of the aorta. The image demonstrates that the patient has
   A. a normal descending aorta.
   B. an intramural hematoma in the descending aorta.
   C. an aortic dissection.
   D. an aortic aneurysm.
   E. atherosclerotic plaque in the descending aorta.

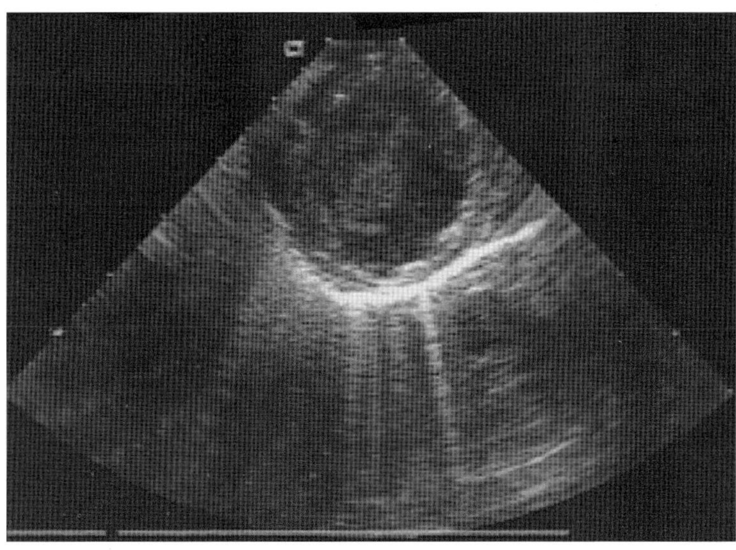

2. Transesophageal echocardiography in another patient reveals the accompanying two-dimensional images in different time frames. The patient with these findings is at serious risk of
   A. mitral regurgitation.
   B. aortic stenosis.
   C. distal embolism.
   D. cardiac tamponade.
   E. none of the above.

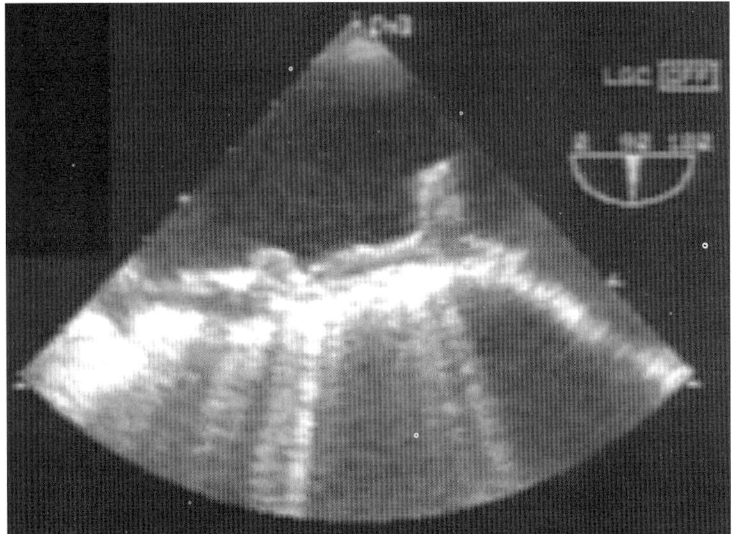

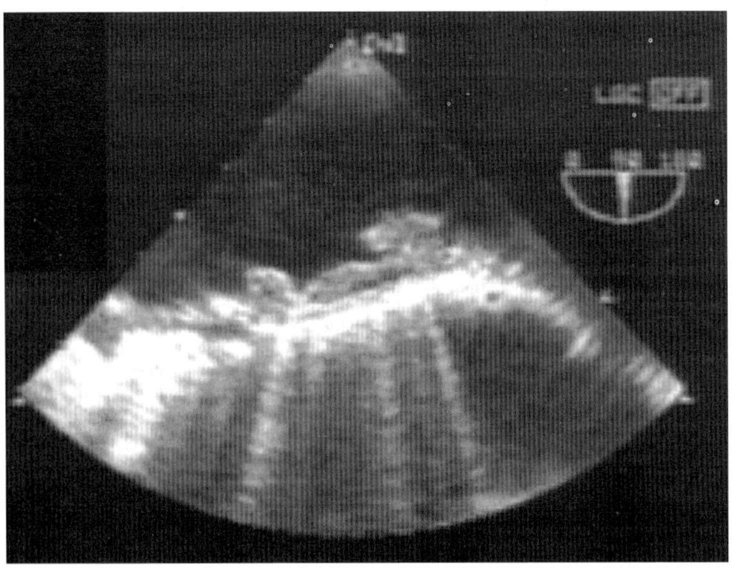

3. The accompanying transesophageal echocardiographic image demonstrates
A. a normal ascending aorta.
B. an ascending aortic dissection.
C. an ascending aortic intramural hematoma.
D. an ascending aortic pseudoaneurysm.
E. an aneurysm of the sinus of Valsalva.

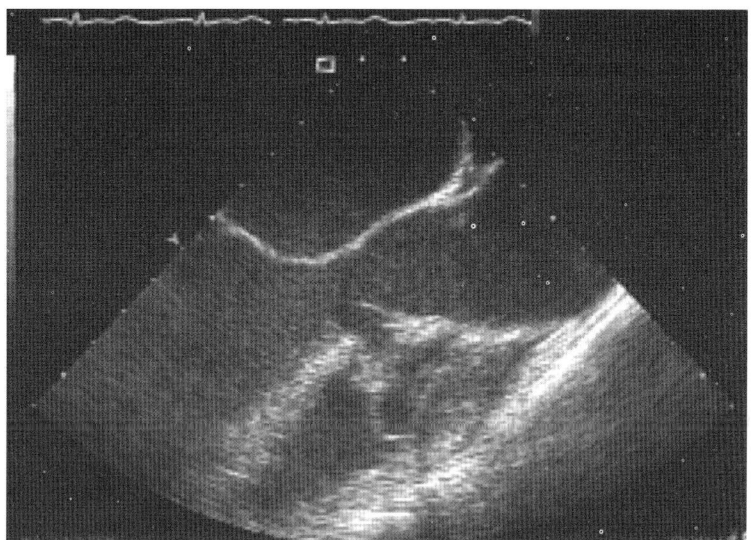

4. A 58-year-old patient with hypertension and morbid obesity develops acute chest pain. In the emergency department, the patient's systolic blood pressure is 81 mm Hg and the heart rate is 81 beats per minute. A chest radiograph shows a widened mediastinum. The most appropriate next step is
A. transthoracic echocardiography.
B. transesophageal echocardiography.
C. angiography.
D. computed tomographic scan with contrast.
E. magnetic resonance imaging.

5. If transesophageal echocardiography reveals the accompanying two-dimensional image in the patient described in Question 4, the diagnosis is
A. a normal aorta with linear reverberation artifact.
B. an ascending aortic aneurysm.
C. Stanford type A aortic dissection.
D. Stanford type B aortic dissection.
E. DeBakey type III aortic dissection.

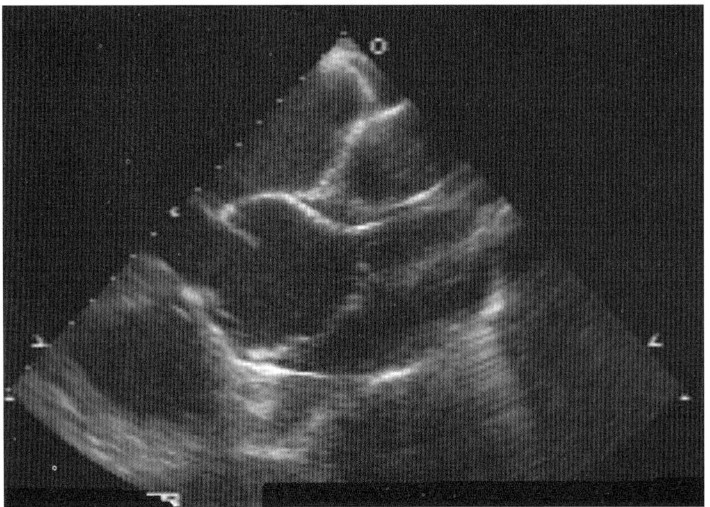

6. On the basis of the two-dimensional image accompanying Question 5, the patient should
A. receive medical therapy with follow-up angiography in 1 week.
B. have follow-up computed tomographic scan with contrast in 2 weeks.
C. be admitted to the intensive care unit for further observation.
D. be discharged after medical management.
E. be taken to the operating room immediately.

7. In hemodynamically stable patients with suspected aortic dissection, which one of the following is the most sensitive and specific method to diagnose aortic dissection?
A. Transthoracic echocardiography.
B. Transesophageal echocardiography.
C. Angiography.
D. Magnetic resonance imaging.
E. Contrast-enhanced x-ray computed tomography.

8. A 54-year-old patient complains of acute back pain. During transesophageal echocardiography, the accompanying two-dimensional and color flow images are obtained. Based on the transesophageal echocardiographic findings, the diagnosis is

A. a normal descending aorta with linear reverberation artifact.
B. Stanford type A dissection.
C. Stanford type B dissection.
D. a descending aortic aneurysm.
E. an intramural hematoma.

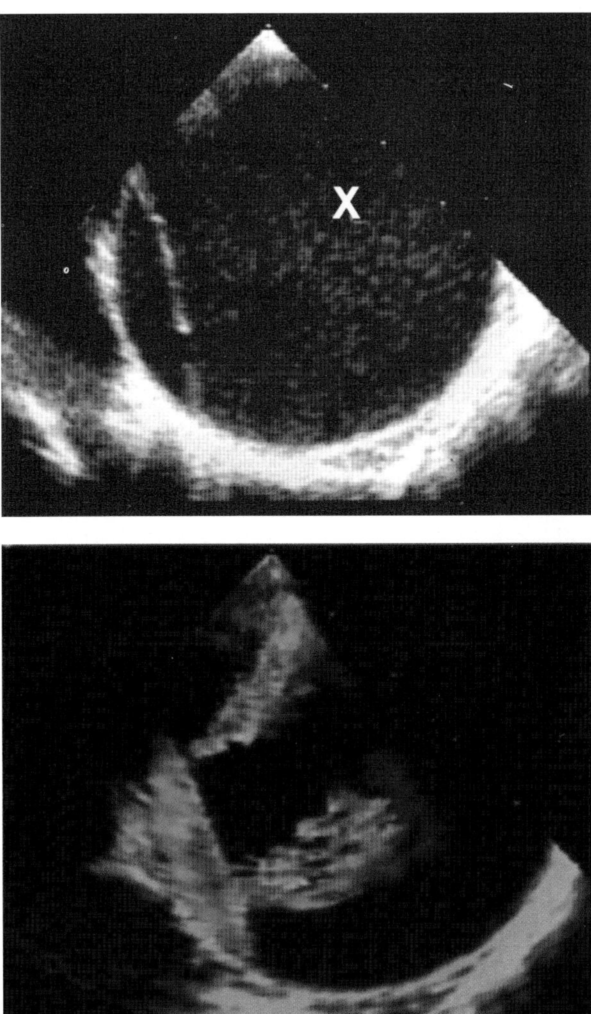

Figure from Freeman et al. (11). Used with permission of Mayo Foundation for Medical Education and Research.

9. The structure labeled by letter X in the image accompanying Question 8 is best described as

A. normal aorta.
B. false lumen.
C. true lumen.
D. aortic intramural hematoma.
E. not determined.

10. Which one of the following statements about echocardiographic findings of aortic dissection is true?

A. The intimal flap moves toward the true lumen during systole.
B. A high-velocity forward systolic flow pattern is seen in the false lumen but not in the true lumen.
C. The hallmark of the echocardiographic diagnosis of aortic dissection is identification of swirling spontaneous echo contrast in the true lumen.
D. Two-dimensional imaging often demonstrates partial thrombosis in the false lumen, but areas of complete thrombosis have never been observed.
E. None of the above.

11. A 72-year-old patient with no previous history of valvular disease is undergoing surgical repair of an acute ascending aortic dissection. Intraoperatively, the cardiologist should especially look for

A. mitral valvular abnormality.
B. tricuspid valvular abnormality.
C. aortic valvular abnormality.
D. coronary artery abnormality.
E. C and D.

12. The accompanying two-dimensional and color flow images show the descending aorta in the long axis view. Which one of the following best describes the diagnosis?

A. A normal descending aorta with reverberation artifact.

B. A mirror image of a normal descending aorta.

C. Congenital double aorta.

D. Dissection of the descending aorta.

E. An intramural hematoma of the descending aorta.

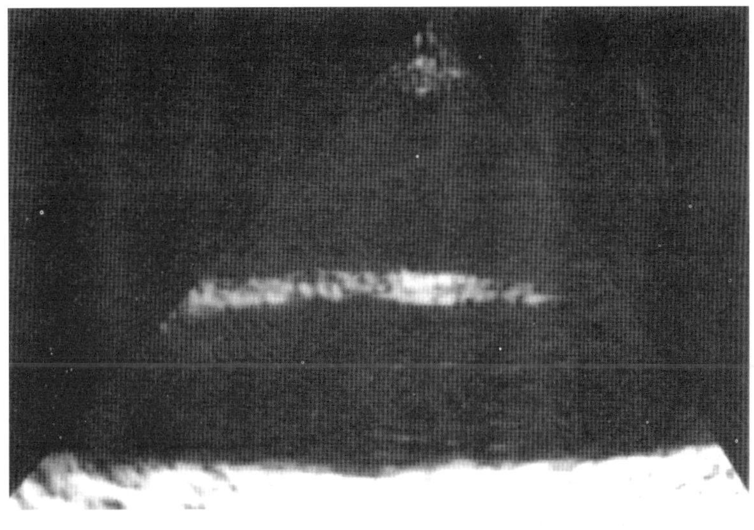

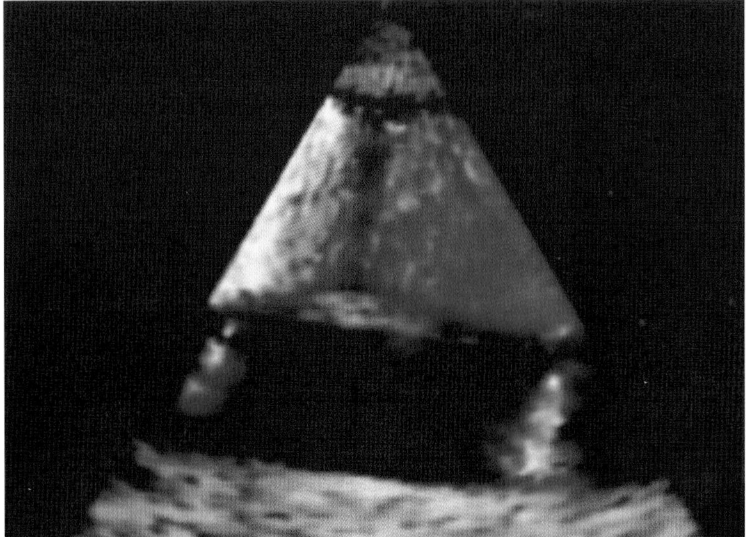

Figure from Freeman et al. (11). Used with permission of Mayo Foundation for Medical Education and Research.

13. A 52-year-old patient with history of hypertension suddenly develops sharp neck pain, radiating to the jaw. Transesophageal echocardiography reveals the accompanying two-dimensional image. No intimal tear is detected during careful transesophageal echocardiography of this patient. The observer's conclusion is

A. a normal aorta with linear reverberation artifact.

B. a penetrating aortic ulcer.

C. an intramural hematoma.

D. an aortic dissection.

E. an aortic aneurysm.

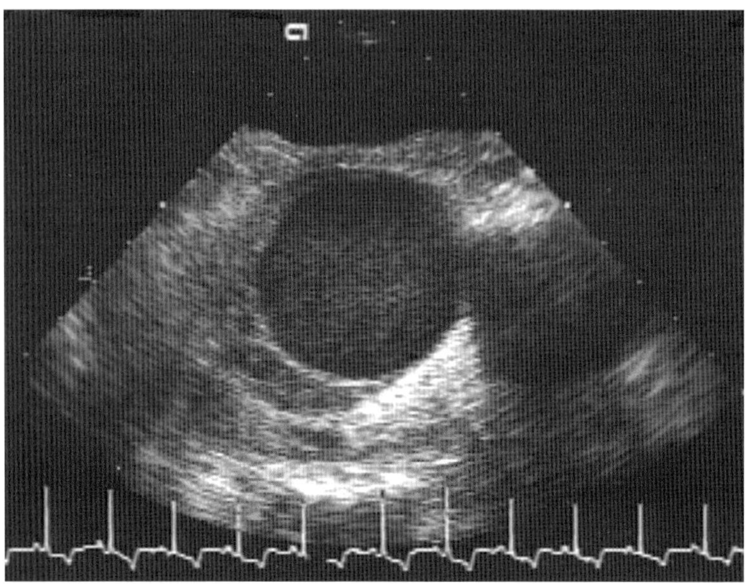

14. Intramural hematoma

A. does not need to be treated surgically.

B. always has an intimal flap with an entry site.

C. is always caused by trauma and, hence, tends to occur in young patients without a history of hypertension.

D. always appears as increased echo density with irregular surface.

E. is none of the above.

15. Which one of the following diagnostic modalities is least valuable in the diagnosis of intramural hematoma?

A. Aortography.

B. Contrast-enhanced computed tomographic scan.

C. Magnetic resonance imaging.

D. Transesophageal echocardiography.

E. B and C.

16. The accompanying two-dimensional image is obtained in a patient with acute back pain. The letter X in the image labels

A. pericardial effusion.
B. peritoneal fluid.
C. pleural fluid.
D. cardiac tamponade.
E. dilated aorta.

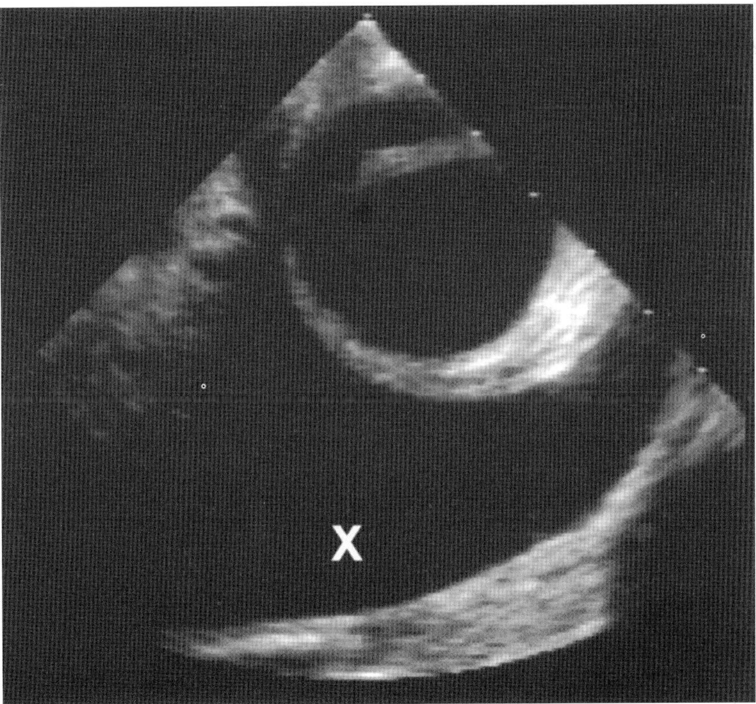

Figure from Freeman et al. (11). Used with permission of Mayo Foundation for Medical Education and Research.

17. A 70-year-old patient with severe coronary artery disease is undergoing coronary artery bypass graft surgery. Intraoperative transesophageal echocardiography is performed during the surgery. Frequently, intraoperative transesophageal echocardiography cannot clearly visualize

A. the aortic cannulation site.
B. the sinotubular junction.
C. the atrial septum.
D. the middle scallop of the posterior mitral leaflet.
E. the descending thoracic aorta.

18. After decannulation, possible aortic dissection or hematoma at the aortic cannulation site is suspected. Which one of the following is the best method to visualize the pathology at the site of aortic cannulation intraoperatively?
A. Transesophageal echocardiography.
B. Transthoracic echocardiography.
C. Epiaortic ultrasonography.
D. Computed tomographic scan with contrast.
E. Magnetic resonance imaging.

19. The hemodynamic characteristics of constrictive pericarditis include
A. dissociation between intrathoracic and intracardiac pressures.
B. exaggerated association between intrathoracic and intracardiac pressures.
C. exaggerated ventricular interdependence in diastolic filling.
D. normal ventricular interdependence in diastolic filling.
E. A and C.

20. Which one of the following Doppler findings is true for patients with constrictive pericarditis?
A. Increased early mitral inflow diastolic velocity during inspiration.
B. Decreased early mitral inflow diastolic velocity during inspiration.
C. Decreased early mitral inflow diastolic velocity during expiration.
D. Decreased early tricuspid inflow diastolic velocity during inspiration.
E. Increased early tricuspid inflow diastolic velocity during expiration.

21. All of the following echocardiographic features are consistent with constrictive pericarditis ***except***
A. abnormal ventricular septal motion.
B. dilated inferior vena cava without respiratory variation.
C. no respiratory variation in ventricular size due to pericardial constriction.
D. flattening of the left ventricular posterior wall during diastole.
E. thickened pericardium.

22. Which one of the following statements about pericardial effusion is true?
A. Pericardial fluid is detected by transesophageal echocardiography as a strong echo reflection.
B. An echo-free space persists throughout the cardiac cycle when pericardial effusion is greater than 25 mL.
C. Pericardial fluid with 5 mm of separation between the parietal and visceral pericardium is considered a large amount of pericardial effusion.
D. Pericardial effusion less than 100 mL cannot be detected by echocardiography.
E. None of the above.

23. The transthoracic echocardiographic image corresponding to the transesophageal echocardiographic mid-esophageal four-chamber view is the apical four-chamber view. The accompanying two-dimensional image is obtained in a patient with hypotension, tachycardia, jugular venous distention, and pulsus paradoxus. The diagnosis is

A. constrictive pericarditis due to thickened pericardium.
B. pericardial tamponade.
C. a small right atrium due to systemic hypovolemia.
D. a large eustachian valve that obstructs venous return.
E. a cardiac cyst.

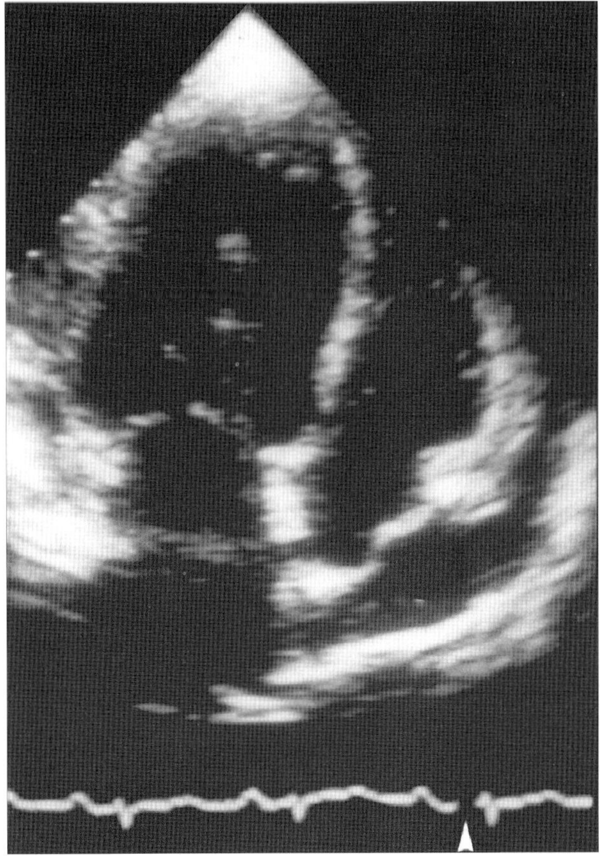

Figure from Oh et al. (23). Used with permission of Mayo Foundation for Medical Education and Research.

24. With progression of the abnormality shown in Question 23, transesophageal echocardiography in this patient most likely will show

A. systolic collapse of the left ventricle.
B. systolic collapse of the right ventricle.
C. diastolic collapse of the right ventricle.
D. diastolic collapse of the left ventricle.
E. diastolic collapse of both the right ventricle and the left ventricle.

25. Other echocardiographic findings in patients with the abnormality described in Questions 23 and 24 include

A. normal ventricular septal motion.
B. a normal inferior vena cava.
C. absence of respiratory variation in ventricular chamber size.
D. all of the above.
E. none of the above.

Answers & Discussion

1. Answer E

2. Answer C

The two-dimensional transesophageal echocardiographic image accompanying Question 1 demonstrates the complex atherosclerotic plaque within the descending thoracic aorta. The images shown in Question 2 and here show systolic and diastolic frames that illustrate the mobility and direction of plaque motion (arrows). Most often, this form of mobile attachment is a primary thrombus complicating an atherosclerotic plaque. Patients with such mobile complex atherosclerotic plaques are at increased risk of a distal embolism. **Reference** 11 *(p 454)*.

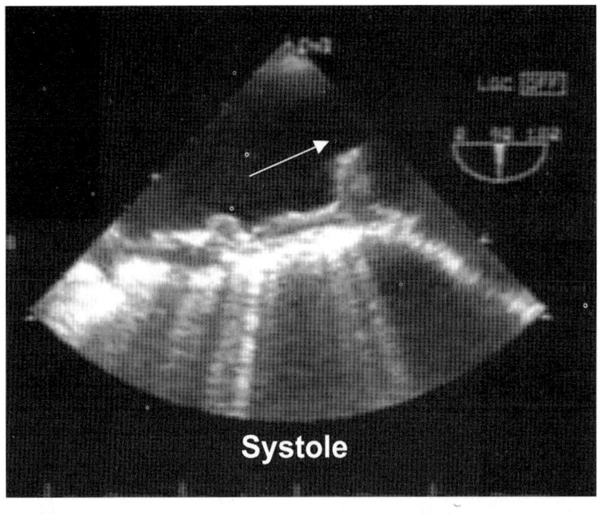

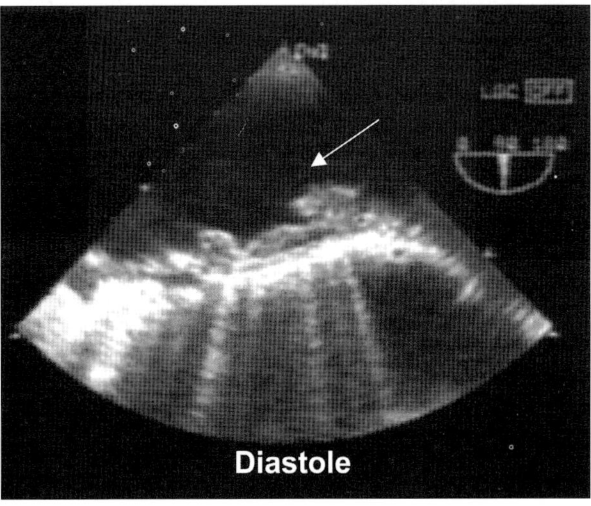

3. Answer E

An aneurysm of the sinus of Valsalva can be seen in the accompanying two-dimensional transesophageal echocardiographic image (AV, atrioventricular valve; LA, left atrium). A sinus of Valsalva aneurysm can be congenital in origin, due to an infectious (such as endocarditis) or inflammatory process. Although it may involve any coronary cusps, it occurs most commonly with the right coronary cusp. Echocardiographically, a dilated and distorted sinus of Valsalva can be seen in the long and short axis views at the aortic valve level. Bulging of the sinus usually does not create symptoms, but it can compress the adjacent structures. Usually, the aneurysm expands in the direction of least resistance, and the most common site of expansion is the right heart chambers. The aneurysm may simply expand into a chamber, or it can rupture and develop communications with that chamber. **References** 10 *(pp 646–647)*; 16 *(pp 140–141)*; 23 *(pp 201–203)*; 26 *(p 386)*; 39 *(pp 448–449)*.

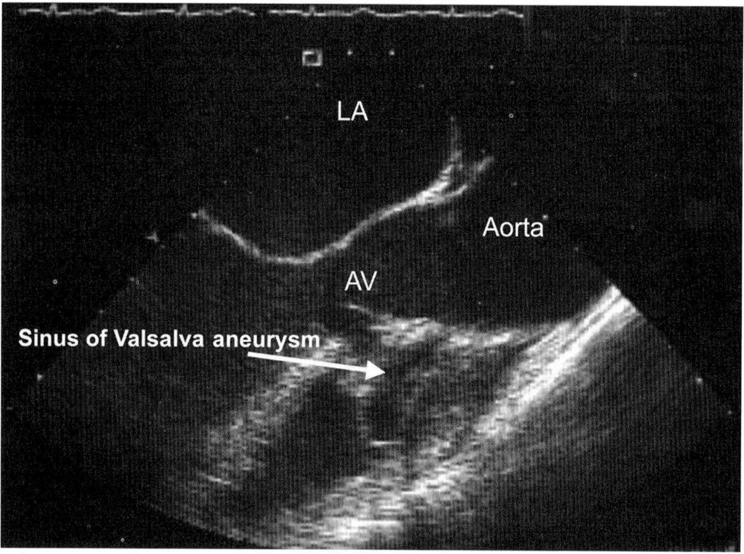

4. Answer B

The patient described in Question 4 with suspected acute aortic dissection is hemodynamically unstable. The optimal diagnostic test for this patient must be accurate, safe, and immediately applicable. Transesophageal echocardiography is portable, can be performed quickly in the emergency department, and provides instant diagnosis of aortic dissection as well as high-quality images of other cardiac and vascular structures at risk. In addition, transesophageal echocardiography avoids the contrast and x-ray exposure associated with computed tomography and angiography and eliminates the time delay and practical encumbrance of magnetic resonance imaging. Transesophageal echocardiography is more sensitive and specific than transthoracic echocardiography in the diagnosis of aortic dissection, especially in patients with morbid obesity. Therefore, immediate diagnosis with transesophageal echocardiography is the most appropriate next step for this hemodynamically unstable patient. **References** 11 *(pp 430–448)*; 23 *(pp 195–199)*; 25 *(pp 547–554)*; 27 *(pp 119–123)*.

5. Answer C

Aortic dissection is classified according to the location of the dissection or intimal tear, as well as the extent of involvement. The two most widely used classifications of aortic dissection are the DeBakey and Stanford classifications.

According to the DeBakey classification, aortic dissections are divided into DeBakey type I, type II, and type III. DeBakey type I aortic dissection has its intimal tear originating in the ascending aorta, and the dissection extends from the ascending aorta into the descending aorta. DeBakey type II aortic dissection is confined to the ascending aorta. DeBakey type III aortic dissection involves the descending aorta, and is further classified into type IIIa and type IIIb; DeBakey type IIIa is confined to the descending thoracic aorta, and DeBakey type IIIb extends into the abdominal aorta and iliac arteries.

The Stanford classification developed from a functional approach based on whether the ascending aorta is involved, regardless of the site of primary intimal tear and irrespective of the extent of distal propagation. On the basis of this classification, aortic dissections are divided into type A and type B. Stanford type A dissection is the aortic dissection with involvement of the ascending aorta (including DeBakey types I and II), and type B dissection is limited to the descending aorta (DeBakey type III). The Stanford classification reflects the clinical observation that the prognosis and management of aortic dissections depend on whether the ascending aorta is involved. The mortality of acute ascending aortic dissections (Stanford type A, DeBakey type I and II) escalates hourly at the rate of 1% per hour for the first 48 hours. Hence, rapid diagnosis and immediate surgical repair are critical for survival in this group of patients. In contrast, descending aortic dissections (Stanford type B or DeBakey type III) are usually managed medically unless there is persistent pain or clinically significant compromise to vital organs. **References** 11 *(pp 430–448)*; 23 *(pp 195–199)*; 25 *(pp 547–554)*; 27 *(pp 119–123)*.

6. Answer E

The two-dimensional image accompanying Question 5 confirms the ascending aortic dissection, which is a surgical emergency. The patient should be taken to the operating room for emergency surgical repair of the ascending aortic dissection. **References** 11 *(pp 430–448)*; 23 *(pp 195–199)*; 25 *(pp 547–554)*; 27 *(pp 119–123)*.

7. Answer D

Among the choices listed in this question, magnetic resonance imaging is the most sensitive and specific diagnostic method for dissection of the thoracic aorta. In a comparison of computed tomographic, transesophageal echocardiographic, and magnetic resonance imaging techniques for aortic dissection, both transesophageal echocardiography and magnetic resonance imaging had excellent sensitivity, but magnetic resonance imaging was the most reliable method of avoiding false-positive findings. Also, magnetic resonance imaging provided the most comprehensive information on associated findings and side branch involvement.

Diagnosis of Thoracic Aortic Dissection: Transesophageal Echocardiography Compared With Computed Tomography and Magnetic Resonance Imaging (N = 110)

OUTCOMES	TEE	CT	MRI
Sensitivity, %	98	94	98
Specificity, %	77	87	98
Accuracy, %	90	91	98
Positive predictive value, %	88	92	98
Negative predictive value, %	95	90	98

CT, computed tomography; MRI, magnetic resonance imaging; TEE, transesophageal echocardiography. Data from Nienaber CA, von Kodolitsch Y, Nicolas V, et al. The diagnosis of thoracic aortic dissection by noninvasive imaging procedures. N Engl J Med 1993;328:1–9.

Transesophageal echocardiography is superior to transthoracic echocardiography for detecting aortic dissection because the esophagus lies close to the thoracic aorta. Even with optimal windows, transthoracic echocardiography is usually limited to the gross detection of dissection. More subtle details of thoracic aortic disease are rarely visualized by the transthoracic approach because resolution is lost with far-field imaging. Transesophageal echocardiography overcomes the multiple problems of acoustic impedance from the thoracic cage, lungs, and other mediastinal structures, vastly improving the image resolution. However, the specificity of transesophageal echocardiography was suboptimal compared with that of magnetic resonance imaging. False-positive findings in the ascending aorta have been reported anecdotally with transesophageal echocardiography, and the explanation has been extensive plaque formation or echo reverberations in an ectatic aorta.

The cumulative results of a European cooperative study group for echocardiography showed the sensitivity and specificity of aortic angiography for dissection were 88% and 94%, respectively. The limited sensitivity and specificity of aortic angiography are caused by false lumen thrombosis, intramural hematoma, and equal flow in true and false lumens. The last cause is also an important limitation for computed tomographic studies, where differential flow may not be detectable even with dynamic computed tomographic imaging. The lower sensitivity of computed tomography reflects its poor definition of the intimal flap and entry tear. Therefore, magnetic resonance imaging has the best sensitivity and specificity among the diagnostic modalities used in detecting dissection of the thoracic aorta.

Although transesophageal echocardiography is less specific than magnetic resonance imaging, it has advantages in hemodynamically unstable patients with suspected aortic dissection. Because transesophageal echocardiography is portable, it can be performed at the bedside of a critically ill patient, without the need to move the patient. Also, transesophageal echocardiography can be performed quickly and provide a diagnosis rapidly, in less time than magnetic resonance imaging. The issues of acutely ill patients with needs for hemodynamic monitoring and infusion of medications or those at risk for hemodynamic collapse continue to make transesophageal echocardiography preferable in many acute settings. A diagnostic strategy using magnetic resonance imaging in hemodynamically stable patients and transesophageal echocardiography in hemodynamically unstable patients may be the optimal approach to detecting dissection of the thoracic aorta. **References** 11 *(pp 425, 441, 443, 447)*; 25 *(pp 569–560)*; 27 *(pp 121–122)*.

8. Answer C

9. Answer B

The accompanying two-dimensional and color flow images demonstrate dissection of the descending aorta in a transverse plane. The intimal flap (arrow, top image) can be observed clearly on the two-dimensional image, separating the small true lumen (left side) from the much larger false lumen (right side), which contains spontaneous echocardiographic contrast. Color flow imaging (bottom image) demonstrates laminar flow in the true lumen (block arrow) and two intimal tears with turbulent jets (small arrows) entering the false lumen. **Reference** 11 *(p 444)*.

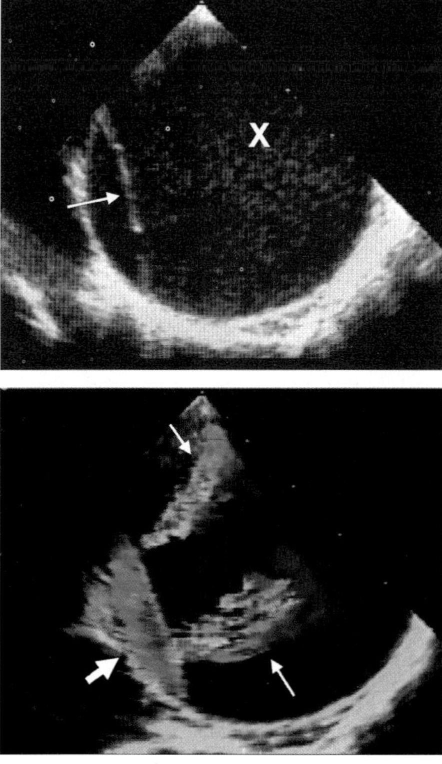

Figure from Freeman et al. (11). Used with permission of Mayo Foundation for Medical Education and Research.

10. Answer E

The hallmark of echocardiographic diagnosis of aortic dissection is identification of an intimal flap, seen as a mobile, linear echo within the vascular lumen, with flow in the true and false lumens on either side of the flap. Another helpful echocardiographic finding of aortic dissection is the pulsatile nature of the true lumen; that is, the perfused true lumen expands in systole and collapses in diastole, resulting in the motion of the intimal flap toward the false lumen during systole. Depending on the size of the intimal tear, turbulent high-velocity flow jets passing through the entry site into the false lumen can be detected by color flow Doppler at the point of communication. When aortic dissection is present, the normal laminar flow within the aorta may be disrupted. The true lumen is compressed by the false lumen, resulting in decreased diameter with high-velocity flow patterns detected during systole. The false lumen contains low-velocity flow, which causes spontaneous echo contrast and various amounts of thrombus. Two-dimensional echocardiography often demonstrates partial thrombosis in the false lumen, and areas of complete thrombosis are also seen. Besides two-dimensional and color flow imaging, M-mode echocardiography may be helpful in showing the oscillations of the intimal flap. **References** 10 *(pp 631–643)*; 11 *(pp 430–443)*; 25 *(pp 552–553)*; 26 *(pp 380–384)*.

11. Answer E

In patients with ascending aortic dissection, the cardiologist should always look for associated aortic regurgitation and coronary artery dissection during transesophageal echocardiography. When the ascending aortic dissection proceeds retrograde from the entry site, the false lumen can cause loss of support of the aortic leaflets with diastolic prolapse or even flail of one or more aortic cusps, leading to severe aortic regurgitation. Also, severe aortic regurgitation in patients with ascending aortic dissection may result from annular dilation with incomplete central cusp coaptation. In addition, diastolic prolapse of the intimal flap into the left ventricular outflow tract has been found to cause severe aortic regurgitation. Transesophageal echocardiography can provide detailed morphologic information about the quality of the leaflet tissue and the mechanism of aortic insufficiency, which helps make the surgical decision about whether aortic valve repair or replacement is needed. Therefore, information about the aortic valve is vital for the surgical management of an ascending aortic dissection.

Another important issue during intraoperative transesophageal echocardiography is the involvement of coronary arteries by aortic dissection. Coronary artery dissection or obstruction due to the intimal flap has been detected in patients with ascending aortic dissection, leading to myocardial ischemia or infarction. Coronary artery ostial occlusion can occur as a result of the dissection flap separating the coronary artery from normal blood flow or by compression of the vessel. Two-dimensional transesophageal echocardiographic imaging is a sensitive method of detecting coronary artery abnormalities associated with ascending aortic dissection. Extension of the dissecting intimal flap into the ostium and lumen of the involved coronary artery has been detected by transesophageal echocardiography with right and left coronary artery dissection of nearly equal frequency. **References** 11 *(p 439)*; 25 *(pp 554–555)*; 26 *(pp 381–382)*.

12. Answer D

The two-dimensional and color flow images demonstrate dissection of the descending aorta. The double-channel aorta is seen in the long axis with the intimal flap separating the true and false lumens. The color Doppler imaging demonstrates the true lumen with laminar flow on the top and the false lumen at the bottom. The laminar flow within the true lumen is orange-red when directed toward the transducer and blue when directed away from the transducer. The color flow imaging also reveals two high-velocity turbulent jets, passing from the true lumen to the false lumen through the entry sites. This is not an intramural hematoma because, by definition, intramural hematoma does not have an intimal tear or an entry site. (See also Questions 11 and 12.) **Reference** 11 *(p 446)*.

13. Answer C

14. Answer E

15. Answer A

Intramural hematoma is also called a noncommunicating variant of aortic dissection. It occurs in the media of the aortic wall without an intimal tear and may progress to a typical aortic dissection or rupture. The pathologic process of intramural hematoma is hemorrhage of the vasa vasorum into the aortic wall, either spontaneously or traumatically (as in closed chest trauma). Usually, intramural hematoma occurs in elderly patients with hypertension.

In all studies, the sensitivity for transesophageal echocardiography, contrast-enhanced computed tomographic scanning, and magnetic resonance imaging exceeded 96%. Contrast aortography is the least sensitive imaging technique for the detection of intramural hematoma because its noncommunicating characteristics make it difficult for differential opacification of the false lumens.

Transesophageal echocardiography in patients with intramural hematoma demonstrates a thickened aortic wall with an intramural space due to fresh blood or with increased echo density along the wall of the aorta, corresponding to thrombus formation between the intima and the adventitia. Because the intima is intact in patients with intramural hematoma, no intimal tear is detectable during transesophageal echocardiography. Typically, intramural hematoma has a crescent appearance in the short axis view, although it may be circumferential. Complications of intramural hematoma readily detected by transesophageal echocardiography include aortic regurgitation, pericardial effusion, pleural effusion, and mediastinal hematoma.

Like aortic dissection, intramural hematomas are classified into type A (involves ascending aorta) and type B (limited to descending aorta). Intramural hematoma should be treated like an aortic dissection because it is a precursor for aortic dissection, leading to typical dissection in up to 30% of cases. Therefore, involvement of the ascending aorta (type A) should prompt urgent surgical repair, while stable patients with intramural hematoma of the descending aorta (type B) can be treated medically. **References** 21; 23 *(p 198)*; 25 *(pp 554–555)*.

16. Answer C

The two-dimensional image accompanying Question 16 shows acute aortic dissection (arrow indicates the dissection flap), complicated by a pleural effusion (Ao indicates the aorta). The letter X labels a left pleural effusion within the posteromedial costophrenic angle, which highlights the dissected descending thoracic aorta. A portion of the left lung (labeled with the letter L) is also noted within the effusion. **Reference** 11 *(p 440)*.

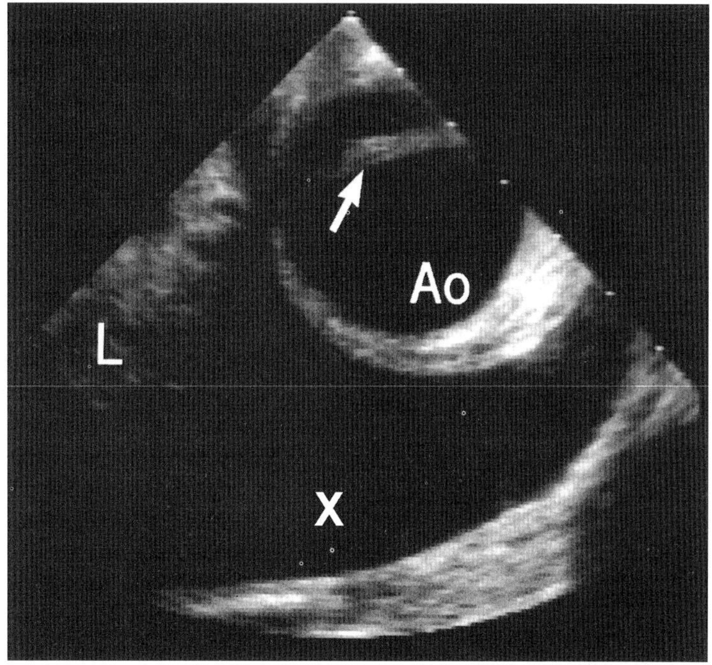

Figure from Freeman et al. (11). Used with permission of Mayo Foundation for Medical Education and Research.

17. Answer A

18. Answer C

Aortic cannulation for cardiopulmonary bypass is usually performed in the distal ascending aorta. Frequently, the aortic cannulation site cannot be visualized well by intraoperative transesophageal echocardiography because the interposition of the trachea between the esophagus and the aorta creates a blind spot that obscures the distal portion of the ascending aorta. In such a situation, direct recording of the aorta with an epiaortic transducer is available for the surgeon. Epiaortic ultrasonography can be performed intraoperatively under sterile conditions, and the surgeon controls exactly what is visualized. With epiaortic ultrasonography, the transesophageal blind spot in the distal ascending aorta can be inspected thoroughly, and the aortic cannulation sites can be evaluated from the exterior aortic surface. In addition, extremely high-resolution images can be recorded by these high-frequency transducers. Hence, epiaortic ultrasonography is superior to transesophageal echocardiography for identifying the aortic pathology at the aortic cannulation site. The major disadvantage of epiaortic ultrasonography is interruption of the surgery. Also, a second person is required to operate the ultrasound machine. **References** 10 *(p 115)*; 16 *(p 223)*; 23 *(pp 197, 242)*; 24 *(p 254)*; 25 *(pp 555–556)*.

19. Answer E

20. Answer B

In constrictive pericarditis, the visceral and parietal layers of the pericardium are adherent, thickened, and fibrotic, resulting in impairment of diastolic ventricular filling. The two hemodynamic characteristics of constrictive pericarditis are dissociation between intrathoracic and intracardiac pressures and exaggerated ventricular interdependence in diastolic filling. Dissociation between intrathoracic and intracardiac pressures occurs when a thickened or inflamed pericardium prevents full transmission of the intrathoracic pressure changes during respiration to the pericardial and intracardiac cavities. The exaggerated ventricular interdependence in diastolic filling is the result of the interrelationship of both ventricular pressures and filling of a heart whose free walls cannot expand because of the constrictive pericarditis.

In normal subjects, intrathoracic pressure declines during inspiration and the pressure in other intrathoracic structures (pulmonary veins, pulmonary capillaries) is reduced to a similar degree; this intrathoracic pressure change during inspiration is transmitted to pericardial and intracardiac cavities. In patients with constrictive pericarditis, the inspiratory pressure change is not fully transmitted to the pericardial and intracardiac cavities, resulting in respiratory variations in the left-sided filling pressure gradient (the pressure difference between the pulmonary vein and the left atrium). Therefore, the driving pressure gradient for left-sided filling decreases during inspiration, leading to reduced mitral inflow with decreased early mitral inflow velocity. Because the overall cardiac volume is relatively fixed within the thickened or noncompliant pericardium and the ventricles rely on each other for diastolic filling, decreased left ventricular diastolic filling during inspiration causes the shift of the ventricular septum toward the left ventricle, which in turn produces increased diastolic filling in the right ventricle with increased early tricuspid inflow velocity. During expiration, the opposite occurs. Increased left ventricular filling produces an increase in early mitral inflow velocity as well as the shift of ventricular septum toward the right ventricle, which limits right ventricular filling and results in decreased early tricuspid inflow velocity during expiration. **References** 10 *(pp 577–583)*; 23 *(p 186)*; 26 *(pp 222–226)* 42 *(pp 1128–1130)*.

21. Answer C

Two-dimensional echocardiographic findings of constrictive pericarditis include thickened pericardium, abnormal ventricular septal motion (septal bounce), reciprocal respiratory variation in the right and left ventricular sizes, and a dilated inferior vena cava without respiratory variation. M-mode echocardiography is helpful for determining constrictive pericarditis. One of the M-mode signs of pericardial constriction is the flattening of the left ventricular posterior wall during diastole. **References** 10 *(pp 577–583)*; 23 *(p 186)*; 26 *(pp 222–226)*; 42 *(pp 1128–1130)*.

22. Answer B

When the potential pericardial space is filled with fluids or blood, it is detected by transesophageal echocardiography as an echo-free space. A pericardial effusion greater than 25 mL can be detected as an echo-free space that persists throughout the cardiac cycle; a smaller amount of pericardial effusion may be detected as a posterior echo-free space that is present only during the systolic phase. Because the amount of pericardial effusion determines the size of the echo-free space surrounding the heart, a semiquantitative approach can be used to judge the amount of pericardial effusion. A large pericardial effusion totally surrounds the heart and is at least 1 cm in width, a moderate pericardial effusion surrounds the heart but is less than 1 cm at its greatest width, and a small pericardial effusion is localized posteriorly. More quantitative measurements of pericardial effusions rarely are needed in the clinical setting. **References** 10 *(pp 559–560)*; 23 *(p 181)*; 26 *(p 217)*.

23. Answer B

24. Answer C

25. Answer E

The accompanying transthoracic echocardiographic apical four-chamber view corresponds to the transesophageal echocardiographic mid-esophageal four-chamber view (LA, left atrium; LV, left ventricle; PE, pericardial effusion; RA, right atrium; RV, right

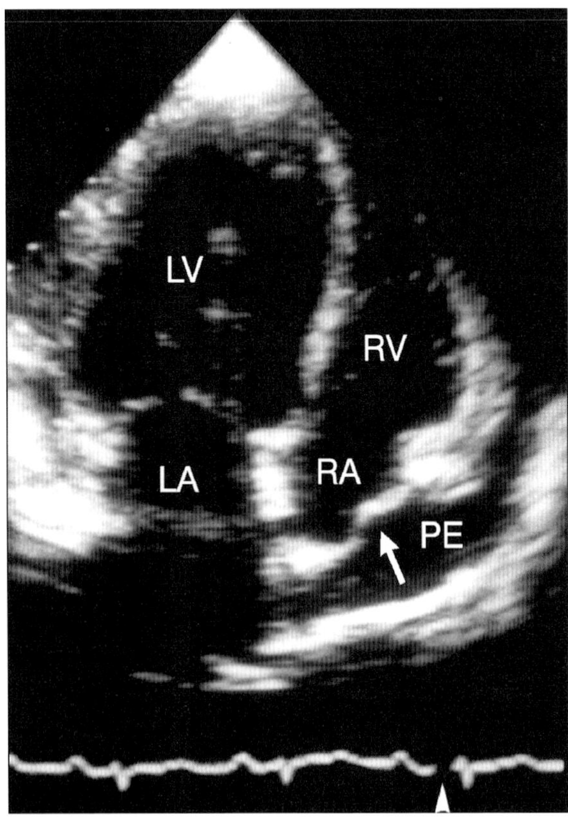

Figure from Oh et al. (23). Used with permission of Mayo Foundation for Medical Education and Research.

ventricle). It demonstrates late diastolic collapse of the right atrial wall (arrow), which is a sensitive sign for cardiac tamponade.

Tamponade physiology occurs when the pressure in the pericardium exceeds the pressure in the cardiac chambers, resulting in impaired cardiac filling. As the pericardial pressure increases, filling of each cardiac chamber is sequentially impaired, with the lower-pressure chambers (atria) affected before the high-pressure chambers (ventricles). Late diastolic right atrial collapse or inversion is a sign of hemodynamically severe pericardial effusion or tamponade, especially when it lasts longer than a third of the RR interval. When intrapericardial pressure exceeds right ventricular diastolic pressure, early diastolic collapse of the right ventricle occurs in patients with previously normal thickness and compliance of the right ventricular free wall. The presence of right ventricular hypertrophy or infiltrative disease of myocardium may allow development of a pressure gradient between the pericardial space and right ventricular chamber without inversion of the normal contour of the free wall. Other two-dimensional and M-mode echocardiographic signs in this life-threatening condition include abnormal ventricular septal motion, respiratory variation in ventricular chamber size, and plethora of the inferior vena cava. Clinically, patients with cardiac tamponade usually present with hypotension, tachycardia, elevated jugular venous pressure, and pulsus paradoxus.
References 10 *(pp 562–565)*; 23 *(pp 181–183)*; 26 *(pp 215–220)*.

Chapter 13

Cardiomyopathies

Questions

Multiple choice (choose the *one* best answer):

1. Which one of the following is true of idiopathic dilated cardiomyopathy?
   A. Spontaneous echo contrast is frequently observed in the left atrium but is never seen in the left ventricle.
   B. Spontaneous echo contrast may be seen in the left ventricle but is never seen in the left atrium.
   C. Mitral regurgitation with an eccentric jet is always present.
   D. The left ventricular dilation is primarily in the long axis rather than in the short axis.
   E. The left ventricular wall thickness typically is within normal limits.

2. Most likely, the accompanying M-mode echocardiogram (ED, end diastolic; ES, end systolic; LV, left ventricular; PW, posterior wall; RV, right ventricular; VS, ventricular septum) at the mid left ventricular level is obtained in a patient with
   A. a normal left ventricle.
   B. restrictive cardiomyopathy.
   C. dilated cardiomyopathy.
   D. arrhythmogenic cardiomyopathy.
   E. hypertrophic cardiomyopathy.

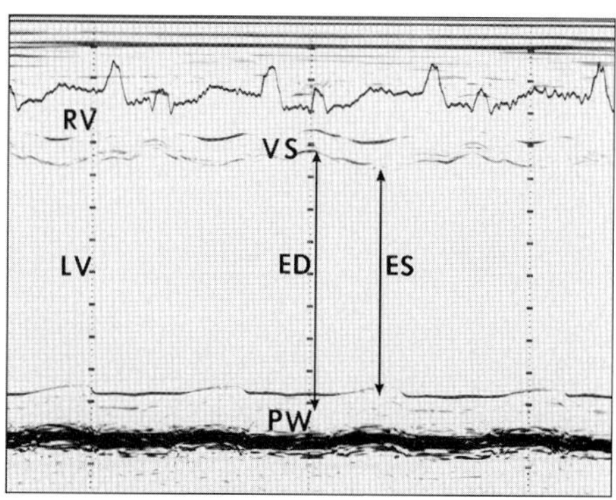

Figure from Oh et al. (23). Used with permission of Mayo Foundation for Medical Education and Research.

3. During transesophageal echocardiography, left ventricular outflow tract flow velocity in patients with hypertrophic cardiomyopathy is best recorded by
   A. a mid-esophageal five-chamber view.
   B. a mid-esophageal four-chamber view.
   C. a mid-esophageal aortic valve long axis view.
   D. a mid-esophageal aortic valve short axis view.
   E. a deep transgastric long axis view.

4. In patients with asymmetric septal hypertrophy, the obstruction occurs at
   A. the posterior mitral leaflet and ventricular septum.
   B. the anterior mitral leaflet and ventricular septum.
   C. the posterior mitral leaflet and left ventricular free wall.
   D. the anterior mitral leaflet and left ventricular free wall.
   E. none of the above.

5. During transesophageal echocardiography in a 32-year-old patient, the accompanying Doppler recording of left ventricular outflow tract velocity is obtained with the transducer placed in the stomach. The Doppler spectrum shown is characteristic of
   A. normal left ventricular outflow tract velocity in a 32-year-old patient.
   B. aortic stenosis.
   C. dynamic left ventricular outflow tract obstruction.
   D. dilated cardiomyopathy.
   E. restrictive cardiomyopathy.

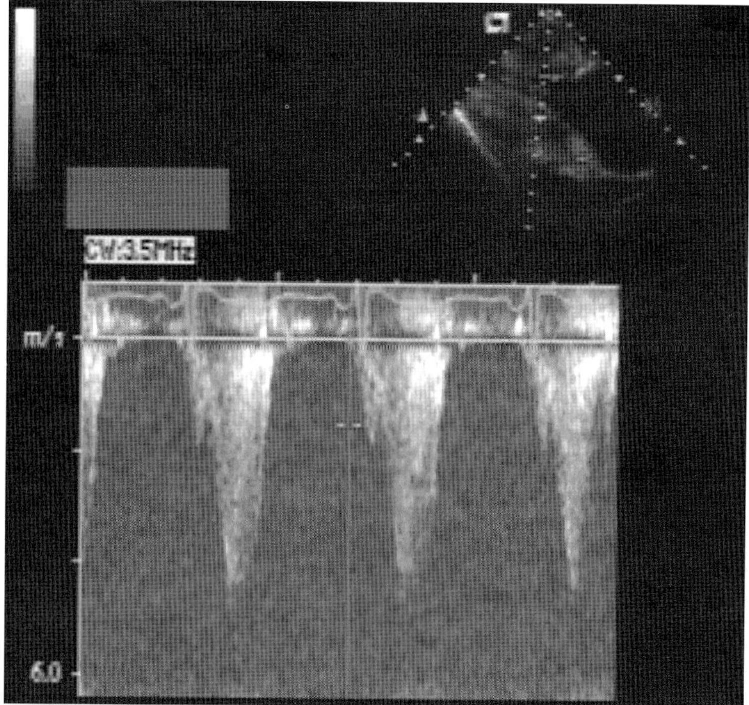

6. If the Doppler spectrum accompanying Question 5 detects the peak velocity of 5 m/s, the pressure gradient across the left ventricular outflow tract in this patient is
   A. 16 mm Hg.
   B. 32 mm Hg.
   C. 36 mm Hg.
   D. 64 mm Hg.
   E. 100 mm Hg

7. Which one of the following statements about hypertrophic obstructive cardiomyopathy is true?
   A. The left ventricular outflow tract is usually obstructed, but the mitral leaflets are always normal.

B. Systolic anterior motion of the anterior mitral leaflet rarely occurs.
C. The point of mitral leaflet coaptation during systole occurs at the tips of the two leaflets in patients with systolic anterior motion.
D. Systolic anterior motion is frequently observed, but mitral regurgitation is rarely seen in patients with hypertrophic obstructive cardiomyopathy.
E. Both the anterior mitral leaflet and the posterior mitral leaflet in patients with hypertrophic obstructive cardiomyopathy are much longer than those in normal subjects.

8. A 48-year-old patient is scheduled for cardiac surgery. The accompanying two-dimensional image is obtained before surgery (LA, left atrium; LV, left ventricle; RA, right atrium; RV, right ventricle). On the basis of this image, the patient most likely has
A. a normal left ventricle.
B. dilated cardiomyopathy.
C. hypertrophic obstructive cardiomyopathy.
D. restrictive cardiomyopathy.
E. arrhythmogenic cardiomyopathy.

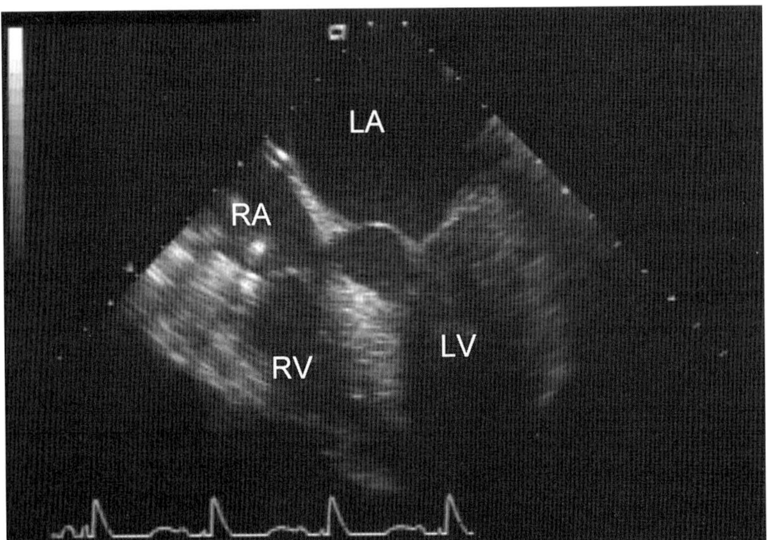

9. After induction, the patient develops severe systemic hypotension. Which one of the following pharmacologic agents should the cardiologist recommend?
A. Ephedrine.
B. Phenylephrine.
C. Dopamine.
D. Dobutamine.
E. Epinephrine.

10. The most likely complication associated with myomectomy surgery for hypertrophic cardiomyopathy is
   A. ventricular septal defect.
   B. atrial septal defect.
   C. mitral regurgitation due to mitral valve prolapse.
   D. tricuspid regurgitation.
   E. a sinus of Valsalva aneurysm.

11. The predominant diastolic filling pattern in patients with hypertrophic cardiomyopathy is
   A. a normal early (E) and late (A) mitral inflow velocity with an E/A ratio of 1.
   B. an increased E/A ratio with prolonged deceleration time and shortened isovolumic relaxation time.
   C. an increased E/A ratio with shortened deceleration time and prolonged isovolumic relaxation time.
   D. a decreased E/A ratio with shortened deceleration time and isovolumic relaxation time.
   E. a decreased E/A ratio with prolonged deceleration time and isovolumic relaxation time.

12. Which one of the following statements about dynamic outflow obstruction is true?
   A. Left ventricular outflow tract obstruction is always present in patients with hypertrophic cardiomyopathy.
   B. Dynamic obstruction of the right ventricular outflow tract is never a component of hypertrophic cardiomyopathy.
   C. Dynamic outflow obstruction only occurs in patients with asymmetric septal hypertrophy.
   D. All of the above.
   E. None of the above.

13. Provocation that brings out systolic anterior motion and dynamic left ventricular outflow tract obstruction includes
   A. amyl nitrite.
   B. isoproterenol.
   C. the Valsalva maneuver.
   D. premature ventricular systole.
   E. all of the above.

14. Which one of the following is observed in patients with dynamic left ventricular outflow tract obstruction?
   A. Partial early systolic closure of the aortic valve.
   B. Partial early diastolic closure of the mitral valve.
   C. Partial mid-diastolic closure of the mitral valve.
   D. Partial mid-systolic closure of the aortic valve.
   E. Partial late diastolic closure of the mitral valve.

15. In comparison with constrictive pericarditis, restrictive cardiomyopathy has
- A. respiratory variation ($\geq$25% change) that is not present in constrictive pericarditis.
- B. systolic dysfunction that is not present in constrictive pericarditis.
- C. normal diastolic function that is not present in constrictive pericarditis.
- D. diastolic heart failure that is not present in constrictive pericarditis.
- E. abnormally slow velocity of anular motion on Doppler imaging, which is not present in constrictive pericarditis.

16. Which one of the following Doppler findings about mitral inflow is commonly seen in a typical case of advanced restrictive cardiomyopathy?
- A. Isovolumic relaxation time is shortened.
- B. Deceleration time is prolonged.
- C. Early mitral inflow velocity is decreased.
- D. Late mitral inflow velocity is normal.
- E. The ratio of early to late mitral inflow velocity is normal or decreased.

Answers & Discussion

1. Answer E

Cardiomyopathies are diseases of the myocardium associated with cardiac dysfunction. Depending on the dominant pathophysiologic mechanism or etiologic or pathogenic factor, cardiomyopathies are classified as dilated cardiomyopathy, hypertrophic cardiomyopathy, restrictive cardiomyopathy, and arrhythmogenic right ventricular cardiomyopathy. Each of these four classes of cardiomyopathy has distinctive morphologic and functional characteristics.

Idiopathic dilated cardiomyopathy is characterized by a dilated, poorly contracting left ventricle with echocardiographic signs of low cardiac output and high intracardiac pressures. Two-dimensional imaging shows a dilated left ventricle with little difference between systole and diastole. The left ventricular dilation is primarily in the short axis rather than in the long axis, and the wall thickness remains within normal limits. With advanced left ventricular dilation, the mitral anulus becomes dilated, leading to incomplete coaptation of the mitral leaflets responsible for the functional mitral regurgitation associated with dilated cardiomyopathy. Generally, the functional mitral regurgitation is moderate and has a central regurgitant jet detected by color flow imaging. Global left ventricular dysfunction is fairly generalized, and all the systolic indices (ejection fraction, fractional shortening, fractional area change, stroke volume, and cardiac output) are uniformly decreased. With a dilated, poorly contracting left ventricle, spontaneous contrast or a swirling pattern of blood flow is frequently observed within the left ventricle, especially in the apical half of the left ventricle. A careful search for an apical mural thrombus is indicated in patients with severe left ventricular systolic dysfunction. In addition, patients with a dilated cardiomyopathy commonly have left atrial enlargement because of increased left ventricular filling pressure and mitral regurgitation. Two-dimensional imaging frequently demonstrates left atrial spontaneous contrast and thrombi in the dilated left atrium. **References** 10 *(pp 526–528)*; 23 *(pp 153–154)*; 26 *(pp 184–186)*; 42 *(pp 804–808)*.

2. Answer C

The image accompanying Question 2 is a typical left ventricular M-mode echocardiogram at the mid-papillary level from a patient with a dilated cardiomyopathy. The left ventricle is dilated with increased end-diastolic and end-systolic dimensions, but the left ventricular wall thickness is within normal limits. Both the septal and posterior ventricular walls move poorly.

Other M-mode findings of dilated cardiomyopathy include increased mitral E point septal separation (EPSS) due to ventricular dilation, "B bump" because of a delayed rate of mitral valve (MV) closure at a higher left ventricular (LV) pressure, and decreased anteroposterior aortic root motion reflecting reduced left atrial filling and emptying (RV, right ventricle). **References** 10 *(pp 199–200, 526–528)*; 23 *(p 154)*; 26 *(pp 184–186)*.

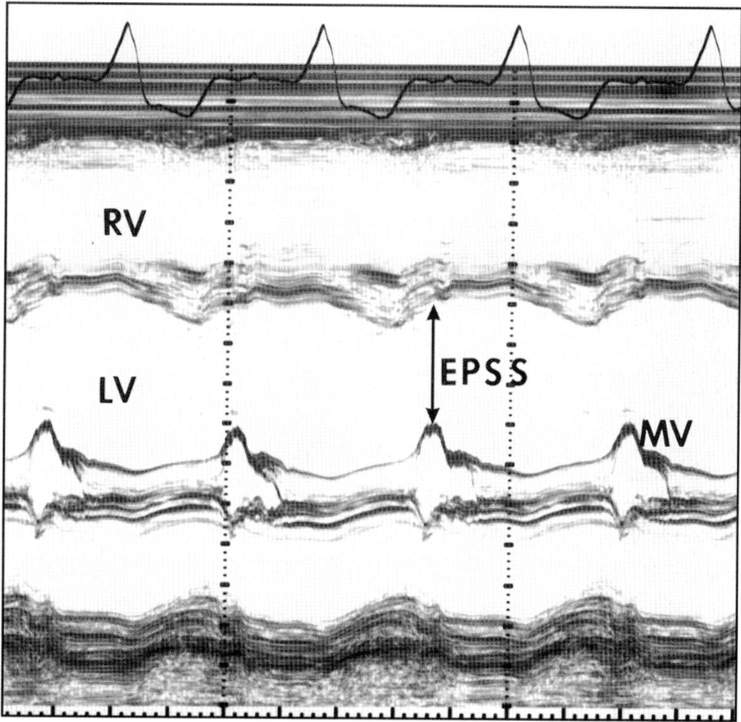

3. Answer E

Among the choices listed in this question, Doppler quantification of blood flow velocity through the left ventricular outflow tract is best performed using the deep transgastric long axis view, shown in the accompanying image (LA, left atrium; LV, left ventricle; LVOT, left ventricular outflow tract). In the transgastric images, the Doppler beam can be directed parallel to flow through the left ventricular outflow tract, providing an accurate measurement of left ventricular outflow tract flow velocity. Although the left ventricular outflow tract can be visualized in the mid-esophageal aortic long axis and five-chamber views, there is an angle between the left ventricular outflow tract and the Doppler beam, resulting in an underestimation of the left ventricular outflow tract velocity. The left ventricular outflow tract cannot be seen in the mid-esophageal atrioventricular short axis and four-chamber views. **References** 28; 37.

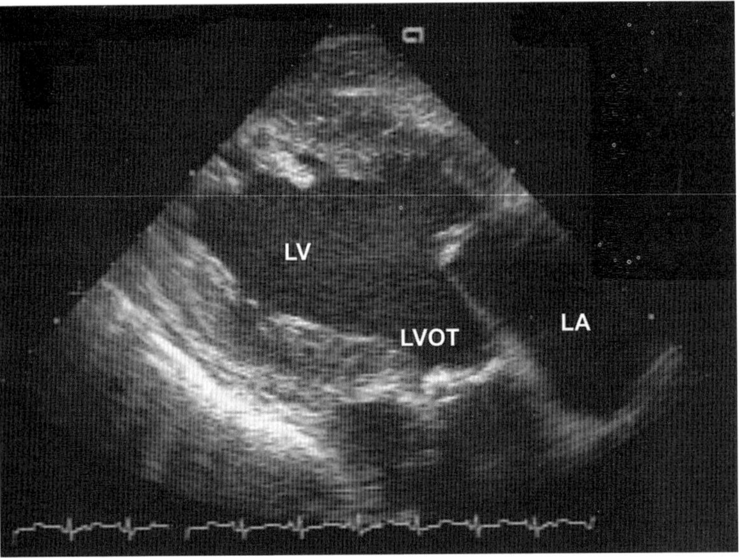

4. Answer B

In patients with asymmetric septal hypertrophy, dynamic obstruction of the left ventricular outflow tract occurs between the anterior mitral leaflet and the ventricular septum. Echocardiography has played an important role in the identification of this dynamic abnormality. When the basal septum is hypertrophied and bulging, the left ventricular outflow tract narrows, providing a substrate for dynamic obstruction. The velocity of blood flow across the narrowed left ventricular outflow tract increases and produces the Venturi effect. As systole progresses, the mitral valve leaflets and support apparatus are drawn toward the ventricular septum, leading to systolic anterior motion of the mitral valve. The anterior mitral leaflet contacts the hypertrophied ventricular septum in late systole, resulting in dynamic obstruction of the left ventricular outflow tract with a late-peaking, dagger-shaped appearance on the Doppler spectrum. Systolic anterior motion of the anterior mitral leaflet is the echocardiographic hallmark of left ventricular outflow tract dynamic obstruction and provides evidence that the mitral valve apparatus plays a role in obliterating the left ventricular outflow tract. The closer the leaflet comes to the ventricular septum and the longer the leaflet is in apposition to the septum, the greater the severity of left ventricular outflow tract obstruction, as shown in the accompanying image (LA, left atrium; LV, left ventricle; MV, mitral valve; RA, right atrium; RV, right ventricle; SAM, systolic anterior motion [arrow]). **References** 10 *(pp 514, 517–518)*; 23 *(p 156)*; 25 *(p 453)*; 26 *(p 102)*.

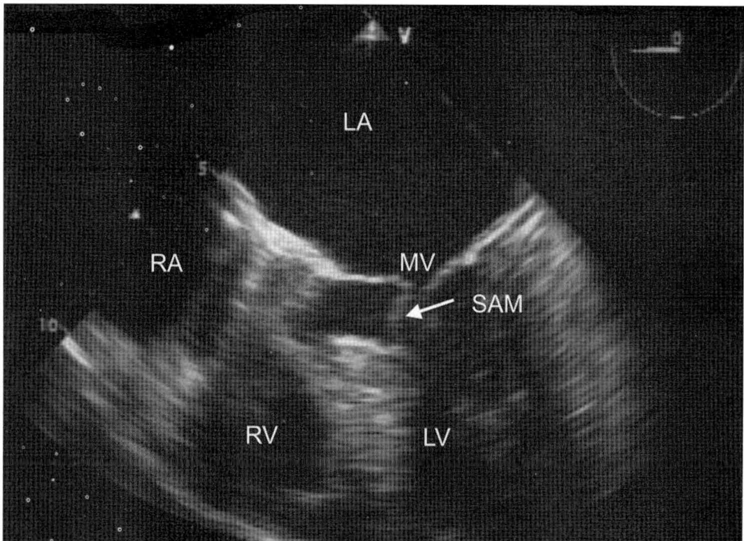

5. Answer C

6. Answer E

In patients with hypertrophic obstructive cardiomyopathy, Doppler echocardiography is the procedure of choice for determining the presence and severity of left ventricular outflow tract obstruction. Increased flow velocity across the left ventricular outflow tract typically is detected from the transesophageal echocardiographic transgastric views. The classic continuous wave Doppler recording of left ventricular outflow tract velocity has a characteristic late-peaking, dagger-shaped appearance. The Doppler spectrum shows a relatively slow increase in velocity in early systole, which then picks up speed and peaks late in systole. This velocity pattern corresponds nicely with the systolic anterior motion of the anterior mitral leaflet.

With the simplified Bernoulli equation, the peak velocity can be converted to the pressure gradient across the left ventricular outflow tract. When Doppler is used to derive pressure gradients, the Doppler sound beam should be oriented as parallel as possible to the flow because even a small error in velocity measurement can lead to serious underestimation of the pressure gradient because of the quadratic relation between velocity and pressure gradient. The peak velocity recorded by Doppler in mid-esophageal atrioventricular long axis view underestimates the true velocity across the left ventricular outflow tract because of the angle between the left ventricular outflow tract and the ultrasound beam. In the transgastric view, the angle between the left ventricular outflow tract and the ultrasound beam is almost zero because the ultrasound beam is parallel to the left ventricular outflow tract. Hence, the peak velocity obtained with the transgastric view is more accurate and should be used to calculate the pressure gradient across the left ventricular outflow tract. According to the simplified Bernoulli equation (LVOT, left ventricular outflow tract),

$$\begin{aligned} \text{Pressure gradient across the LVOT} &= 4 \times (\text{LVOT velocity})^2 \\ &= 4 \times (5)^2 \\ &= 4 \times 25 \\ &= 100 \text{ mm Hg} \end{aligned}$$

Using a simplified Bernoulli equation, the calculated pressure gradient across the left ventricular outflow tract in this patient is 100 mm Hg. Studies have shown that the correlation between the Doppler-derived and catheter-derived pressure gradients is good. **References** 8 *(pp 185–187, 194–196)*; 10 *(p 523)*; 23 *(p 158)*; 37; 42 *(pp 791–797)*.

7. Answer E

The pathophysiology of mitral leaflet malcoaptation and mitral regurgitation in patients with hypertrophic obstructive cardiomyopathy has been studied in great detail. Normally, the point of mitral leaflet coaptation occurs within 3 mm of the distal tip of the two leaflets. In comparison with normal subjects, in patients with hypertrophic obstructive cardiomyopathy, the anterior mitral leaflet and the posterior mitral leaflet have an increased surface area and are longer, particularly the anterior mitral leaflet; the coaptation between the mitral leaflets occurs in the body of the leaflet instead of at the leaflet tips. Systolic anterior motion of the anterior mitral leaflet is commonly seen in patients with hypertrophic obstructive cardiomyopathy. Systolic anterior motion produces mitral leaflet–septal contact and results in failure of coaptation with the posterior mitral leaflet, leading to mitral regurgitation in mid to late systole. The amount of mitral regurgitation is related to the degree of left ventricular outflow tract obstruction and is usually moderate in severity. **References** 23 *(pp 156–163, 239–241)*; 25 *(pp 453, 455)*; 26 *(p 194)*; 42 *(pp 781–804)*.

8. Answer C
9. Answer B
10. Answer A

The image accompanying Question 8 shows the hypertrophied ventricular septum and systolic anterior motion of the anterior mitral leaflet, resulting in dynamic obstruction of the left ventricular outflow tract in mid and late systole. Therefore, this patient has asymmetric septal hypertrophy, the most common form of hypertrophic obstructive cardiomyopathy. The left ventricular outflow tract obstruction in patients with asymmetric septal hypertrophy is dynamic, depending on the loading condition, left ventricular size, and contractility. Decreased volume with small left ventricular size and increased contractility worsen the left ventricular outflow tract obstruction, while volume loading and increased left ventricular size reduce the obstruction. When hypotension occurs in patients with dynamic left ventricular outflow tract obstruction, prompt management includes fluids, a β-blocker, or a pure α-agonist such as phenylephrine. After myomectomy, intraoperative transesophageal echocardiography is used to evaluate residual left ventricular outflow tract obstruction and detect postmyomectomy complications. Ventricular septal defect at the site of the myomectomy is the most likely complication associated with the surgical resection of the hypertrophied ventricular septum. **References** 23 *(pp 156–157, 239–240)*; 26 *(p 195)*; 42 *(pp 781–783, 788–791, 799–803)*.

11. Answer E

Patients with hypertrophic cardiomyopathy usually have diastolic dysfunction with preserved systolic function. The predominant diastolic abnormality is impaired myocardial relaxation due to the hypertrophic myocardium. Delayed left ventricular relaxation results in a slower decline in left ventricular pressure after aortic valve closure. Consequently, the isovolumic relaxation time between aortic valve closure and mitral valve opening is prolonged. Increased duration of the atrioventricular pressure gradient prolongs the deceleration time of the early (E) mitral inflow velocity. In addition, delayed ventricular relaxation and increased chamber stiffness elevate the left ventricular diastolic pressure and thus diminish the pressure gradient between the left atrium and the left ventricle, resulting in decreased velocity of early mitral inflow (the E wave). The velocity of late diastolic filling after atrial contraction (the A wave) is increased because the left atrium has failed to empty in early diastole and is at a higher point in its Starling curve in late diastole. The net result is a decrease in the ratio of the peak E wave to peak A wave velocities (the E/A ratio). Therefore, the Doppler spectrum of mitral inflow in patients with hypertrophic cardiomyopathy typically shows impaired diastolic filling pattern with decreased E velocity, increased A velocity, decreased E/A ratio, and prolonged deceleration time and isovolumic relaxation time. **References** 23 *(p 160)*; 42 *(pp 797–798)*.

12. Answer E

13. Answer E

Left ventricular outflow tract obstruction in patients with hypertrophic cardiomyopathy is dynamic and may not always be present at rest. Provocation that brings out systolic anterior motion of the mitral valve with left ventricular outflow tract obstruction includes the Valsalva maneuver, amyl nitrite, intravenous isoproterenol, and noninvasively induced premature ventricular systole. One of the recognized features of hypertrophic obstructive cardiomyopathy is that patients with grossly normal mitral leaflet motion during a sinus beat may develop systolic anterior motion after the compensatory pause following a premature ventricular systole. The right ventricle may also be involved with hypertrophic cardiomyopathy. Dynamic obstruction in the right ventricular outflow can produce a late-peaking velocity on Doppler recording.

Dynamic left ventricular outflow tract obstruction does not occur only with asymmetric septal hypertrophy. Other clinical settings may be associated with dynamic left ventricular outflow tract obstruction. For any given ejection velocity, dynamic left ventricular outflow tract obstruction or functional subvalvular obstruction occurs any time the distance between the interventricular septum and the anterior mitral leaflet reaches a critical point if there is sufficient flexibility of the mitral valve apparatus to permit anterior leaflet motion. Given these relationships, any factor that increases ejection velocity, decreases the space between the anterior mitral leaflet and septum, or increases leaflet redundancy should increase the tendency for obstruction. In elderly patients with concentric left ventricular hypertrophy secondary to hypertension, hypovolemia resulting from excessive diuresis and treatment with afterload-reducing agents may produce systolic anterior motion with dynamic left ventricular outflow tract obstruction. In the postoperative period, dynamic left ventricular outflow tract obstruction may occur when the intravascular volume is depleted and the patient is receiving treatment with an inotropic agent. In patients with anteroapical myocardial infarction, acute left ventricular outflow tract obstruction may occur because compensatory hyperdynamic motion of the inferobasal myocardium may result in systolic anterior motion of the mitral valve. Also, left ventricular outflow tract obstruction may be an initial presentation of cardiac amyloidosis. **References** 10 *(pp 518–519, 524)*; 23 *(p 162)*; 42 *(pp 803–804)*.

14. Answer D

Aortic valve motion can indicate an alteration in aortic blood flow. When aortic blood flow is abruptly decreased due to dynamic obstruction of the left ventricular outflow tract, the aortic valve partially closes in mid systole. Usually, only one or two cusps exhibit this partial mid-systolic closure, which may be explained by an asymmetric poststenotic outflow tract jet that maintains the opening of the cusps against which it is directed and fails to support the others. Partial mid-systolic closure of the aortic valve can be identified using M-mode echocardiography. The accompanying M-mode echocardiogram was obtained in a patient with systolic anterior motion and left ventricular outflow tract obstruction (AV, atrioventricular valve; LA, left atrium; RV, right ventricle). When obstruction to left ventricular ejection occurs, the aortic valve partially closes and produces mid-systolic aortic valve notching as indicated by the arrows. **References** 10 *(p 522)*; 23 *(pp 156, 158)*; 42 *(p 791)*.

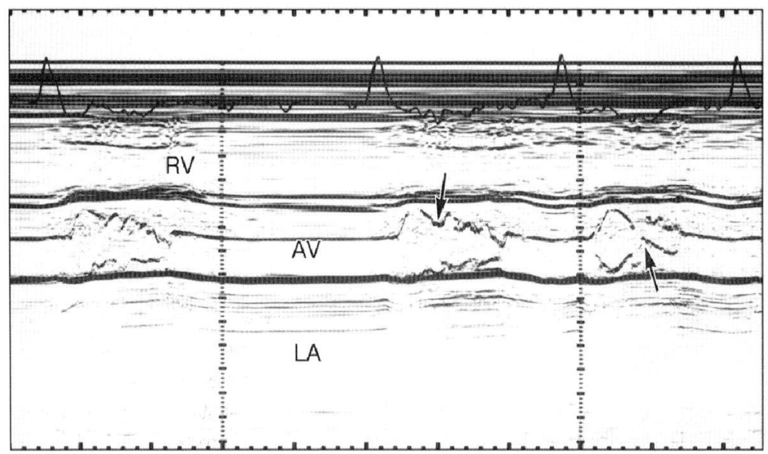

Figure from Oh et al. (23). Used with permission of Mayo Foundation for Medical Education and Research.

15. Answer E

The differentiation of restriction and constriction remains challenging. Although the pathophysiologic mechanisms of restrictive cardiomyopathy and constrictive pericarditis are distinctly different, they have many clinical and hemodynamic similarities. Both disease processes limit diastolic filling and may result in diastolic heart failure, with relatively preserved global systolic function. Diastolic dysfunction in restrictive cardiomyopathy is the result of a stiff and noncompliant ventricular myocardium, but in constrictive pericarditis, it is caused by a thickened, noncompliant pericardium.

Several echocardiographic approaches have been advocated to differentiate restriction and constriction. Patients with pure restrictive cardiomyopathy have minimal respiratory variation in mitral and tricuspid flow velocities. In contrast, respiratory variation is one of the main characteristic features of constrictive pericarditis. Because the total intrapericardial volume is fixed in patients with constrictive pericarditis, any change in right ventricular filling, as with respiration, is accompanied by an opposite change in left ventricular filling. Doppler tissue imaging is the new technology in the differentiation of restriction and constriction. The velocity of mitral anular motion is markedly decreased in restrictive cardiomyopathy, whereas it is abnormally elevated in constrictive pericarditis. In addition, color Doppler M-mode velocity propagation across the mitral valve is abnormally slow in restrictive cardiomyopathy because of delayed relaxation, whereas it is abnormally rapid in constrictive pericarditis. (See also Chapter 12, Questions 19–21.) **References** 10 *(pp 528–532)*; 23 *(pp 191–192)*; 42 *(pp 816–817)*.

16. Answer A

The hallmark of restrictive physiology is abnormal compliance of the left ventricle with elevated ventricular filling pressures and normal or nearly normal systolic function. Ventricular pressure in such conditions declines prominently at the onset of diastole and then rises abruptly because of decreased chamber compliance. This hemodynamic feature produces a "dip-and-plateau" pattern or a "square-root sign" appearance in the ventricular diastolic pressure waveform. Such a distinctive pattern of ventricular filling has its counterpart in the Doppler recordings of mitral and tricuspid inflow velocities. In a typical case of advanced restrictive cardiomyopathy, Doppler echocardiography records restrictive diastolic filling pattern. With the increase in left atrial pressure, the mitral valve opens at a higher pressure, resulting in a shortened isovolumic relaxation time. In addition, high left atrial pressure also results in an elevated transmitral pressure gradient, leading to increased early (E) mitral inflow velocity. Because of elevated ventricular end-diastolic pressure, there is rapid equalization of pressures across the atrioventricular valves in diastole with little further flow during atrial contraction, resulting in a shortened E wave deceleration time (<150 ms) and greatly diminished late (A) mitral inflow wave. As a result, the E/A ratio is increased markedly (more than twofold). This characteristic morphology of a Doppler recording is analogous to the "dip-and-plateau" pattern in the ventricular diastolic pressure waveform. **References** 10 *(pp 528–532)*; 23 *(pp 164–165)*; 25 *(p 475)*; 42 *(pp 814–816)*.

Chapter 14

Recognizing Intracavitary Contents and Source of Emboli

Questions

Multiple choice (choose the *one* best answer):

1. The most common primary cardiac tumor is
   A. lipoma.
   B. myosarcoma.
   C. myxoma.
   D. papillary fibroelastoma.
   E. fibroma.

2. The most common location of myxomas is
   A. the right atrium.
   B. the left atrium.
   C. the right ventricle.
   D. the left ventricle.
   E. the right atrial appendage.

3. The most common attachment of myxomas is
   A. the left atrial free wall.
   B. the right atrial free wall.
   C. the ventricular free wall.
   D. the interventricular septum.
   E. the interatrial septum.

4. Which one of the following statements about myxomas is true?
   A. Myxomas are not deformable throughout the cardiac cycle.
   B. Cystic echolucent vacuolations are never seen with myxomas.
   C. Myxomas are friable but do not embolize.
   D. Myxomas never cause atrioventricular valve incompetence, damage, or obstruction.
   E. Echo-free spaces may be present within myxomas, which correspond to hemorrhage and necrosis.

5. The accompanying transesophageal echocardiographic two-dimensional images are obtained during systole and diastole. Most likely, the patient has

A. a papillary fibroelastoma.

B. a myxoma.

C. a large atrial thrombus.

D. a large vegetation of mitral valve.

E. metastasis of renal cell carcinoma.

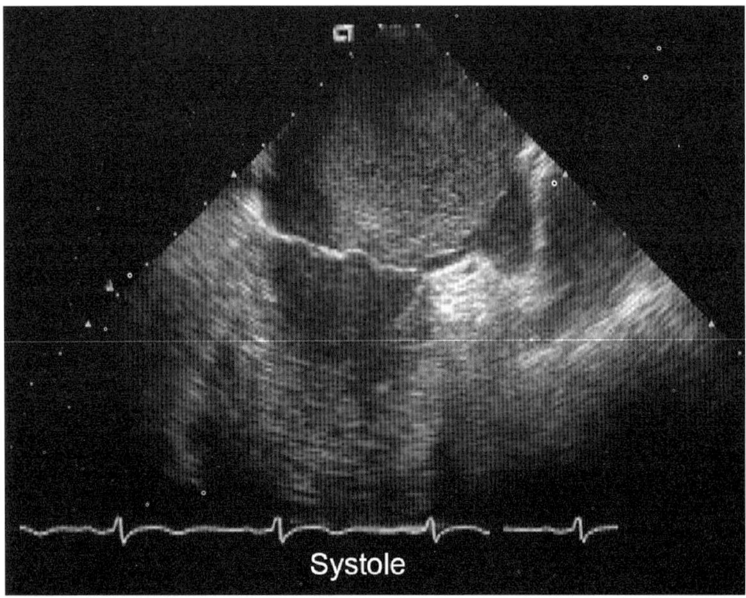

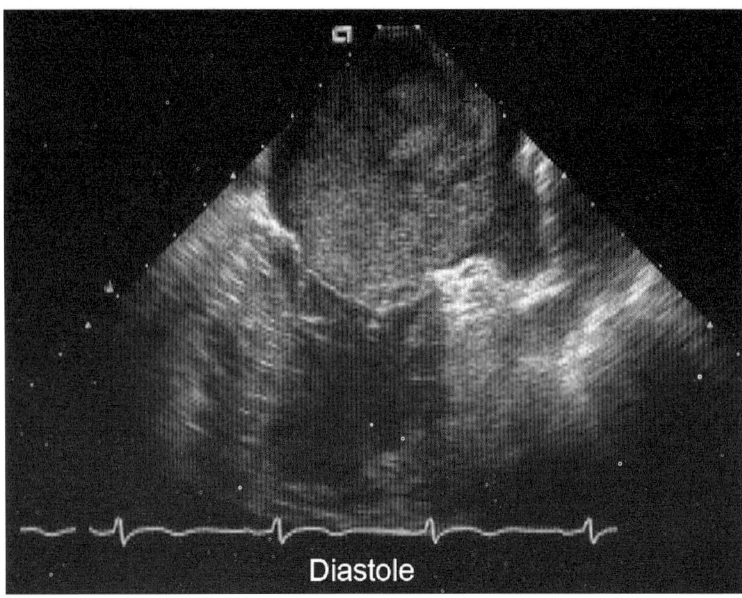

6. The most common location for a papillary fibroelastoma is
   A. the eustachian valve.
   B. the tricuspid valve.
   C. the pulmonic valve.
   D. the mitral valve.
   E. the aortic valve.

7. A 63-year-old afebrile patient with coronary artery disease is scheduled for elective off-pump coronary artery bypass graft surgery. His left ventricular ejection fraction is 55% according to the cardiac catheterization report. The accompanying two-dimensional image is obtained at the beginning of the surgery. Color flow Doppler does not reveal any valvular regurgitation. Most likely, the patient has
   A. a small myxoma.
   B. a papilloma.
   C. a thrombus.
   D. a vegetation.
   E. a normal aortic valve.

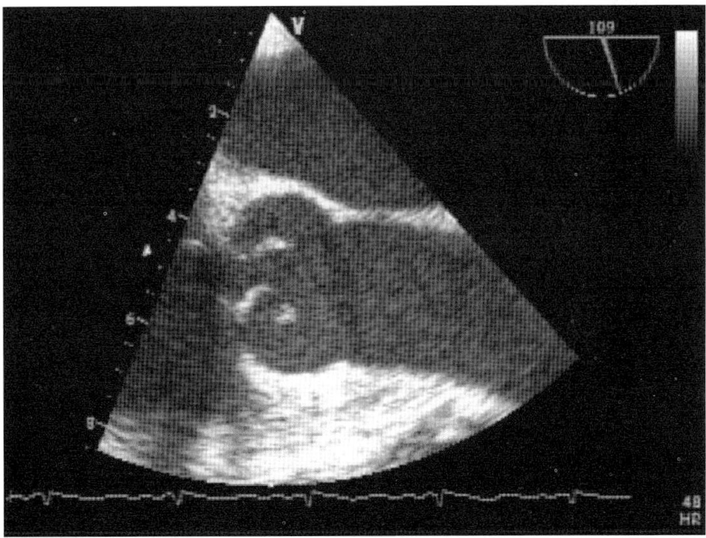

8. The most serious complication for the patient described in Question 7 is most likely to be
   A. left ventricular outflow tract obstruction with hemodynamic instability.
   B. metastasis.
   C. a stroke.
   D. abscess formation.
   E. none of the above because the aortic valve is normal.

9. The usual recommendation for such an asymptomatic patient, as in Question 7, is to
   A. proceed with the scheduled off-pump coronary artery bypass graft surgery.
   B. cancel the procedure, wake up the patient, and call for an oncology consultation.
   C. treat the patient with an anticoagulant and reschedule the surgery in 6 months.
   D. treat the patient with antibiotics and reschedule the surgery in 6 months.
   E. put the patient on cardiopulmonary bypass and remove the mass even though the patient is asymptomatic.

10. A left ventricular thrombus may be differentiated from a tumor because a thrombus
   A. is relatively small in size.
   B. has a relatively rough surface.
   C. is almost always associated with akinetic to dyskinetic myocardium underlying the thrombus.
   D. is almost never located at the ventricular apex.
   E. is always better visualized in a four-chamber view by transesophageal echocardiography than by transthoracic echocardiography.

11. Echocardiographic findings indicating increased risk for left ventricular thrombus formation include
   A. echocardiographic contrast seen after the injection of agitated saline.
   B. spontaneous echocardiographic contrast in the left ventricle.
   C. a negative echocardiographic contrast effect.
   D. a positive echocardiographic contrast effect.
   E. none of the above.

12. The accompanying two-dimensional transesophageal echocardiographic image is obtained in a patient with a history of atrial fibrillation and an embolic event. Spontaneous echocardiographic contrast is observed in the left atrium. Most likely, this patient has

A. a normal left atrium.

B. normal pectinate muscle in the left atrial appendage.

C. hypertrophied pectinate muscle in the left atrial appendage with spontaneous echo contrast in the left atrium.

D. a ligated left atrial appendage.

E. a thrombus in the left atrial appendage.

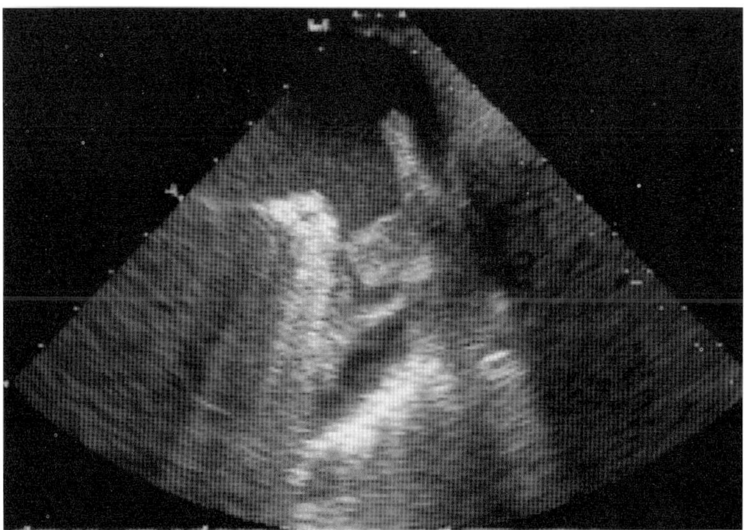

13. Patients with a patent foramen ovale are at increased risk for paradoxical embolism. In patients without a history of cardiac disease, the incidence of probe-patent foramen ovale is

A. less than 1%.

B. about 1% to 2%.

C. about 5% to 10%.

D. about 30%.

E. greater than 50%.

14. A 58-year-old patient has transesophageal echocardiography to rule out any cardiac source of embolism. Agitated saline is injected into the right atrium through an arm vein. Which one of the following statements characterizes the presence of patent foramen ovale?

A. The appearance of contrast bubbles in the left atrium is delayed more then 10 cardiac cycles after being seen in the right atrium.
B. The appearance of contrast bubbles is seen in the right ventricle immediately after being seen in the right atrium.
C. The appearance of contrast bubbles is seen in the right ventricle between five and 10 cardiac cycles after being seen in the right atrium.
D. The appearance of contrast bubbles is seen in the left atrium between five and 10 cardiac cycles after being seen in the right atrium.
E. None of the above.

15. For a consciously sedated patient who breathes spontaneously, a patent foramen ovale is best detected using agitated saline

A. at the end of inspiration.
B. at the end of expiration.
C. at the beginning of inspiration.
D. at the release phase of a Valsalva maneuver.
E. at the beginning of a cough.

16. Studies have shown that, during mechanical ventilation, a patent foramen ovale is best detected

A. at the release of positive end-expiratory pressure.
B. at the beginning of inspiration.
C. at the end of inspiration.
D. at the end of expiration.
E. any time during positive pressure ventilation.

17. All of the following echocardiographic findings in patients with atrial fibrillation have been associated with thromboembolism ***except***

A. impaired left ventricular function.
B. dense spontaneous echocardiographic contrast.
C. left atrial appendage velocity of 0.6 m/s.
D. a complex atheromatous plaque in the thoracic aorta.
E. a left atrial or left atrial appendage thrombus.

18. After cardiac transplantation, the structure that looks different from a normal heart on two-dimensional transesophageal echocardiography is

A. the left atrium.
B. the left ventricle.
C. the mitral valve.
D. the tricuspid valve.
E. the pulmonary veins.

19. The accompanying two-dimensional image is obtained during cardiac surgery. The arrow points to

A. a venous cannula.

B. an arterial cannula.

C. a pulmonary artery catheter.

D. an intra-aortic balloon pump.

E. the cardiac surgeon's fingers.

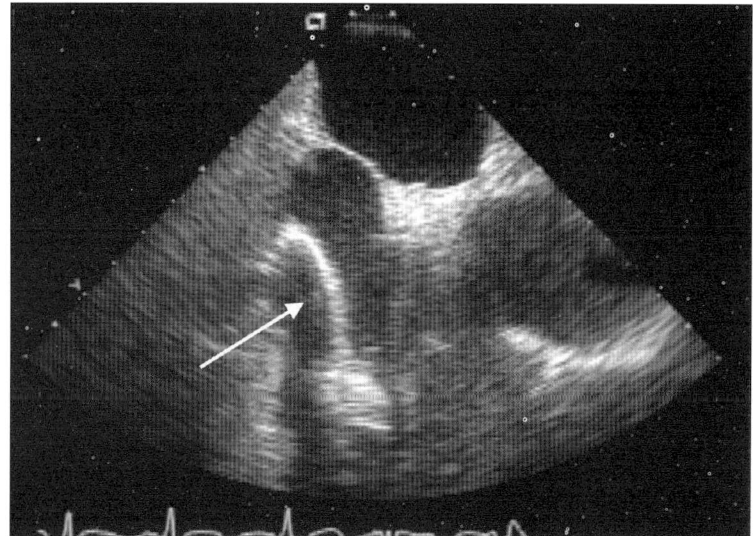

20. The accompanying transesophageal echocardiographic image is obtained immediately after the patient's chest is closed. Which one of the following best describes what the image shows?

A. A normal left ventricle with good contractility.
B. A foreign body in the left ventricle.
C. A dislodged mitral annular ring.
D. A left ventricular assist device.
E. An intra-aortic balloon counterpulsation device.

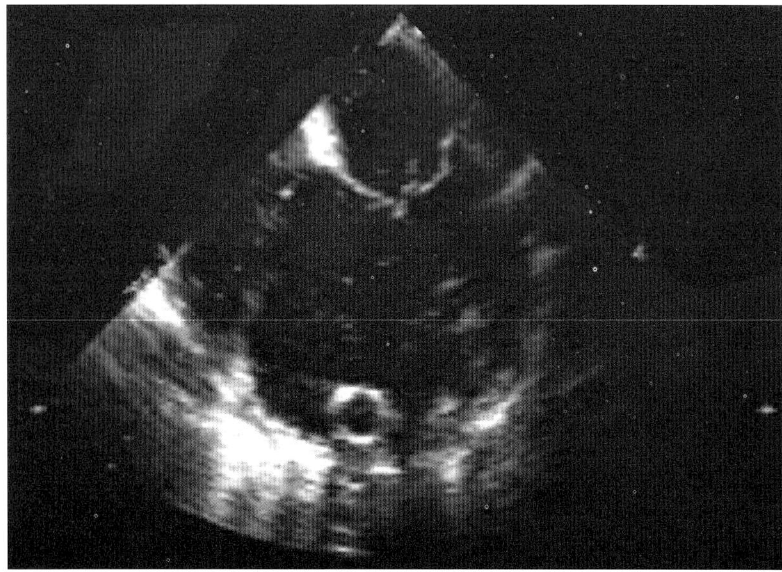

21. In addition to the image accompanying Question 20, the aortic valve is closed during systole. Based on this finding, the cardiologist tells the surgeon

A. to replace the aortic valve.
B. to repair the aortic valve.
C. this finding is expected for the patient.
D. the finding is abnormal for this patient.
E. to open the chest again and put the patient on cardiopulmonary bypass.

22. Optimal placement of the intra-aortic balloon pump requires that

A. the tip be positioned just inferior to the origin of the left subclavian artery.
B. the tip be positioned in the ascending aorta.
C. the tip be positioned in the descending aorta, 10 cm away from the left subclavian artery.
D. the balloon be positioned in the aorta with the tip near the aortic valve.
E. the tip be positioned anywhere as long as the balloon is in the aorta.

23. A 72-year-old patient undergoes coronary artery bypass grafting. The accompanying image is obtained before cardiopulmonary bypass. The arrow in the image points to

A. dissection of the descending aorta.

B. dissection of the aortic arch.

C. an intra-aortic balloon pump.

D. an arterial cannula.

E. an artifact.

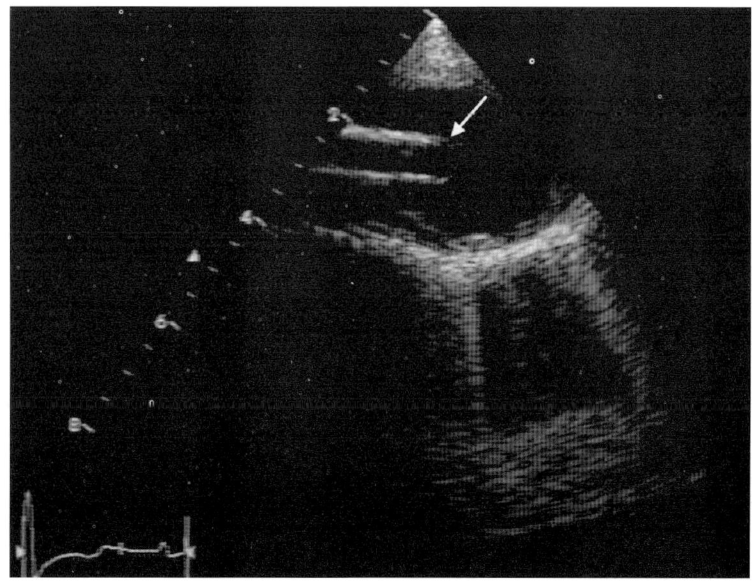

24. In the accompanying image from the same patient shown in Question 23 (LA, left atrium; RA, right atrium), the arrow points to

A. an artifact.
B. a left ventricular assist device.
C. an automatic implantable cardioverter-defibrillator wire.
D. a permanent pacemaker wire.
E. a venous cannula.

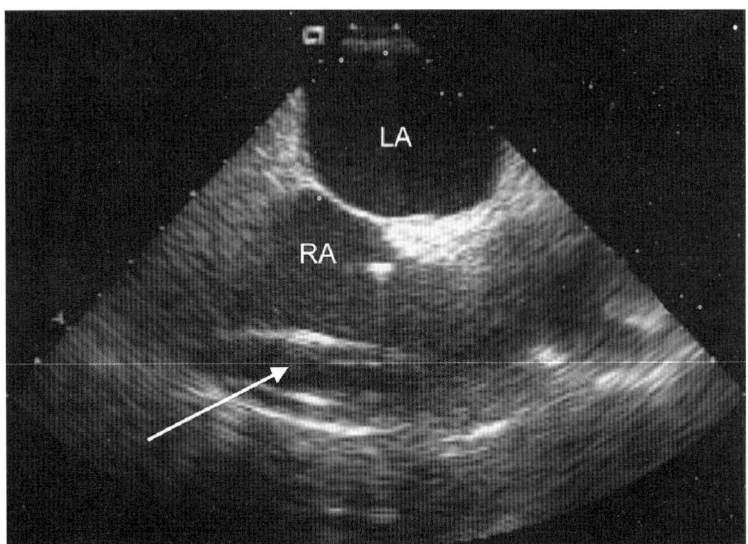

Answers & Discussion

1. Answer C
2. Answer B
3. Answer E

In adults, the most common primary cardiac tumor is a myxoma, which accounts for 90% of surgically excised cardiac neoplasms and about 50% of intracardiac tumors diagnosed at autopsy. The most common location of myxomas is the left atrium (87%), and the second most common location for myxomas is the right atrium. The most common attachment site of myxomas is the interatrial septum in the region of the fossa ovalis (70%–80%). As an atrial myxoma grows, it characteristically expands into the atrial cavity but remains attached to the septum by a stalk, as shown in the accompanying figure (LV, left ventricle; RA, right atrium; RV, right ventricle). The large block arrow indicates the attachment site of myxoma on the atrial septum, and the small arrows show the myxoma in the left atrium. A small percentage of atrial myxomas originate from any location in the atrium, including the atrial free walls and the atrial appendage. Ventricular myxomas may arise from the ventricular free wall or interventricular septum. Syndrome myxoma represents about 3% of cases and usually occurs in younger patients in a familial pattern, along with cutaneous lesions and endocrine neoplasms. Since syndrome myxoma is characterized by multiple myxomas with atypical locations, complete examination of all four chambers is warranted in each patient. In addition, the postoperative recurrence rate is high in patients with syndrome myxoma. Recurrence can occur at the site of the original tumor or at multiple intracardiac sites. Serial echocardiographic studies provide the best means of screening for the recurrence of myxomas. **References** 10 *(pp 599–604)*; 11 *(pp 340–347)*; 23 *(p 205)*; 26 *(pp 358–360)*; 42 *(pp 1135–1142)*.

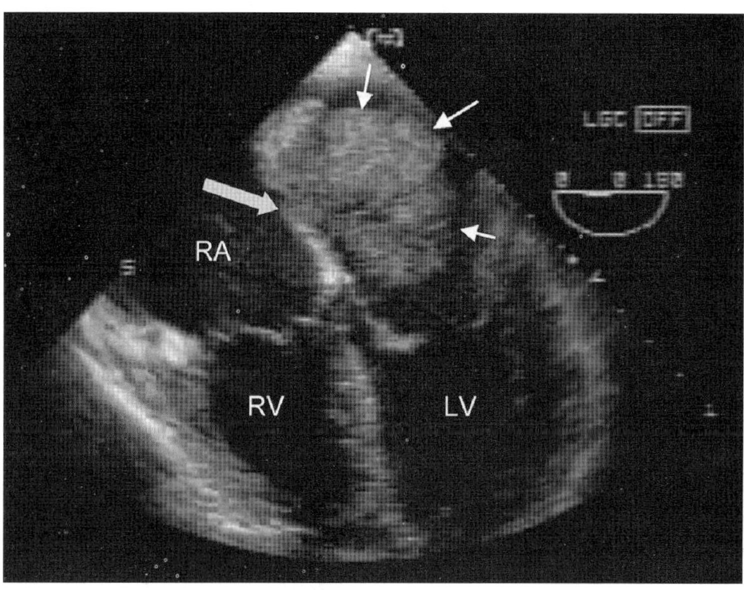

4. Answer E

On gross examination, myxomas often appear polypoid, gelatinous, and friable, with some lobulation and occasional central necrosis. They may contain areas of hemorrhage and calcification. Echocardiographically, myxomas typically appear as a "grape cluster" echo mass in a cardiac chamber, as seen in the figure accompanying Answers 1–3. Echo-free spaces within the mass correspond to areas of hemorrhage or necrosis. Cystic echolucent vacuolations may give the myxoma a "mottled" appearance in contrast to thrombus, vegetation, or other neoplasms. Areas of calcification may also appear within the tumor mass. Most myxomas are pedunculated with a stalk, although they may occasionally be sessile. Usually, the tumor is deformable throughout the cardiac cycle. A large atrial myxoma can cause various degrees of tumor prolapse, resulting in atrioventricular valve incompetence, damage, or obstruction, with a tumor plop on auscultation.

The effects of an atrial myxoma on mitral or tricuspid valve function and competency are best examined by transesophageal echocardiography. After a myxoma resection, the valve leaflets, anulus, and residual regurgitation can be evaluated by intraoperative transesophageal echocardiography to determine whether additional valvular repair is necessary before the operation is complete. A ventricular myxoma may produce obstruction of the outflow tract, which can be demonstrated by turbulent mosaic inflow signals on color Doppler images. In addition, myxomas have embolic potential and may be the source of emboli. **References** 10 *(pp 599–604)*; 11 *(pp 340–347, 476)*; 23 *(p 205)*; 42 *(pp 1135–1142)*.

5. Answer B

The accompanying two-dimensional images demonstrate systolic and diastolic frames of a transesophageal view of a large left atrial myxoma attached to the atrial septum. In systole, the tumor appears as an echogenic mass that almost completely fills the left atrium. During diastole, the left atrial myxoma prolapses into the left ventricle through the mitral orifice, resulting in obstruction of the mitral inflow with increased pressure gradient across the valve as well as impaired left ventricular filling. Quantitation of mitral inflow gradient is possible with Doppler echocardiography. Because of mitral orifice obstruction produced by the large atrial myxoma, an increased mean pressure gradient (14 mm Hg) across the mitral valve was detected using continuous wave Doppler.

Generally, the characteristic appearance, motion, and site of origin of most myxomas distinguishes them from the majority of atrial and valvular masses. Clinical settings often aid in the distinction of atrial myxoma from other atrial masses. For example, atrial thrombi tend to occur in the setting of mitral valve disease, atrial fibrillation, or dilated cardiomyopathy and are frequently localized in the left atrial appendage.

Important goals of intraoperative transesophageal echocardiography are to identify the site of tumor attachment, to ensure that the tumor does not involve the valve leaflets, and to exclude the possibility of multiple masses. After surgical excision, intraoperative transesophageal echocardiography is used to document complete excision of the myxoma and to rule out surgical complications. It is important to emphasize that the diagnosis of myxoma is only presumptive until confirmed histologically. On pathologic examination, a "typical" myxoma may actually be a primary cardiac malignancy or metastasis. **References** 11 *(pp 340–347)*; 23 *(p 206)*; 42 *(pp 1135–1142)*.

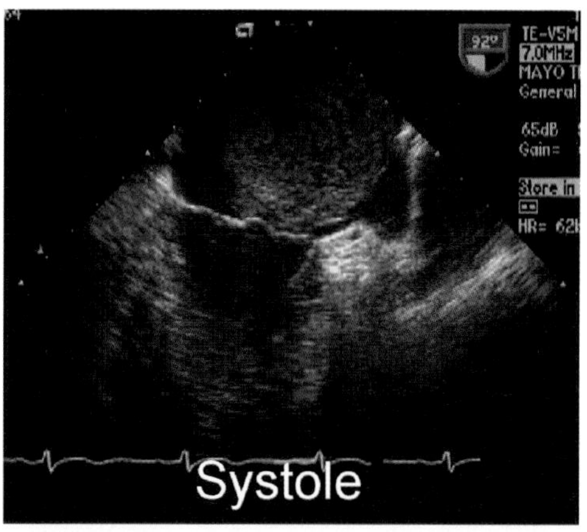
Systole

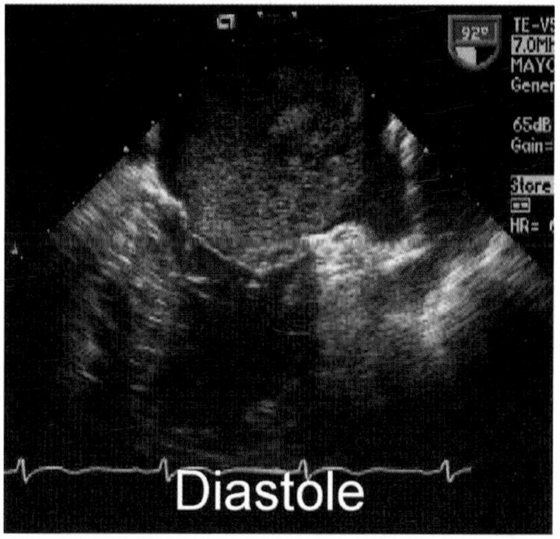
Diastole

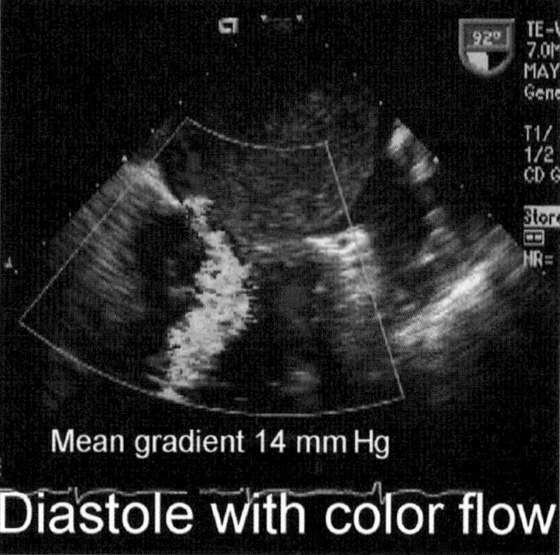
Mean gradient 14 mm Hg
Diastole with color flow

6. Answer E

Papillary fibroelastomas are also called papillomas. They are small, benign cardiac tumors that most frequently arise from valvular endocardium. The aortic valve is most frequently involved in adults, and the tricuspid valve in children. Less commonly, these tumors may arise from mural endocardium and be attached to the ventricular septum or near the left ventricular outflow tract. Occasionally, papillary fibroelastomas are multiple. (See also Questions 7–9.) **References** 10 *(pp 604–605, 607)*; 11 *(pp 348, 350–351)*; 14; 23 *(pp 209–210)*; 26 *(p 360)*; 32 *(p 204)*; 42 *(pp 1144–1145)*.

7. Answer B
8. Answer C
9. Answer E

Echocardiographically, papillomas or papillary fibroelastomas usually appear as small round homogeneous masses or pom-pom–like masses with a diameter about 1 cm or less. The attachment to the cardiac valves can be visualized, and the aortic valve has been reported to be involved most frequently. Although papillary fibroelastomas may occur in all age groups, they are most commonly seen in patients more than 60 years of age. Before the introduction of two-dimensional echocardiography, papillary fibroelastomas were incidental findings at autopsy or during open heart surgery. With the development of ultrasound techniques, papillary fibroelastomas have been identified with increasing frequency. Historically, papillary fibroelastomas were considered to have no clinical importance. Recent evidence suggests these tumors have the potential to cause cerebral or coronary embolization, occlusion of the coronary ostium, and sudden death. The reports of symptomatic cases of papillary fibroelastomas have led this small benign tumor to be considered a potentially dangerous lesion. Surgical removal of a papillary fibroelastoma is safe, simple, effective, and permanent. It has been recommended that all symptomatic papillary fibroelastomas should be removed unless there are compelling contraindications. Asymptomatic lesions of the left side of the heart should be removed

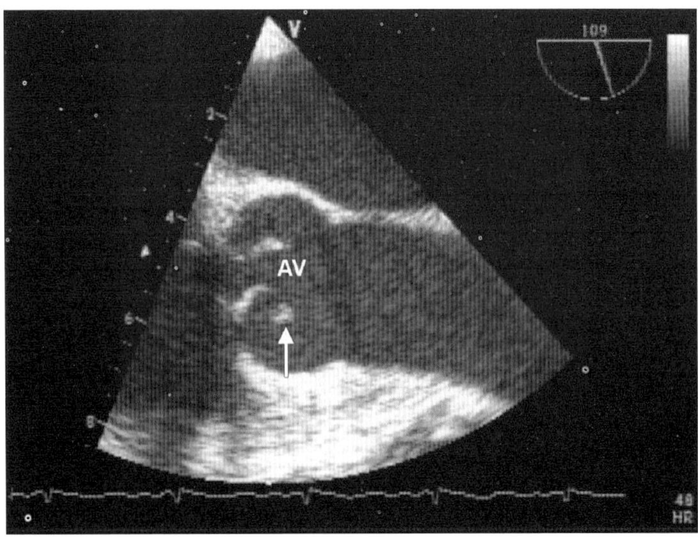

because of their potentially serious or fatal consequences, whereas those arising from the right side of the heart may be observed.

The incidental transesophageal echocardiographic finding in the 63-year-old patient shown in the accompanying image is consistent with papillary fibroelastoma or papilloma on the aortic valve (AV). The arrow indicates the aortic valve fibroelastoma. Because of the potential for complications, the papillary fibroelastoma should be removed surgically even though the patient is asymptomatic and is scheduled for off-pump coronary artery bypass graft surgery.

Echocardiographically, aortic vegetations appear as masses or clumps of echoes attached to the ventricular surface of the leaflets. The characteristic valve involvement of this echo mass is not consistent with vegetation. In addition, the patient does not have any symptoms and signs of endocarditis, and the clinical setting makes the diagnosis of vegetation unlikely for this afebrile patient. (See also Question 6.) **References** 10 *(pp 604–605, 607)*; 11 *(pp 348, 350–351)*; 14; 23 *(pp 209–210)*; 26 *(p 350)*; 36; 38; 42 *(pp 1144–1145, 1189)*.

10. Answer C

Left ventricular thrombi nearly always occur in patients with severe regional or global left ventricular dysfunction, which results in a low blood flow state or blood stasis. Hence, akinetic to dyskinetic myocardium is usually found underlying the thrombus. Left ventricular mural thrombi are a complication of acute infarction. The incidence of left ventricular thrombi is related to the size and location of the infarct, as well as the presence of akinesis, hypokinesis, or dyskinesis. A left ventricular thrombus can complicate 30% to 40% of acute anterior myocardial infarctions, which is especially common in patients with infarction involving the cardiac apex. It occurs in less than 5% of patients with inferior infarctions. Diagnosis of a left ventricular thrombus is most certain when an echogenic mass is located in a region of abnormal wall motion. An exception is apical thrombus formation in hypereosinophilic cardiomyopathy, which obliterates the ventricular apex and does not have underlying impaired apical motion.

Echocardiographically, left ventricular thrombi appear as a mass of echoes superimposed on and interrupting the normal endocardial contour of the ventricle in regions of depressed wall motion. These thrombi are most commonly located in the apex. The size and surface of a thrombus are not characteristics used to differentiate a thrombus from a tumor. Some studies have suggested that recent thrombi may be more shaggy and irregular in configuration, whereas organized thrombi may be more circumscribed and immobile. Sometimes, transesophageal echocardiographic visualization of left ventricular apical thrombi may be difficult because the imaging plane may truncate the true apex, especially in the mid-esophageal four-chamber view (foreshortening). In addition, the left ventricular apex is located at considerable distance from the transducer; this far-field location of the left ventricular apex limits resolution of structural detail. In such a situation, a transthoracic apical four-chamber view may be a better approach for identification of left ventricular apical thrombi. **References** 11 *(pp 376–378)*; 23 *(p 212)*; 26 *(pp 362–363)*; 42 *(pp 1162–1164)*.

11. Answer B

Echocardiographic findings indicating increased risk for left ventricular thrombus formation include left ventricular aneurysm, apical akinesis, severe left ventricular systolic dysfunction with an ejection fraction less than 20%, and spontaneous echocardiographic contrast. Spontaneous echocardiographic contrast is the smoke-like appearance of swirling blood seen in low blood flow states. It is seen in the left ventricle in dilated cardiomyopathy and severely reduced left ventricular function. Thrombus formation in the left ventricle tends to occur in regions of blood stasis with spontaneous echocardiographic contrast. Evidence of apical flow stasis or continuous swirling of flow around the apex identifies patients at particular high risk for apical thrombosis. Several studies have found the association between spontaneous echocardiographic contrast and embolic events. **References** 10 *(pp 476–478, 612–613, 615)*; 11 *(pp 474–475)*; 26 *(pp 361–362)*; 42 *(pp 1162–1164)*.

12. Answer E

In patients referred for determination of the cardiac source of an embolism, a frequent positive finding is a thrombus in the left atrium or left atrial appendage. It has been reported that about 30% to 50% of left atrial thrombi are located in the atrial appendage. One of the major advantages of transesophageal echocardiography in the evaluation of a suspected cardiac source of embolism is the ability to better visualize the left atrium and left atrial appendage contents because of the unique position of the probe behind the left atrium.

The accompanying two-dimensional image is a transverse view of the left atrium and its appendage (LA, left atrium; LAA, left atrial appendage; LUPV, left upper pulmonary vein). An echogenic mass can be visualized in the left atrial appendage (arrow). This mass has a relatively well-circumscribed, defined border with acoustic density that differs from adjacent myocardium. The patient's history of atrial fibrillation and the presence of spontaneous echocardiographic contrast in the left atrium predispose the patient to increased risk of left atrial thrombus formation. Therefore, both the clinical setting and the echocardiographic findings are consistent with the diagnosis of a thrombus in the left atrial appendage, which most likely is the source of the embolic event in this patient. **References** 11 *(pp 471–474)*; 23 *(p 211)*; 42 *(pp 1164–1165)*.

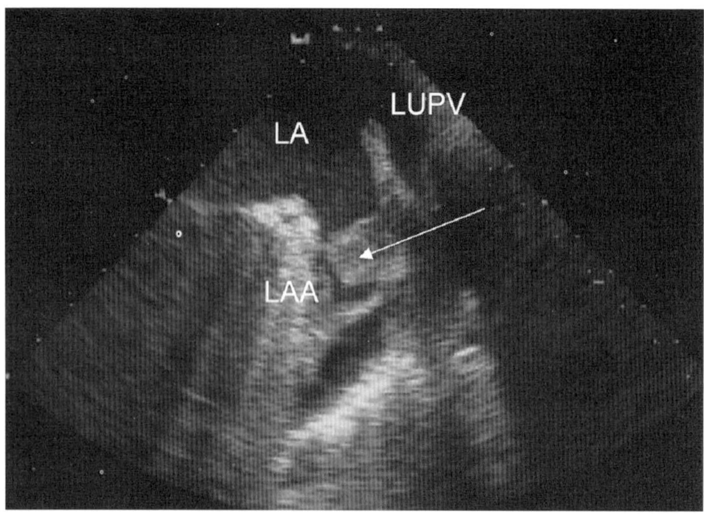

13. Answer D

The foramen ovale is an opening in the mid portion of the fetal atrial septum at the junction of the septum primum and septum secundum. It is normally covered by a thin flap of septum primum. Before birth, the foramen ovale is kept open by blood flow from the right atrium to the left atrium. After birth, the establishment of normal pulmonary circulation increases the left atrial pressure, presses the flap of septum primum against the foramen ovale, and hence closes the opening. The flap may fuse with the septum secundum to close the orifice permanently or may remain separate as a patent foramen ovale. In patients with a patent foramen ovale, the orifice can reopen if the right atrial pressure is higher than the left atrial pressure, predisposing these patients to paradoxical embolization. A patent foramen ovale has been demonstrated at autopsy in 25% to 34% of individuals with no history of cardiac disease. During echocardiographic examination, a patent foramen ovale can be detected by color flow imaging, as shown in the accompanying figure (LA, left atrium; L → R flow, left atrium to right atrium flow seen as a blue color jet [arrow]; PFO, patent foramen ovale; RA, right atrium), or contrast echocardiography with provocative maneuvers, such as the Valsalva maneuver and cough. Compared with transthoracic echocardiography, transesophageal echocardiography has the advantage of superior visualization of the atrial septum and the fossa ovalis membrane, especially in the longitudinal view. The prevalence of a patent foramen ovale has been studied using contrast transesophageal echocardiography. The overall prevalence of a patent foramen ovale was 17.8% at rest and 35.9% with the Valsalva maneuver. The vast majority of these abnormalities remain clinically silent and undetected; however, they have the potential for paradoxical embolization. **References** 3; 11 *(pp 478–485)*; 42 *(p 931)*.

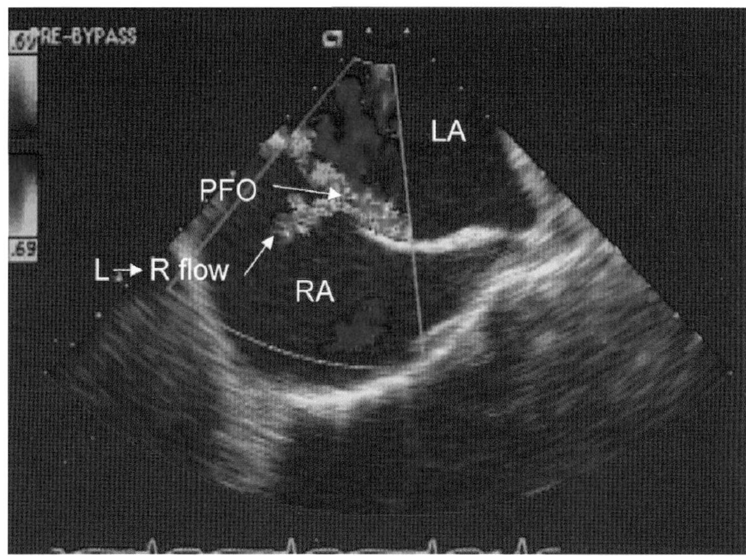

14. Answer E

Contrast echocardiography with agitated saline is useful in the identification of an intracardiac shunt, such as a patent foramen ovale. Because agitated saline has air-filled microbubbles with an acoustic reflectivity different from that of cardiovascular structures, it allows visualization of intracardiac structures containing air bubbles. In normal subjects without a patent foramen ovale, the agitated saline injected into an arm vein is expected to be seen in the right atrium, the right ventricle, and then the pulmonary artery. In case of an intracardiac shunt at the level of the atrium, such as a patent foramen ovale, the contrast bubbles appear in the left atrium immediately after being seen in the right atrium. The appearance of contrast bubbles in the left atrium within three to five cardiac cycles indicates the presence of an intrapulmonary shunt such as a pulmonary arteriovenous fistula. **References** 23 *(p 245)*; 42 *(p 316)*.

15. Answer D

16. Answer A

The sensitivity of contrast echocardiography using a Valsalva maneuver or cough in detecting a known patent foramen ovale has been reported to range between 64% and 100%. In awake or sedated patients with spontaneous breathing, increased right-to-left shunting was observed at the release phase of a Valsalva maneuver or following a cough during contrast echocardiography. During mechanical ventilation, a patent foramen ovale is best detected at the release of positive end-expiratory pressure. It has been suggested that with increased intrathoracic pressure, systemic venous return is impeded; with the discontinuation of positive end-expiratory pressure or a Valsalva maneuver, the sudden increase in systemic venous return to the right atrium would increase right atrial pressure at the time when venous return to the left atrium remained lower. This transiently increased atrial pressure gradient influences the occurrence of right-to-left shunting through a patent foramen ovale. During the strain phase of the Valsalva maneuver or positive end-expiratory pressure, the increased intrathoracic pressure does not alter the atrial pressure gradient across the patent foramen ovale, and hence does not increase the right to left shunt through a patent foramen ovale. **References** 3; 23 *(p 245)*; 42 *(p 316)*.

17. Answer C

Patients with atrial fibrillation are at high risk for thromboembolism. Echocardiographic findings associated with thromboembolism include impaired left ventricular systolic function, left atrial or left atrial appendage thrombus, dense spontaneous echo contrast, complex atheromatous plaque in the thoracic aorta, and reduced velocity of blood flow in the left atrial appendage. Transesophageal echocardiography is the most sensitive and specific imaging technique for detection of left atrial and left atrial appendage thrombus, far surpassing transthoracic echocardiography. This modality also permits superior evaluation for other causes of cardiogenic embolism, as well as a means of measuring left atrial appendage function. Contraction and relaxation of the left atrial appendage produce flow velocities that can be detected at the mouth of the appendage. The normal left atrial appendage velocity is greater than 50 cm/s (or 0.5 m/s). With the loss of sinus rhythm, the left atrial appendage velocity decreases. Generally, patients with left atrial appendage velocities less than 20 cm/s are more likely to develop left atrial appendage thrombus and systemic thromboembolism. Other echocardiographic signs, such as the diameter of the left atrium and fibrocalcific endocardial abnormalities, have been variably associated with thromboembolism and may interact with other factors. **References** 12; 23 *(p 256)*.

18. Answer A

The echocardiographic appearance of the heart after transplantation is most easily appreciated with an understanding of the surgical procedure. The original failing heart is excised from the recipient by incisions through the pulmonary artery, the aorta, and the posterior walls of the right and left atria. The inflow portions of the superior vena cava, inferior vena cava, and pulmonary veins are not disturbed. The donor heart is transplanted to the recipient by suturing the heart to remnants of the recipient atria, proximal pulmonary artery, and proximal ascending aorta. Because patients with cardiac transplantation have atria from both donor and recipient hearts, the long axis of the atria appears larger. The suture lines within the left and right atria appear prominently as an echo-dense ridge between the donor and recipient atria. The structure that looks different from a normal heart after cardiac transplantation is the left atrium. The suture lines at the junction between the donor and recipient left atria produce prominent echoes in four-chamber and two-chamber views. Occasionally, these echoes can be fairly large and simulate a pathologic mass. The pulmonary artery anastomosis site is also represented as a ridge in the main pulmonary artery. The anastomosis of the donor heart to the aorta is the least consistent finding because of the variations in its position within the aorta. **References** 10 *(pp 542–543, 599)*, 42 *(pp 1231–1238)*.

19. Answer E

The transesophageal echocardiographic bicaval view accompanying this question reveals the surgeon's fingers (as shown also in the accompanying figure; LA, left atrium; RA, right atrium) that push on the free wall of the right atrium toward the atrial septum, leading to the invagination of the right atrial free wall. During open-heart surgery, cardiac surgeons may grab, lift, or push on the heart for different reasons. On the

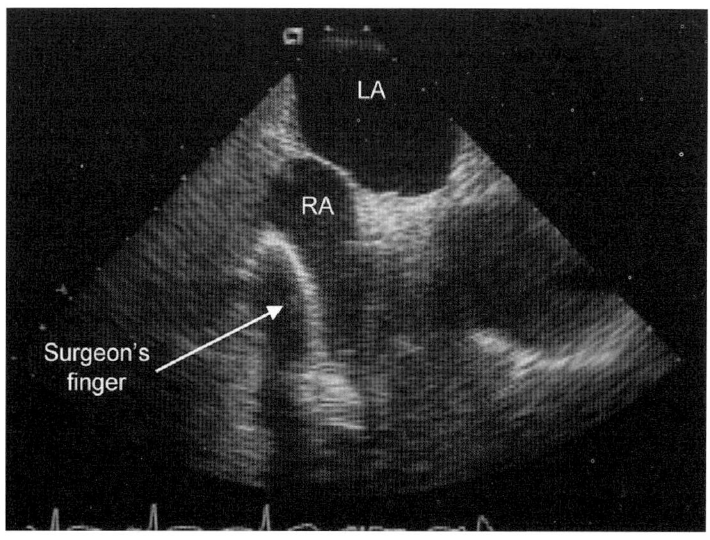

two-dimensional image, a surgeon's finger can be differentiated from a venous cannula because the dome-shaped echo density of the fingertip continues with the linear echo density of both sides of the finger. In contrast, the linear echo density of a cannula is discontinued at the tip of the cannula. Also, a cannula has a different texture, i.e., the ultrasound reflection of a plastic cannula is usually stronger (more echo dense) than that of a surgeon's finger. In addition, when the surgeon pushes on the free wall of the right atrium, more than one finger may be observed with transesophageal echocardiography. Usually, only one venous cannula can be seen in the right atrium. An aortic cannula is placed in the distal ascending aorta, not in the right atrium. A pulmonary artery catheter is seen in the bicaval view as a linear echo from the superior vena cava to the right atrium, not through the free wall of the right atrium. An intra-aortic balloon pump is found in the descending aorta, distal to the left subclavian artery. (See also Questions 23 and 24.)

20. Answer D

21. Answer C

Ventricular assist devices are used as temporary circulatory support in patients with ventricular failure and maximum intravenous inotropic support and who cannot be weaned from cardiopulmonary bypass after a technically successful operation. These devices support the circulation and perfusion as a bridge to cardiac transplantation or patients in whom the recovery of considerable myocardial function is expected. Some ventricular assist devices are designed only for left ventricular support, whereas others may be used for right ventricular or biventricular support. Usually, left ventricular assist devices have the inflow cannula placed in the left ventricular apex and the outflow conduit is anastomosed to the ascending aorta. One type of the left ventricular assist device (Thoratec) may have its inflow cannula placed in the left atrium or in the left ventricular apex (as shown in the accompanying schematic; LVAD, left ventricular assist device; RVAD, right ventricular assist device).

The two-dimensional image accompanying this question is a mid-esophageal four-chamber view obtained in a patient with a left ventricular assist device (LA, left atrium; LV, left ventricle; LVAD, left ventricular assist device). The inflow cannula inserted into the left ventricular apex appears as a circular echo reflector in the mid-esophageal four-chamber view. During normal operation, the left ventricular assist device completely unloads the left ventricle and supports cardiac output at physiologic levels. The blood flow in the left ventricle enters the inflow cannula to the device pump, which then pumps the blood into the ascending aorta through the outflow conduit. Since the blood flow bypasses the aortic valve, it is expected that the aortic valve is normally closed during systole in patients with a left ventricular assist device. To maintain satisfactory flow through the ventricular assist device, it is important to have good drainage of blood by both drainage cannulas. Doppler echocardiography can determine the velocity of the inflow cannula. In patients with obstruction of the inflow cannula, Doppler recording reveals increased velocity of antegrade flow, and color flow imaging demonstrates turbulence caused by high-velocity flow. In addition, two-dimensional imaging may reveal increased angulation of the inflow cannula as well as increased left ventricular size. After placement of a left ventricular assist device, intraoperative transesophageal echocardiography can be used to assess left ventricular volume, and hence ventricular distention can be prevented by adjusting flow rates of the pump. **References** 15; 24 *(pp 269–271)*.

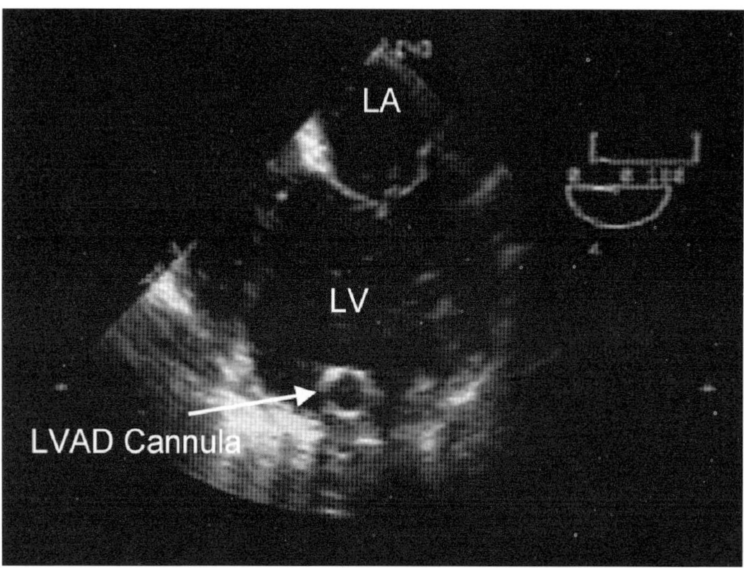

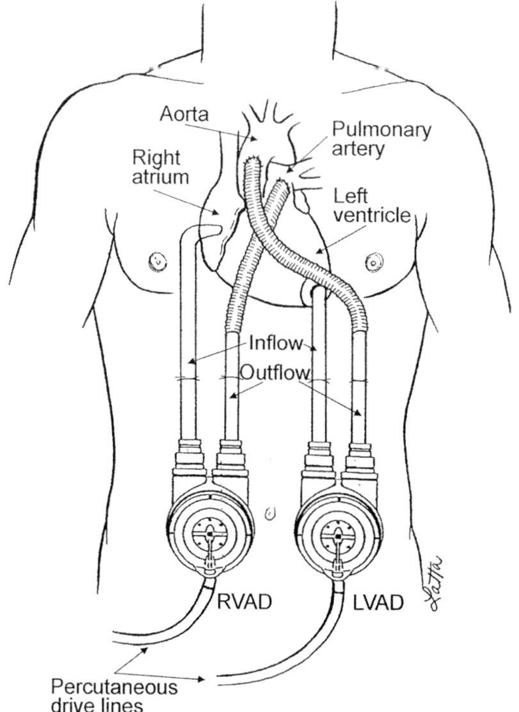

Figure from Hunt and Frazier (15). Used with permission.

22. Answer A

The optimal position of the intra-aortic balloon pump can be readily imaged by transesophageal echocardiography, which is a useful technique for confirmation of the position of the intra-aortic balloon pump tip when fluoroscopy is not readily available or is impractical, such as in the operating room setting. Optimal placement of an intra-aortic balloon pump requires that the tip be positioned just inferior to the origin of the left subclavian artery. If it is placed too proximally, the left carotid or the innominate artery may be occluded; if it is placed too distally, the renal and celiac arteries may be obstructed. In addition, the degree of diastolic augmentation and cardiac unloading provided by an intra-aortic balloon pump would be compromised if the device is not positioned properly. Transesophageal echocardiography can also be used to monitor the pulsatile function of the intra-aortic balloon pump during surgery. Balloon inflation and deflation can be easily visualized in the descending thoracic aorta. Loss of intra-aortic balloon pump pulsation in the descending aorta suggests possible catheter kinking, rupture of the balloon, or system failure. **References** 24 *(pp 262, 266–269)*; 29 *(pp 128–130)*.

23. Answer D

The image accompanying Question 23 was obtained with the transesophageal echocardiographic probe placed in the upper esophagus, at the level of the aortic arch. The arrow points to the tip of the arterial cannula in the aortic arch. During coronary artery bypass grafting, the distal ascending aorta is commonly used for arterial cannulation because of ease of placement and fewer complications than with other sites. Usually, the aortic cannula is inserted 1 to 2 cm in the distal ascending aorta and positioned to direct flow distally. A few surgeons prefer a long arterial cannula with the tip placed at the level of the aortic arch. The tip of the arterial cannula may be malpositioned against the aortic wall or in an arch vessel, leading to inadequate or excessive cerebral perfusion. Therefore, it is essential to monitor and observe the aorta for possible cannula-related complications. Intraoperative transesophageal echocardiography can help detect malposition of the arterial cannula at the level of aortic arch.

24. Answer E

The image accompanying Question 24 is a view of the right atrium (LA, left atrium; RA, right atrium). The arrow points to a venous cannula inserted through the right atrial appendage, with its tip directed inferiorly into the inferior vena cava. For standard coronary artery bypass grafting, venous cannulation is commonly performed with a two-stage venous cannula, which is a single cannula using a dual drainage system. Usually, this type of venous cannula is inserted in the right atrial appendage, with the proximal drainage port positioned within the right atrium and the distal port advanced into the inferior vena cava. Advantages of the two-stage venous cannula include the need for only a single atriotomy, and during cardiopulmonary bypass, blood entering the right atrium via the coronary sinus and/or persistent left superior vena cava (0.5% of patients) is drained. Malposition of the venous cannula may result in incomplete venous drainage to the cardiopulmonary bypass pump so that either the right ventricle continues to receive blood or the venous return is partially obstructed. A major disadvantage of a two-stage venous cannula is limited access to the right atrium. **References** 3 *(pp 1027–1029, 1061–1110)*; 15 *(pp 320–321, 590–591)*; 24 *(pp 254–256)*.

References

1. Ammash NM, Seward JB, Warnes CA, et al. Partial anomalous pulmonary venous connection: diagnosis by transesophageal echocardiography. *J Am Coll Cardiol* 1997;29:1351–1358.
2. Baim DS, Grossman W, eds. *Grossman's cardiac catheterization, angiography, and intervention*, 6th ed. Philadelphia: Lippincott Williams & Wilkins, 2000.
3. Black S, Cucchiara RF, Nishimura RA, et al. Parameters affecting occurrence of paradoxical air embolism. *Anesthesiology* 1989;71:235–241.
4. Block M, Hourigan L, Bellows WH, et al. Comparison of left atrial dimensions by transesophageal and transthoracic echocardiography. *J Am Soc Echocardiogr* 2002;15:143–149.
5. Bonow RO, Carabello B, de Leon AC Jr., et al. ACC/AHA guidelines for the management of patients with valvular heart disease: a report of the American College of Cardiology/American Heart Association. Task Force on Practice Guidelines (Committee on Management of Patients with Valvular Heart Disease). *J Am Coll Cardiol* 1998;32:1486–1588.
6. Click RL, Oh JK. Intraoperative echocardiography. In: Oh JK, Seward JB, Tajik AJ, eds. *The Echo Manual*, 3rd ed. Philadelphia: Lippincott Williams & Wilkins, 2006;368–382.
7. Dajani AS, Taubert KA, Wilson W, et al. Prevention of bacterial endocarditis: recommendations by the American Heart Association. *JAMA* 1997;277:1794–1801.
8. de Bruijn NP, Clements FM, eds. *Intraoperative Use of Echocardiography*. Philadelphia: Lippincott, 1991.
9. Edelman SK. *Understanding Ultrasound Physics: Fundamentals and Exam Review*, 2nd ed. ESP, 1994.
10. Feigenbaum H. *Echocardiography*, 5th ed. Philadelphia: Lea & Febiger, 1994.
11. Freeman WK, Seward JB, Khandheria BK, et al. *Transesophageal Echocardiography*. Boston: Little, Brown, 1994.
12. Fuster V, Rydén LE, Asinger RW, et al. ACC/AHA/ESC guidelines for the management of patients with atrial fibrillation: executive summary: a report of the American College of Cardiology/American Heart Association Task Force on Practice Guidelines and the European Society of Cardiology Committee for Practice Guidelines and Policy Conferences (Committee to Develop Guidelines for the Management of Patients With Atrial Fibrillation). *J Am Coll Cardiol* 2001;38:1231–1265.
13. García-Fernández MA, Zamorano J, Azevedo J. *Doppler Tissue Imaging Echocardiography*. Madrid: McGraw-Hill, 1998.
14. Heath D. Pathology of cardiac tumors. *Am J Cardiol* 1968;21:315–327.
15. Hunt SA, Frazier OH. Mechanical circulatory support and cardiac transplantation. *Circulation* 1998;97:2079–2090.
16. Izzat MB, Sanderson JE, St. John Sutton MG, eds. *Echocardiography in Adult Cardiac Surgery*. Oxford: ISIS Medical Media, 1999.
17. Kerut EK, McIlwain EF, Plotnick GD. *Handbook of Echo-Doppler Interpretation*. Armonk (NY): Futura Publishing, 1996.
18. Labovitz AJ, Williams GA. *Doppler Echocardiography: The Quantitative Approach*, 3rd ed. Philadelphia: Lea & Febiger, 1992.

19. Lambert AS, Miller JP, Merrick SH, et al. Improved evaluation of the location and mechanism of mitral valve regurgitation with a systematic transesophageal echocardiography examination. *Anesth Analg* 1999;88:1205–1212.
20. Nanda NC, Domanski MJ. *Atlas of Transesophageal Echocardiography*. Baltimore: Williams & Wilkins, 1998.
21. O'Gara PT, DeSanctis RW. Acute aortic dissection and its variants: toward a common diagnostic and therapeutic approach. *Circulation* 1995;92:1376–1378.
22. O'Leary PW, Hagler DJ, Seward JB, et al. Biplane intraoperative transesophageal echocardiography in congenital heart disease. *Mayo Clin Proc* 1995;70:317–326.
23. Oh JK, Seward JB, Tajik AJ. *The Echo Manual*, 2nd ed. Philadelphia: Lippincott-Raven, 1999.
24. Oka Y, Konstadt SN, eds. *Clinical Transesophageal Echocardiography: A Problem-Oriented Approach*. Philadelphia: Lippincott-Raven, 1996.
25. Otto CM, ed. *The Practice of Clinical Echocardiography*. Philadelphia: WB Saunders, 1997.
26. Otto CM. *Textbook of Clinical Echocardiography*, 2nd ed. Philadelphia: Saunders, 2000.
27. Poelaert J, Skarvan K, eds. *Transoesophageal Echocardiography in Anaesthesia*. London: BMJ, 2000.
28. Quinones MA, Otto CM, Stoddard M, et al. Doppler Quantification Task Force of the Nomenclature and Standards Committee of the American Society of Echocardiography. Recommendations for quantification of Doppler echocardiography: a report from the Doppler Quantification Task Force of the Nomenclature and Standards Committee of the American Society of Echocardiography. *J Am Soc Echocardiogr* 2002;15:167–184.
29. Rafferty TD. *Basics of Transesophageal Echocardiography*. New York: Churchill Livingstone, 1995.
30. Randolph GR, Hagler DJ, Connolly HM, et al. Intraoperative transesophageal echocardiography during surgery for congenital heart defects. *J Thorac Cardiovasc Surg* 2002;124:1176–1182.
31. Reynolds T. *Ultrasound Physics: A Registry Exam Preparation Guide*. School of Cardiac Ultrasound Arizona Heart Institute Foundation. Phoenix: Arizona Heart Institute Foundation, 1996.
32. Roelandt JRTC, Padian NG, eds. *Multiplane Transesophageal Echocardiography*. New York: Churchill Livingstone, 1996.
33. Schiller NB, Shah PM, Crawford M, et al. American Society of Echocardiography Committee on Standards, Subcommittee on Quantitation of Two-Dimensional Echocardiograms. Recommendations for quantitation of the left ventricle by two-dimensional echocardiography. *J Am Soc Echocardiogr* 1989;2:358–367.
34. Seward JB, Khandheria BK, Freeman WK, et al. Multiplane transesophageal echocardiography: image orientation, examination technique, anatomic correlations, and clinical applications. *Mayo Clin Proc* 1993;68:523–551.
35. Seward JB, Khandheria BK, Oh JK, et al. Critical appraisal of transesophageal echocardiography: limitations, pitfalls, and complications. *J Am Soc Echocardiogr* 1992;5:288–305.
36. Shahian DM. Papillary fibroelastomas. *Semin Thorac Cardiovasc Surg* 2000;12:101–110.
37. Shanewise JS, Cheung AT, Aronson S, et al. ASE/SCA guidelines for performing a comprehensive intraoperative multiplane transesophageal echocardiography examination: recommendations of the American Society of Echocardiography Council for Intraoperative Echocardiography and the Society of Cardiovascular Anesthesiologists Task Force for Certification in Perioperative Transesophageal Echocardiography. *Anesth Analg* 1999;89:870–884.
38. Shub C, Tajik AJ, Seward JB, et al. Cardiac papillary fibroelastomas: two-dimensional echocardiographic recognition. *Mayo Clin Proc* 1981;56:629–633.

39. Snider AR, Serwer GA, Ritter SB. *Echocardiography in Pediatric Heart Disease*, 2nd ed. St. Louis: Mosby, 1997.
40. Stümper O, Sutherland GR. *Transesophageal Echocardiography in Congenital Heart Disease*. London: Edward Arnold, 1994.
41. Thys DM, Abel M, Bollen BA, et al. Task Force on Perioperative Transesophageal Echocardiography. Practice guidelines for perioperative transesophageal echocardiography: a report by the American Society of Anesthesiologists and the Society of Cardiovascular Anesthesiologists Task Force on Transesophageal Echocardiography. *Anesthesiology* 1996;84:986–1006.
42. Weyman AE. *Principles and Practice of Echocardiography*, 2nd ed. Philadelphia: Lea & Febiger, 1994.

Index

$$\Delta F = \frac{2 V f \cos \Theta}{C}$$